Methods in Molecular Biology™

Series Editor
John M. Walker
School of Life Sciences
University of Hertfordshire
Hatfield, Hertfordshire, AL10 9AB, UK

For further volumes:
http://www.springer.com/series/7651

Haemostasis

Methods and Protocols

Edited by

Paul Monagle

Department of Paediatrics, University of Melbourne, Parkville, VIC, Australia

Humana Press

Editor
Paul Monagle
Department of Paediatrics
University of Melbourne
Parkville, VIC, Australia

ISSN 1064-3745 ISSN 1940-6029 (electronic)
ISBN 978-1-4939-6102-3 ISBN 978-1-62703-339-8 (eBook)
DOI 10.1007/978-1-62703-339-8
Springer New York Heidelberg Dordrecht London

Softcover re-print of the Hardcover 1st edition 2013

Printed on acid-free paper

Humana Press is a brand of Springer
Springer is part of Springer Science+Business Media (www.springer.com)

Preface

The haemostatic system is one the most important physiological systems for maintaining health and well-being. Disturbances of the haemostatic system, in the broader sense (e.g., heart disease, strokes), arguably constitute the single greatest contribution to non-infectious mortality in the world today. Bleeding and clotting problems are also major causes of morbidity and mortality in patients with primary underlying diseases such as cancer, whether secondary to the disease or the therapy. In this context, understanding the laboratory methods to assess the haemostatic system is vital for the practice of complex clinical medicine. Perhaps even more importantly, the investigation of the haemostatic system remains a research priority.

This book provides a basic description of the major components of haemostatic system in the introductory part. The general principles of haemostatic testing are described in the second part, and subsequent chapters describe many of the common techniques used to assess various aspects of the haemostatic system, grouped according to their functional indications.

The techniques vary from biological clot-based assays to chromogenic assays and immunological measurements of proteins. The obvious link between all these assays is that they are all in vitro tests that do not really measure the haemostatic system in its functional reality. Thus no test can claim to truly measure the overall functionality of the haemostatic system. Rather each test provides a result which can, in the light of previous clinical research, hopefully predict something useful about the patient's current status or likely outcome.

There remains an urgent need for further research to develop better methods of assessing the haemostatic system in humans, and perhaps through reading this book, which highlights the benefits and shortcomings of most major tests currently available, a young scientist will spark an interest that will lead to that discovery.

Parkville, VIC, Australia *Paul Monagle*

Contents

Part IV Examples of Tests for Bleeding Disorders

Part V Examples of Specific Assays Related to Anticoagulant Activity

Part VI Examples of Tests for Inhibitors of Coagulation

Contributors

MANUELA ALBISETTI • *Division of Haematology, University Children's Hospital, Zurich, Switzerland*
SIMON AUGUSTIN • *Department of Cardiac Surgery, Royal Children's Hospital, Melbourne, Australia*
LESLIE R. BERRY • *Thrombosis and Atherosclerosis Research Institute (TaARI), McMaster University, Hamilton, ON, Canada*
JENNY BUTLER • *Haematology Laboratory, Monash Medical Centre, Clayton, VIC, Australia*
ANTHONY K.C. CHAN • *Thrombosis and Atherosclerosis Research Institute (TaARI), McMaster University, Hamilton, ON, Canada*
MARGARET COLLECUTT • *Alfred Pathology Service, The Alfred Hospital, Melbourne, Australia*
GEMMA CRIGHTON • *Department of Haematology, Royal Children's Hospital, Melbourne, Australia*
MARK CROWTHER • *Division of Hematology and Thromboembolism, McMaster University and St Joseph's Hospital, Hamilton, ON, Canada*
JONAS DENECKE • *Department of Paediatrics, University Hospital Hamburg-Eppendorf, Hamburg-Eppendorf, Germany*
ELIZABETH DUNCAN • *Division of Haematology, Institute of Medical and Veterinary Science, Adelaide, SA, Australia*
ODILE FENNETEAU • *Biological Hematology Department, National French Reference Center on Inherited Platelet Disorders (CRPP), Robert Debré Hospital, AP-HP and Paris 7 Denis Diderot University, Paris, France*
JUAN PABLO FRONTROTH • *Laboratorio de Hemostasia y Trombosis, Hospital de Pediatría, "Prof. Dr. Juan P. Garrahan", Buenos Aires, Argentina*
BIRGITT FÜRLL • *Institute for Immunology and Transfusion Medicine, Ernst-Moritz-Arndt-University, Greifswald, Germany*
ANDREAS GREINACHER • *Institute for Immunology and Transfusion Medicine, Ernst-Moritz-Arndt-University, Greifswald, Germany*
MIRTA HEPNER • *Laboratorio de Hemostasia y Trombosis, Hospital de Pediatría "Prof. Dr. Juan P. Garrahan", Buenos Aires, Argentina*
STEPHEN HORTON • *Department of Cardiac Surgery, Royal Children's Hospital, Melbourne, Australia*
VERA IGNJATOVIC • *Haematology Research Laboratory, Murdoch Childrens Research Institute, Melbourne, Australia; Department of Paediatrics, The University of Melbourne, Melbourne, Australia*
HRATSCH KARAPETIAN • *Division of Paediatric Cardiology, Department of Paediatric and Adolescent Medicine, Medical University of Vienna, Vienna, Austria*
VASILIKI KARLAFTIS • *Haematology Research Laboratory, Murdoch Children's Research Institute, Melbourne, Australia*
CLAUS LANGER • *Department of Laboratory Medicine, University Hospital, Munster, Germany*

VÉRONIQUE LATGER-CANNARD • *Hematology Department and Grand East Competence Center on Inherited Platelet Disorders, CHU Nancy, Nancy, France*
THOMAS PIERRE LECOMPTE • *Département des Spécialités de Médecine, Service d'Hématologie, Hôpitaux Universitaires de Genève (HUG), Geneva, Switzerland*
MATTHEW D. LINDEN • *Centre for Microscopy, Characterisation and Analysis, University of Western Australia, Crawley, WA, Australia*
ERICA MALAN • *Haematology Laboratory, Monash Medical Centre, Clayton, VIC, Australia*
CLAUDIA METZGER • *Division of Haematology, University Children's Hospital, Zurich, Switzerland*
LESLEY G. MITCHELL • *Hematology/Oncology, Department of Pediatrics, University of Alberta, Edmonton, AB, Canada, T6G 2S2*
KAREN MOFFAT • *Department of Medicine, McMaster University, Hamilton, ON, Canada; Hamilton Regional Laboratory Medicine Program, Hamilton, ON, Canada*
FIONA NEWALL • *Department of Clinical Haematology, The Royal Children's Hospital, Melbourne, Australia; Department of Paediatrics, The University of Melbourne, Melbourne, Australia; Department of Nursing, The University of Melbourne, Melbourne, Australia*
ULRIKE NOWAK-GÖTTL • *Thrombosis and Hemostasis Treatment Center, University Hospital Schleswig-Holstein, Kiel, Germany*
STEPHEN OPAT • *Department of Haematology, Monash Medical Centre, Clayton, VIC, Australia*
NETHNAPHA PAREDES • *Thrombosis and Atherosclerosis Research Institute (TaARI), McMaster University, Hamilton, ON, Canada*
ANNE RABY • *External Quality Assessment, Quality Management Program – Laboratory Services, Toronto, ON, Canada*
KOTTAYAM RADHAKRISHNAN • *Department of Clinical Haematology, Royal Children's Hospital, Melbourne, Australia*
SYLVAIN SALIGNAC • *Hematology Department and Grand East Competence Center on Inherited Platelet Disorders, CHU Nancy, Nancy, France*
NICOLE SCHLEGEL • *Biological Hematology Department, National French Reference Center on Inherited Platelet Disorders (CRPP), Robert Debre´ Hospital, AP-HP and Paris 7 Denis Diderot University, Paris, France*
MARKUS SCHMUGGE • *Division of Haematology, University Children's Hospital, Zurich, Switzerland*
SIXTEN SELLENG • *Klinik für Anaesthesie und Intensivmedizin, Ernst-Moritz-Arndt-University, Greifswald, Germany*
OLIVER SPEER • *Division of Haematology, University Children's Hospital, Zurich, Switzerland*
LINDA J. STANG • *Department of Laboratory Medicine and Pathology, University of Alberta Hospital, Edmonton, AB, Canada*
ALISON STREET • *Department of Haematology, The Alfred Hospital, Melbourne, Australia*
ROBYN SUMMERHAYES • *Haematology Research Laboratory, Murdoch Children's Research Institute, Melbourne, Australia*
BERTRAM TAMBYRAYAH • *Hemostasis and Thrombosis Unit, University Hospital Schleswig-Holstein, Kiel, Germany*
HUYEN A.M. TRAN • *Department of Haematology, Monash Medical Centre, Clayton, VIC, Australia*

Part I

The Haemostatic System

Chapter 1

The Coagulation System in Humans

Anthony K.C. Chan and Nethnapha Paredes

Abstract

Complex, interrelated systems exist to maintain the fluidity of the blood in the vascular system while allowing for the rapid formation of a solid blood clot to prevent hemorrhaging subsequent to blood vessel injury. These interrelated systems are collectively referred to as haemostasis. The components involved in the haemostatic mechanism consist of vessel walls, platelets, coagulation factors, inhibitors, and the fibrinolytic system. In the broadest sense, a series of cascades involving coagulation proteins and enzymes, as well as cell surfaces (platelets and endothelial cells), work together to generate thrombin, the key enzyme in coagulation, subsequently leading to the formation of a fibrin clot. However, there also exist direct and indirect inhibitors of thrombin to ensure that clot formation does not go uncontrolled. Once the fibrin clot is formed, the fibrinolytic system ensures that the clot is lysed so that it does not become a pathological complication. Taken together, the systems exist to balance each other and maintain order. The balance of coagulation and fibrinolysis keeps the haemostatic system functioning efficiently.

Key words Haemostasis, Coagulation, Fibrinolysis, Thrombin generation, Coagulant inhibitors

1 Introduction

The study into the individual components of haemostasis has revealed that the haemostatic system in infants and children are profoundly different from adults. The pioneering work of Andrew et al. in the 1980s established that the haemostatic system in adults and children are compositionally different (1–4). It is a widely accepted view that the haemostatic system in the young is an evolving, dynamic system with the concentration of coagulation proteins varying significantly with age. The young are not "little adults" in terms of their haemostatic composition and these publications set the clinical reference ranges for fetuses, premature and full-term infants, and children (ages 1–16 years). The development of microassays (5), requiring a smaller volume of blood for testing, allowed researchers to delineate age-dependent reference ranges for coagulation parameters for healthy children from preterm infants to adolescents (1–4).

Paul Monagle (ed.), *Haemostasis: Methods and Protocols*, Methods in Molecular Biology, vol. 992,
DOI 10.1007/978-1-62703-339-8_1, © Springer Science+Business Media New York 2013

The coagulation system of children provides an innate protection from thrombosis without an increased risk of bleeding (6). Children with inherited prothrombotic states, such as factor V Leiden, prothrombin gene mutation, and deficiency of natural inhibitors of the coagulation system, do not usually develop thrombosis until early adulthood (6, 7). Also, children undergoing surgery or prolonged immobilization have a significantly lower incidence of thrombotic disease when compared to the adult population facing similar thrombotic challenges (6, 7). However, when children are diagnosed with thromboembolic disease, it is almost always associated with a higher rate of morbidity and mortality (8). When an infant has congenital or acquired haemostatic defects, they are more vulnerable to hemorrhagic disorders than older patients or adults (9). However, in the absence of any disorders, children seem to be protected from thrombosis but the mechanism by which this protection is exerted is not fully understood. The differences in coagulation parameters may be explained by decreased synthesis, accelerated clearance, and consumption at birth (9).

The haemostatic system of the young is considered physiologic because it provides protection from hemorrhagic and thrombotic complications in healthy children (10). The neonatal coagulation system gradually matures to the adult form and is complete by the late teenage years (4). Understanding the ontogeny of haemostasis will provide new insights into the pathophysiology of hemorrhagic and thrombotic complications for all ages, leading to better prevention, diagnosis, and treatment of haemostatic diseases. The following is a general overview of haemostasis with some emphasis on the developmental aspects of each component of coagulation and fibrinolysis.

2 Coagulant Proteins

When there is an assault, the coagulation system is activated to stem the flow of blood. Damage to vessel walls initiates processes whereby platelets, plasma proteins, and damaged surfaces contribute to the formation and regulation of haemostatic plugs. Thrombosis is a complicated process where fibrin clots appear as a result of reactions within the coagulation cascade, in which formation of thrombin is the key point in the coagulant process.

The assembly of factor (F) IXa and FVIIIa on phospholipids surfaces or tissue factor (TF)/FVIIa, in the presence of calcium, results in the generation of FXa from surface-bound FX (11, 12). FXa, in turn, converts prothrombin to thrombin in the presence of FVa, calcium, and a phospholipid surface (the prothrombinase complex). Physiological activation of coagulation occurs mainly due to TF/FVIIa activity (13, 14). Once the initial amounts of thrombin are generated, thrombin causes feedback activation of its own formation (from prothrombin) by proteolytic cleavage of FV, FVIII, and FXI to produce the active form FVa, FVIIIa, and FXIa, respectively (15–17). Thrombin's coagulant activity also includes cleaving fibrinopeptide A and fibrinopeptide B from fibrinogen resulting in fibrin formation and activation of FXIII to FXIIIa leading to fibrin cross-linking, resulting in a fibrin clot and platelet activation.

The placental barrier does not allow for maternal coagulation factors to pass (18). Fetal synthesis of coagulation factors, as in the case of fibrinogen (19), starts as early as 5.5 weeks, and fetal blood is able to clot at 11 weeks gestational period (20). Compared to preterm and term neonates, fetal plasma coagulation factors were consistently lower (2, 3).

Procoagulant factors, including vitamin K-dependent coagulation factors (thrombin, FVII, FIX, FX) and contact factors (FXI, FXII, prekallikrein, and high-molecular-weight kininogen), in healthy newborns are about one-half of adult values (1–3). The plasma levels continue to rise as the infant ages to approximately 80% of normal adult values by 6 months of life and remains decreased throughout childhood (4, 21). Clinically, during the first 6 months of life, the decreased levels of vitamin K-dependent coagulation factors result in a slight prolongation of the prothrombin time (PT) or international normalized ratio (INR) and the low levels of contact factors contribute to a prolongation of the activated partial thromboplastin time (aPTT) (2, 22, 23).

Some coagulation factors in newborns, such as fibrinogen, FV, FVIII, and FXIII, are similar to adult levels and remain so throughout childhood (1, 2, 21). In fact, plasma levels of von Willebrand factor (vWF), important in the binding/stabilization of circulating FVIII as well as binding to platelets and endothelial cells, are elevated in fetuses and may contribute to haemostasis in utero (24). vWF levels in newborns are about twice that of adult levels and gradually decrease over the first 6 months of life (2–4). Also, the fetal form of fibrinogen, although at the same plasma levels as adults, contains more sialic acid content compared to adult fibrinogen (25, 26), resulting in prolonged thrombin clotting time (TCT) in newborns if the test is performed in the absence of calcium. However, the significance of increased sialic acid content in fetal fibrinogen remains unclear.

3 Coagulant Inhibitors

3.1 Direct Thrombin Inhibitors

Once thrombin is generated, regulation of thrombin occurs either through direct inhibition or indirect inhibition by limitation of thrombin generation. Active thrombin is ultimately neutralized over time by direct complexation with either α_2-macroglobulin (α_2M) (27), antithrombin (AT, catalyzed by heparin) (28), or heparin cofactor II (HCII, catalyzed by dermatan sulfate) (29, 30) to form inert 1:1 covalent complexes with thrombin. While all of the direct inhibitor can neutralize free thrombin effectively, thrombin bound to fibrin is resistant to inactivation. Clot propagation is due, in part, to the activity of this clot-bound thrombin (31–33). AT–heparin complex is ineffective at inactivating thrombin bound to fibrin (33, 34) and FXa bound to phospholipids (31, 32). In addition, HCII–dermatan sulfate has significantly reduced activity against fibrin-bound thrombin (35). Summarily, there are significant biophysical limitations to antithrombotic therapies that function through the native plasma thrombin inhibitors.

Inhibitors of the clotting cascade are one-half normal adult levels at birth and in early childhood, but will continue to rise throughout infancy and childhood (4). Plasma concentrations of direct coagulation inhibitors AT and HCII in the fetus were approximately 20% and 37% of adult levels, respectively (21). Fetal plasma levels of AT and HCII increase to about 50% of adult levels at birth (21), similar to plasma levels of heterozygote adults who develop spontaneous thrombotic complications (1, 2, 36), and reach adult levels by 6 months of life. Another direct thrombin inhibitor, α_2M, is elevated at birth and increases to about twice adult values at 6 months of life. α_2M remains elevated throughout childhood and partially compensates for the reduced thrombin inhibition by AT in the young until AT levels reach adult concentrations (37–39).

3.2 Indirect Thrombin Inhibitors

Alternatively, fibrin formation can be prevented by inhibition of thrombin generation. The two mechanisms by which thrombin formation is shut down are the protein C (PC) and tissue factor pathway inhibitor (TFPI) pathways. Inhibition of thrombin generation through PC is a pathway in which conversion of PC to activated PC (APC) is cell membrane-mediated. When thrombin is bound to endothelial cell-associated thrombomodulin (TM), it can activate PC (especially when bound to the endothelial PC receptor (EPCR)), the active form of which (in association with protein S (PS)) inactivates FVIIIa and FVa, which constrains thrombin production (40).

At birth, levels of PC and PS are significantly lower and PC eventually increases to adult levels by adolescence and PS by 3 months of age (1–4, 21, 41). The influence of age on the expression of TM on endothelial cell surfaces has not been assessed. However, plasma concentrations of TM are increased at birth and gradually decreased during childhood (4, 42, 43). Although the concentrations of the individual components vary with age, it is unclear whether the overall activity of the PC/PS system is age-dependent.

3.3 Tissue Factor Pathway Inhibitor

TFPI can combine with FXa, FVIIa, and TF to form a quaternary complex in which FXa's activity is inhibited (44, 45). The TFPI–FXa complex inhibits FVIIa, thereby inhibiting the generation of thrombin. However, while TFPI has been shown to exert a significant effect on the inhibition of thrombin generation (46–48), the relative involvement of TFPI is somewhat obscured by the fact that elevation in activity requires displacement of vessel wall-bound TFPI (50–80% of total) (47) and in the fluid phase >85% of TFPI is present as lipoprotein complexes with low anticoagulant activity (49).

Plasma concentrations of TFPI are 20% lower at birth compared with adults (50). Cord plasma values of TFPI are 64% of adult values (50). Limited information is available on the influence of age on TFPI.

4 Thrombin Generation and Inhibition

Chromogenic assays on plasmas from newborns have shown that thrombin generation is delayed and decreased by ~50% compared to adults (1, 51). The capacity to generate thrombin increases throughout childhood but remains ~20% less than adults (1, 51). In these sets of experiments, the amount of thrombin generated is related to the lower prothrombin plasma concentrations in the young compared to adults (52). Inhibition of thrombin is slower in newborn plasma compared to adult plasma (37, 51). However, the overall capacity of newborn plasma to inhibit thrombin is similar to adult plasma due to increased binding of thrombin by α_2M (53). Additionally, circulating dermatan sulfate proteoglycan (DSPG) in newborn plasma catalyzes the inhibition of thrombin by HCII, thus enhancing in the inhibition of thrombin (54).

The overall capacity to generate and inhibit thrombin can be assessed by thrombin generation assays in vitro and further quantified in vivo by measuring prothrombin fragment F1.2 (PF1.2) and thrombin–AT (TAT) inhibitor complexes. At birth, levels of PF1.2 and TAT are increased indicative of activation of coagulation (43, 55) but plasma coagulation proteins are not significantly consumed during the birth process. The plasma concentrations of PF1.2 and TAT in children and young adults (20–40 years old) are similar (4) but levels of PF1.2 are increased in those over 40 years old (56). The increase in plasma concentration of PF1.2 parallels an increased risk of thrombotic complications observed in the older population. In the young, the decreased levels of prothrombin translate into decreased capacity to generate thrombin, whereby this may be another mechanism for protection against thromboembolic complications during childhood (52, 57).

5 Fibrinolytic System

Once the fibrin clot has formed in vivo, the fibrinolytic system alters the clot and plays an important role in the dissolution of the clot (58). In the fibrinolytic system, like thrombin in the coagulation system, plasmin regulation is of central importance, thus leading to the mediation of fibrin degradation. A series of serine proteases interact to ultimately cleave insoluble fibrin into fibrin degradation products (FDP). Plasminogen is converted into its active form, plasmin, by tissue-type plasminogen activator (tPA) and urokinase-type plasminogen activator (uPA). The activators of plasminogen are inhibited by plasminogen activator inhibitor-1 (PAI-1) (59). α_2-Antiplasmin (α_2AP) and, to a lesser extent, α_2M and thrombin activatable fibrinolysis inhibitor (TAFI) are the primary inhibitors of plasmin (59–61).

As with the coagulation system, the fibrinolytic system has components that are age-dependent (1, 2). The capacity to generate and inhibit plasmin during infancy and throughout childhood is very similar to adults (1). There are significant differences in the levels of the fibrinolytic components between children and adults. Some fibrinolytic components are lower at birth when compared to adults, especially plasminogen (75% and 50% of adult values for the healthy premature and full-term newborns, respectively) and the primary inhibitor of plasmin, α_2AP (at 80% of adult values) (1–3). However, the levels of fibrinolytic activators such as tPA and uPA and regulators such as PAI-1 are elevated at birth compared with adults (1, 62, 63). Although α_2M has a major role in the inhibition of thrombin in coagulation during infancy and childhood, the importance of α_2M in plasmin inhibition in the fibrinolytic system in the young is unclear (4, 37, 39).

TAFI is a plasma zymogen that can be activated by thrombin, the thrombin–TM complex, or plasmin (61). The activated form of TAFI removes C-terminal lysine residues of plasmin-modified fibrin that mediates a positive feedback mechanism in plasminogen activation, thereby attenuating fibrinolysis (61, 64). The TAFI pathway is active in vivo and most likely provides the proper balance between fibrin deposition and fibrin degradation.

Overall, the fibrinolytic potential in children is depressed most likely due to the limited amounts of fibrinogen (1, 2, 62, 63, 65), but the fibrinolytic system in the newborn is very effective despite the lower levels of fibrinolytic components compared to adult values. It is still unclear whether the fibrinolytic system contributes to the protection from thromboembolic complications during childhood.

6 Summary

When the haemostatic system is challenged, the coagulation and fibrinolytic components work together to stem the flow of blood by forming a fibrin clot and subsequent lysis of the clot ensures that the fluidity of blood is maintained. Haemostasis is a complicated, but efficient process, and the plasma concentration of various components have been shown to vary with age. The haemostatic system is a dynamic, evolving system in the fetal/neonatal stage that eventually matures into the adult version by the late teenage years (4). Much progress has been achieved through research in delineating the differences between children and adults, thanks to the milestone work of Andrew et al. (1–4) who was one of the first to publish clinical reference ranges for children. Prior to this, most clinical guidelines for diagnosing and/or treating children with thrombotic or hemorrhagic disease were extrapolated from adult data. Given that the plasma levels of procoagulant and anticoagulant factors are lower in neonates and children compared to adults, differences in their haemostatic composition can lead to incorrect diagnosis or treatment regimens in the young. Thus, establishing age-dependent reference ranges is critical and necessary.

Although the landmark publications of Andrew et al. paved the way for research into developmental haemostasis, the reference ranges set out in these publications may not be relevant in modern coagulation laboratories. It is known that coagulation testing is dependent upon the type of analyzer and reagent systems used (60). Each coagulation laboratory has their own testing system and since the 1980s, technology has advanced and coagulation analyzers and reagent systems have significantly changed (66). Different individual reagents and analyzers used by different laboratories for coagulation testing give varying results depending on the testing system used (60, 67–70), thus past reference ranges may not be applicable to present-day coagulation testing. A recent study (67) has shown that the absolute values of reference ranges for coagulation assays in neonates and children vary with analyzer and reagent systems. As a result, it is imperative that each coagulation laboratory develop their own age-related reference ranges for their own testing system in order to effectively diagnose and manage neonates and children with suspected bleeding or clotting disorders, and should not rely on published data as it may not be relevant to their laboratory analyzer and reagent system.

Acknowledgments

Anthony Chan is supported by the Bayer Thrombosis and Haemostasis Research Grant.

References

1. Andrew M, Paes B, Johnston M (1990) Development of the hemostatic system in the neonate and young infant. Am J Pediatr Hematol Oncol 12:95–104
2. Andrew M, Paes B, Milner R, Johnston M, Mitchell L, Tollefsen DM, Powers P (1987) Development of the human coagulation system in the full-term infant. Blood 70:165–172
3. Andrew M, Paes B, Milner R, Johnston M, Mitchell L, Tollefsen DM, Castle V, Powers P (1988) Development of the human coagulation system in the healthy premature infant. Blood 72:1651–1657
4. Andrew M, Vegh P, Johnston M, Bowker J, Ofosu F, Mitchell L (1992) Maturation of the hemostatic system during childhood. Blood 80:1998–2005
5. JohnstonM,ZipurskyA(1980)Microtechnology for the study of the blood coagulation system in newborn infants. Can J Med Technol 42: 159–164
6. Andrew M (1995) Developmental hemostasis: relevance to thromboembolic complications in pediatric patients. Thromb Haemost 74: 415–425
7. Monagle P, Chan A, Massicotte P, Chalmers E, Michelson AD (2004) Antithrombotic therapy in children: the Seventh ACCP Conference on Antithrombotic and Thrombolytic Therapy. Chest 126:645S–687S
8. Andrew M, David M, Adams M, Ali K, Anderson R, Barnard D, Mernstein M, Brisson L, Cairney B, DeSai D, Grant R, Isreals S, Jardine L, Luke B, Massicotte P, Silva M (1994) Venous thromboembolic complications (VTE) in children: first analyses of the Canadian Registry of VTE. Blood 83:1251–1257
9. Andrew M (1997) The relevance of developmental hemostasis to hemorrhagic disorders of newborns. Semin Perinatol 21:70–85
10. Sutor A (1992) Thrombosis in the newborn and infants. In: Poller L, Thomson J (eds) Thrombosis and its management. Churchill Livingstone, Edinburgh, pp 126–133
11. Kurachi K, Davie EW (1977) Activation of human factor XI (plasma thromboplastin antecedent) by factor XIIa (activated Hageman factor). Biochemistry 16:5831–5839
12. Nemerson Y (1966) The reaction between bovine brain tissue factor and factors VII and X. Biochemistry 5:601–608
13. Hoffman M, Monroe DM, Oliver JA, Roberts HR (1995) Factors IXa and Xa play distinct roles in tissue factor-dependent initiation of coagulation. Blood 86:1794–1801
14. Nemerson Y (2007) Tissue factor and hemostasis. Blood 71:1–8
15. Naito K, Fujikawa K (1991) Activation of human blood coagulation factor XI independent of factor XII. Factor XI is activated by thrombin and factor XIa in the presence of negatively charged surfaces. J Biol Chem 266:7353–7358
16. Ofosu FA, Sie P, Modi GJ, Fernandez F, Buchanan MR, Blajchman MA, Boneu B, Hirsh J (1987) The inhibition of thrombin-dependent positive-feedback reactions is critical to the expression of the anticoagulant effect of heparin. Biochem J 243:579–588
17. Ofosu FA, Liu L, Freedman J (1996) Control mechanisms in thrombin generation. Semin Thromb Hemost 22:303–308
18. Cade JF, Hirsh J, Martin M (1969) Placental barrier to coagulation factors: its relevance to the coagulation defect at birth and to haemorrhage in the newborn. Br Med J 2:281–283
19. Gitlin D, Biasucci A (1969) Development of gamma G, gamma A, gamma M, beta IC-beta IA, C 1 esterase inhibitor, ceruloplasmin, transferrin, hemopexin, haptoglobin, fibrinogen, plasminogen, alpha 1-antitrypsin, orosomucoid, beta-lipoprotein, alpha 2-macroglobulin, and prealbumin in the human conceptus. J Clin Invest 48:1433–1446
20. Zilliacus H, Ottelin AM, Mattsson T (1966) Blood clotting and fibrinolysis in human foetuses. Biol Neonat 10:108–112
21. Reverdiau-Moalic P, Delahousse B, Body G, Bardos P, Leroy J, Gruel Y (1996) Evolution of blood coagulation activators and inhibitors in the healthy human fetus. Blood 88:900–906
22. Andrew M, Karpatkin M (1982) A simple screening test for evaluating prolonged partial thromboplastin times in newborn infants. J Pediatr 101:610–612
23. Gordon EM, Ratnoff OD, Saito H, Gross S, Jones PK (1980) Studies on some coagulation factors (Hageman factor, plasma prekallikrein, and high molecular weight kininogen) in the normal newborn. Am J Pediatr Hematol Oncol 2:213–216
24. Mazurier C, Daffos F, Forestier F (1992) Electrophoretic and functional characteristics of the von Willebrand factor in human fetal plasma. Br J Haematol 81:263–270
25. Witt I, Müller H, Künzer W (1969) Evidence for the existence of foetal fibrinogen. Thromb Diath Haemorrh 22:101–109
26. Francis JL, Armstrong DJ (1982) Sialic acid and enzymatic desialation of cord blood fibrinogen. Haemostasis 11:223–228
27. Lerant I, Kovacs T, Papp B, Mandl J, Lambin P, Machovich R (1990) Interaction of thrombin with endothelial cells in the presence of fibrinogen and alpha 2-macroglobulin. Haematologia (Budap) 23:161–169

28. Sie P, Ofosu F, Fernandez F, Buchanan MR, Petitou M, Boneu B (1986) Respective role of antithrombin III and heparin cofactor II in the in vitro anticoagulant effect of heparin and of various sulphated polysaccharides. Br J Haematol 64:707–714
29. Tollefsen DM, Pestka CA, Monafo WJ (1983) Activation of heparin cofactor II by dermatan sulfate. J Biol Chem 258:6713–6716
30. Mascellani G, Liverani L, Bianchini P, Parma B, Torri G, Bisio A, Guerrini M, Casu B (1993) Structure and contribution to the heparin cofactor II-mediated inhibition of thrombin of naturally oversulphated sequences of dermatan sulphate. Biochem J 296:639–648
31. Eisenberg PR, Siegel JE, Abendschein DR, Miletich JP (1993) Importance of factor Xa in determining the procoagulant activity of whole-blood clots. J Clin Invest 91:1877–1883
32. Prager NA, Abendschein DR, McKenzie CR, Eisenberg PR (1995) Role of thrombin compared with factor Xa in the procoagulant activity of whole blood clots. Circulation 92:962–967
33. Weitz JI, Hudoba M, Massel D, Maraganore J, Hirsh J (1990) Clot-bound thrombin is protected from inhibition by heparin-antithrombin III but is susceptible to inactivation by antithrombin III-independent inhibitors. J Clin Invest 86:385–391
34. Hogg PJ, Jackson CM (1989) Fibrin monomer protects thrombin from inactivation by heparin-antithrombin III: implications for heparin efficacy. Proc Natl Acad Sci U S A 86:3619–3623
35. Bendayan P, Boccalon H, Dupouy D, Boneu B (1994) Dermatan sulfate is a more potent inhibitor of clot-bound thrombin than unfractionated and low molecular weight heparins. Thromb Haemost 71:576–580
36. Monagle PT, Andrew M (2000) Hemorrhagic and thromboembolic complications during infancy and childhood. In: Colman RW, Hirsh J, Marder VJ, Clowes AW, George JN (eds) Hemostasis and thrombosis: basic principles and clinical practice. Lippincott Williams & Wilkins, Philadelphia, PA, pp 1053–1070
37. Schmidt B, Mitchell L, Ofosu FA, Andrew M (1989) Alpha-2-macroglobulin is an important progressive inhibitor of thrombin in neonatal and infant plasma. Thromb Haemost 62:1074–1077
38. Levine JJ, Udall JN Jr, Evernden BA, Epstein MF, Bloch KJ (1987) Elevated levels of alpha 2-macroglobulin-protease complexes in infants. Biol Neonate 51:149–155
39. Mitchell L, Piovella F, Ofosu F, Andrew M (1991) Alpha-2-macroglobulin may provide protection from thromboembolic events in antithrombin III-deficient children. Blood 78:2299–2304
40. Dahlback B (1995) The protein C anticoagulant system: inherited defects as basis for venous thrombosis. Thromb Res 77:1–43
41. Schwarz HP, Mutean W, Watzke H, Richter B, Griffin JH (1988) Low total protein S antigen but high protein S activity due to decreased C4b-binding protein in neonates. Blood 71:562–565
42. Menashi S, Aurousseau MH, Gozin D, Daffos F, D'Angelo A, Forestier F, Boffa MC (1999) High levels of circulating thrombomodulin in human foetuses and children. Thromb Haemost 81:906–909
43. Knöfler R, Hofmann S, Weissbach G, Kuhlisch E, Neef B, Otte M, Pargac N, Nachtrodt G (1998) Molecular markers of the endothelium, the coagulation and the fibrinolytic systems in healthy newborns. Semin Thromb Hemost 24:453–461
44. Girard TJ, Warren LA, Novotny WF, Likert KM, Brown SG, Miletich JP, Broze GJ Jr (1989) Functional significance of the Kunitz-type inhibitory domains of lipoprotein-associated coagulation inhibitor. Nature 338:518–520
45. Broze GJ Jr (1995) Tissue factor pathway inhibitor. Thromb Haemost 74:90–93
46. Lindahl AK (1997) Tissue factor pathway inhibitor: from unknown coagulation inhibitor to major antithrombotic principle. Cardiovasc Res 33:286–291
47. Sandset PM (1996) Tissue factor pathway inhibitor (TFPI)—an update. Haemostasis 26: 156–165
48. Camici M, Sagripanti A (1999) Tissue factor pathway inhibitor. Minerva Med 90:25–32
49. Lindahl AK, Jacobsen PB, Sandset PM, Abildgaard U (1991) Tissue factor pathway inhibitor with high anticoagulant activity is increased in post-heparin plasma and in plasma from cancer patients. Blood Coagul Fibrinolysis 2:713–721
50. Weissbach G, Harenberg J, Wendisch J, Pargac N, Thomas K (1994) Tissue factor pathway inhibitor in infants and children. Thromb Res 73:441–446
51. Shah JK, Mitchell LG, Paes B, Ofosu FA, Schmidt B, Andrew M (1992) Thrombin inhibition is impaired in plasma of sick neonates. Pediatr Res 31:391–395
52. Andrew M, Schmidt B, Mitchell L, Paes B, Ofosu F (1990) Thrombin generation in newborn plasma is critically dependent on the concentration of prothrombin. Thromb Haemost 63:27–30
53. Fischer AM, Tapon-Bretaudiere J, Bros A, Josso F (1981) Respective roles of antithrombin III and alpha 2 macroglobulin in thrombin inactivation. Thromb Haemost 45:51–54
54. Andrew M, Mitchell L, Berry L, Paes B, Delorme M, Ofosu F, Burrows R, Khambalia B

(1992) An anticoagulant dermatan sulfate proteoglycan circulates in the pregnant woman and her fetus. J Clin Invest 89:321–326
55. Suarez CR, Menendez CE, Walenga JM, Fareed J (1984) Neonatal and maternal hemostasis: value of molecular markers in the assessment of hemostatic status. Semin Thromb Hemost 10:280–284
56. Bauer KA, Weiss LM, Sparrow D, Vokonas PS, Rosenberg RD (1987) Aging-associated changes in indices of thrombin generation and protein C activation in humans. Normative Aging Study. J Clin Invest 80:1527–1534
57. Andrew M, Mitchell L, Vegh P, Ofosu F (1994) Thrombin regulation in children differs from adults in the absence and presence of heparin. Thromb Haemost 72:836–842
58. Collen D, Lijnen HR (1991) Basic and clinical aspects of fibrinolysis and thrombolysis. Blood 78:3114–3124
59. Francis CW, Marder VJ (1992) Physiologic regulation and pathologic disorders of fibrinolysis. In: Colman RW, Hirsh J, Marder VJ, Salzman EW (eds) Hemostasis and thrombosis: basic principles and clinical practice. JB Lippincott, Philadelphia, PA, pp 1076–1103
60. Barrett AJ (1981) Alpha 2-macroglobulin. Methods Enzymol 80:737–754
61. Bajzar L (2000) Thrombin activatable fibrinolysis inhibitor and an antifibrinolytic pathway. Arterioscler Thromb Vasc Biol 20:2511–2518
62. Corrigan JJ Jr, Sleeth JJ, Jeter M, Lox CD (1989) Newborn's fibrinolytic mechanism: components and plasmin generation. Am J Hematol 32:273–278
63. Ginsberg JS, Hirsh J, Rainbow AJ, Coates G (1989) Risks to the fetus of radiologic procedures used in the diagnosis of maternal venous thromboembolic disease. Thromb Haemost 61:189–196
64. Nesheim M (2003) Thrombin and fibrinolysis. Chest 124:33S–39S
65. Andrew M, Brooker L, Leaker M, Paes B, Weitz J (1992) Fibrin clot lysis by thrombolytic agents is impaired in newborns due to a low plasminogen concentration. Thromb Haemost 68:325–330
66. Hirsh J, Raschke R (2004) Heparin and low-molecular-weight heparin: the Seventh ACCP Conference on Antithrombotic and Thrombolytic Therapy. Chest 126: 188S–203S
67. Declerck PJ, Moreau H, Jespersen J, Gram J, Kluft C (1993) Multicenter evaluation of commercially available methods for the immunological determination of plasminogen activator inhibitor-1 (PAI-1). Thromb Haemost 70: 858–863
68. Gram J, Declerck PJ, Sidelmann J, Jespersen J, Kluft C (1993) Multicentre evaluation of commercial kit methods: plasminogen activator inhibitor activity. Thromb Haemost 70: 852–857
69. Stevenson KJ, Easton AC, Curry A, Thomson JM, Poller L (1986) The reliability of activated partial thromboplastin time methods and the relationship to lipid composition and ultrastructure. Thromb Haemost 55: 250–258
70. D'Angelo A, Seveso MP, D'Angelo SV, Gilardoni F, Dettori AG, Bonini P (1990) Effect of clot-detection methods and reagents on activated partial thromboplastin time (APTT). Implications in heparin monitoring by APTT. Am J Clin Pathol 94:297–306

Chapter 2

Platelet Physiology

Matthew D. Linden

Abstract

Platelets are cell fragments which circulate in blood. They are of pivotal importance in blood clot formation, affecting thrombosis and haemostasis. By rapidly altering the activation and expression of surface receptors, platelets are able to quickly undergo structural and phenotypic changes in response to stimulation, such as collagen exposure on injured vascular endothelium. This response to stimulation allows platelets to become adhesive, aggregate to form a thrombus, and release a variety of mediators affecting coagulation, inflammation, and chemotaxis at the site of injury. Therefore, in addition to their critical role in thrombosis and haemostasis, platelets also play a role in immunity, inflammation, wound healing, haematologic malignancies, and metabolic disorders. The role of platelets in disease, particularly in atherothrombosis, is increasingly the focus of current research and antiplatelet therapy plays a significant role in the prevention and treatment of atherothrombotic and inflammatory diseases.

Key words Platelet physiology, Platelet structure, Granules, Platelet activation, Platelet receptors

1 Introduction

Platelets are small cells of large importance in medicine. They are involved in many pathophysiological processes, such as thrombosis, haemorrhage, inflammation, and cancer. The involvement of platelets in disease may be a direct primary disorder of platelet number and function, or an indirect result of the critical role of platelets in thrombosis, such as with coronary artery disease, stroke, peripheral vascular disease, and diabetes.

2 Platelet Structure

Platelets are subcellular fragments released from megakaryocytes that circulate in blood as small, granular, anuclear discs. These 3.0 by 0.5 μm discoid cells circulate in laminar blood flow near the apical surface of the endothelium for about 7 days or until they become activated, whereupon they undergo rapid metamorphic

Paul Monagle (ed.), *Haemostasis: Methods and Protocols*, Methods in Molecular Biology, vol. 992,
DOI 10.1007/978-1-62703-339-8_2, © Springer Science+Business Media New York 2013

changes to spread and adhere to damaged endothelial surfaces, release granules and aggregate with other platelets (1).

Platelets have a dynamic glycocalyx covered with glycoprotein receptors necessary to facilitate platelet adhesion, aggregation, and signal activation, principally the mobile receptors glycoprotein (GP) Ib–IX–V complex and integrin $\alpha_{IIb}\beta_3$ (the GPIIb–IIIa complex) (2). Anionic phospholipid, phosphatidylserine from the platelet membrane facilitates and acts as the site of formation of the prothrombinase complex of coagulation, and contains tissue factors—exposed on activation and decrypted with the release of microparticles—which also contributes to coagulation.

Below the plasma membrane of platelets lies a complex microtubule and microfilament cytoskeleton capable of dynamically changing platelet cell shape and surface area with activation (2). They contain many granules and bodies with haemostatic mediators, adhesion molecules, signaling molecules, calcium, ATP, ADP, and serotonin which can be released to the site of clot formation or expressed on the platelet surface in response to platelet activation (3).

2.1 The Platelet Cytoskeleton

The cytoskeleton of platelets is a spectrin mesh reinforced by a microtubule core and a rigid network of cross-linked actin filaments which maintains the discoid shape and maintains cell integrity against high shear forces as blood flow forces platelets against endothelium, and allows for transformation of the platelet shape with activation (1).

The spectrin membrane of platelets is a two-dimensional assembly of spectrin strands interconnected to each other in a mesh by actin filaments (4). Each molecular end of the spectrin molecule has an actin-binding site. Actin is the most abundant molecule in platelets; much of it is cross-linked into a rigid cytoplasmic network by homodimeric filamin (FLNa and FLNb) and α-actinin (5). These proteins act as "scaffolding molecules" which bind, via the carboxyl terminus, and localize molecules such as GTPase, sal A, sac, rho, cdc42, Trio and Toll, kinases, phosphatases, and transmembrane proteins, particularly the glycoprotein Ib_{α} subunit of the von Willebrand factor (vWF) receptor, adjacent to the plasma membrane (6).

A single coiled microtubule core, which sits in the cytoplasm, just beneath the plasma membrane, along the thin edge of the platelet, is responsible for the characteristic discoid shape of resting platelets (7).

When activated, the platelet cytoskeleton undergoes significant alteration to facilitate shape change, attachment to and spreading of platelets over the damaged endothelium. Activation also initiates other platelet responses such as secretion of granules (see Subheading 2.2) which moves adhesion receptors to the cell surface and releases agonists and mediators to the circulation, activates biochemical pathways—such as stimulating the synthesis and release of thromboxane, and causes conformational changes in platelet surface receptors—such as activation of the $\alpha_{IIb}\beta_3$ integrin to allow fibrinogen and vWF binding and thus platelet aggregation (8).

Platelet shape change is a complex, actin-dependent process that involves reorganization of the platelet cytoskeleton and assembly of new actin filaments. This process follows a reproducible sequence as the platelet activates and spreads, beginning with sphering as a result of a transient rise in cytosolic calcium concentration in response to activation of phospholipase C secondary to platelet receptor binding (9). Phospholipase C hydrolyzes membrane-bound polyphosphoinositide P_2 (PIP_2) into inositol triphosphate (IP_3) (9). IP_3 then binds to dense granules, releasing the calcium stored in them (9). Furthermore, active transport of extracellular calcium across the plasma membrane by calcium channels occurs (10). The increased intracellular calcium causes a conformational change in gelsolin, allowing it to bind and F-actin and cleave filaments, resulting in the loss of normal discoid platelet shape and sphering of the cell (10).

New actin filaments are assembled from unpolymerized pools of actin in the cytoplasm and attach to the barbed end of the filaments fragmented by gelsolin (11). These filaments extend, causing lamellar spreading of the platelet, before the actin is capped by CapZ, preventing further filament assembly (11, 12). This extension unfolds invaginations of the plasma membrane- and surface-connected open canalicular system to increase surface area of the platelet. During activation, underlying actin filaments also become tethered to integrin $\alpha_{IIb}\beta_3$. Through calcium- and rho kinase-stimulated phosphorylation of platelet myosin, contractile force is applied to the actin, $\alpha_{IIb}\beta_3$, and the fibrinogen bound to it, causing clot retraction (13). The action of myosin phosphorylation is also involved in the secretion of granules and the modulation of platelet surface receptors, such as the down-regulation of glycoprotein Ib (GPIb)–IX–V complex from the surface after activation (1).

2.2 Platelet Granules and Secretion

Platelets contain α-granules, dense granules, and lysosomes (3). Secretion of granule contents releases haemostatic mediators at the site of vascular injury, or causes expression of surface molecules which facilitate cellular adhesion. α-granules are the most numerous of the platelet organelles, and are 200–500 nm in diameter with a highly organized interior substructure divided into different zones. They contain a variety of adhesion molecules, chemokines, coagulation and fibrinolysis proteins, growth factors, immunologic molecules, and other proteins (Table 1) (3, 14). Dense granules contain ionic calcium, magnesium, phosphate, and pyrophosphate as well as ATP, GTP, ADP, and GDP nucleotides and the transmitter serotonin (15). Platelet lysosomes, though few in number,

Table 1
Components of alpha granules

Adhesion molecules	Fibronectin, fibrinogen, integrin $\alpha_{IIb}\beta_3$, integrin $\alpha_v\beta$ P-selectin, von Willebrand factor
Chemokines	β-Thromboglobulin, growth-regulated oncogene α, interleukin 8, macrophage inflammatory protein 1α, monocyte chemotactic protein 3, neutrophil-activating protein, platelet factor 4, RANTES
Coagulation proteins	Factor V, factor VIII, high-molecular-weight kininogen, multimerin
Fibrinolysis proteins	α_2-Macroglobulin, plasminogen, plasminogen activator inhibitor 1
Growth factors	Basic fibroblast growth factor, epidermal growth factor, hepatocyte growth factor, insulin-like growth factor 1, platelet-derived growth factor, transforming growth factor β, vascular endothelial growth factor
Immunologic molecules	B1H globulin, c1 inhibitor, factor D, IgG
Other proteins	α_1 antitrypsin, albumin, osteonectin

contain acid hydrolases, cathepsins, and lysosomal membrane proteins similar to lysosomes in other cells (3).

Exocytosis of platelet granules and secretion of granular contents occur after cells are activated by specific ligands that interact with platelet membrane receptors through G-protein couple signaling. Diglycerol, which results from the cleavage of membrane phosphatidylinositol 4,5 bisphosphate (PIP_2) to IP_3, activates protein kinase C (PKC) which acts in synergy with calcium ions released from dense granules by IP_3 to amplify the secretion of granules (see Subheading 4). Changes to the cytoskeleton associated with platelet activation facilitate the development, targeting, and exocytosis of secretory granules (16, 17). Platelet shape change can occur without secretion, particularly when signaling via the G_i but not G_q pathways takes place, but secretion cannot take place if the cytoskeletal rearrangement is inhibited (18).

2.3 Microparticles

Activated platelets release two types of membrane vesicles: (1) platelet-derived microparticles (PMPs) budded from the plasma membrane, and (2) exosomes, which are smaller than PMP and released from α-granules during secretion (19).

Signal transduction resulting from agonists such as thrombin or collagen-binding receptors on the surface of platelets, and the resulting elevation of intracellular calcium, results in the activation of several enzymes, such as calpain and PKC, which facilitate PMP production by degrading structural proteins including actin-binding protein, talin, and the heavy chain of myosin (20, 21). Concurrently, the platelet cell membrane loses its organized asymmetrical distribution and negatively charged aminophospholipids phosphatidylserine (PS) and phosphatidylethanolamine (PE) become expressed on the surface, facilitating interaction with the coagulation system and the tenase complex (see Subheading 5). PS and PE are therefore also expressed on the PMPs which bud off from the platelet, and thus PMPs are procoagulant particles (22, 23). Furthermore, platelets and PMPs share glycoprotein receptors such as GPIb, PECAM-1, and integrin $\alpha_{IIb}\beta_3$, and subpopulations may express P-selectin from platelet granules, suggesting that PMPs can participate in cellular interactions, adhesion, and aggregation (19).

In addition to being formed as a result of agonist-induced platelet activation, PMPs may form as a result of complement activation/damage to platelets, and platelet aging and destruction, and may be released directly from megakaryocytes in platelet genesis (19).

3 Platelet Receptors

Platelets express a variety of different receptors on their surface, most having a direct role in haemostasis by activating the platelet in response to agonists, as adhesive receptors interacting with the damaged cell wall, or aggregating with other platelets and other cells to contribute to thrombus formation (24). By changing the expression and activation status of these surface molecules, platelets are able to markedly change their phenotype to carry out physiological functions or deal with pathological events. Table 2 summarizes the known platelet receptors, their structural family, function, and importance. A number of the more major receptors are discussed in detail.

3.1 GPIb–IX–V

GPIb is a heterodimeric transmembrane protein consisting of a disulfide-linked 140 kDa alpha chain and 22 kDa beta chain (25, 26). It exists on the platelet surface in complex non-covalent association with GPIX and platelet GPV to form the receptor for vWF and mediates platelet adhesion to the arterial circulation (27). vWF, which is present in blood, must undergo conformational alterations through binding to collagen prior to being recognized and bound by the GPIb alpha chain of the receptor complex on platelets. Furthermore, this process is much more efficient when high shear stress exerts conformational changes on both the vWF and the GPIb–IX–V complex (27).

Interaction between the GPIb–IX–V complex on the surface of platelets and vWF bound to collagen, while insufficient to firmly adhere platelets to the matrix, allows them to roll along the matrix and facilitates firm adhesion via other surface proteins. However, binding of vWF to the receptor complex causes transmembrane signaling through phosphorylation of the intracellular chain of GPIb beta, resulting in activation of $\alpha_{IIb}\beta_3$ to its ligand-receptive state (see Subheading 3.2), and acts synergistically with signals generated from the binding of collagen to GPVI and $\alpha_2\beta_1$ (Table 2) (28, 29).

In addition to binding collagen–vWF and causing platelet activation, GPIb–IX–V also acts as a receptor for Mac-1 on leukocytes (30). Leukocytes and activated platelets bind primarily through interaction of P-selectin on the activated platelet to constitutively express P-selectin glycoprotein ligand 1 (PSGL-1) on the leukocyte (31). This proximity and heterotypic aggregation of cells allow the N-terminal region globular region of GPIb alpha to recognize the alpha chain of activated Mac-1 (25, 32). This process is thought to mediate firm aggregation of the platelet and

Table 2
Platelet membrane receptors

Class	Family	Receptor	Function
Integrins	β_3	$\alpha_{IIb}\beta_3$	The glycoprotein IIb–IIIa complex, also CD61/CD41. A unique platelet receptor that is essential for fibrinogen binding and platelet aggregation
		$\alpha_v\beta_3$	Vitronectin receptor of low importance and low expression on platelets
	β_1	$\alpha_2\beta_1$	The glycoprotein Ia–IIa complex, also CD49b. A major collagen adhesion receptor on platelets. In combination with GPIb–IX–V complex, allows firm adhesion and platelet activation in response to collagen stimulation
		$\alpha_5\beta_1$	Fibronectin receptor with a supplementary role in platelet adhesion at injury sites
		$\alpha_6\beta_1$	Laminin receptor with a supplementary role in platelet adhesion at injury sites
	β_2	$\alpha_L\beta_2$	May play a role in regulation or caspase activation. Expressed in platelet granules and only found on the surface of platelets that have undergone activation and secretion
Leucine-rich repeat (LRR)		GPIb–IX–V	Pivotal platelet receptor in initiating and propagating haemostasis and thrombosis with a number of ligands including collagen, von Willebrand Factor (vWF), thrombospondin, P-selectin, and leukocyte integrin Mac-1
	Toll-like receptors	TLR1 TLR2 TLR4 TLR6 TLR9	Lipopolysaccharide receptors which increase platelet adhesion to fibrinogen and increase platelet activation to agonists such as thrombin. Present on about 40% of human platelets

(continued)

Table 2 (continued)

Class	Family	Receptor	Function
Seven-transmembrane receptors	Thrombin receptors	PAR1 PAR4	After cleavage by thrombin acts as a ligand and receptor signaling platelet activation
	ADP receptors	$P2Y_1$	Mediates transient platelet shape change and aggregation by ADP binding via G_q signaling leading to calcium release and activation of phospholipase C
		$P2Y_{12}$	Inhibits adenylyl cyclase by ADP binding via $G_{\alpha i2}$ signaling and amplified mobilization of cytoplasmic calcium by $P2Y_1$
	Prostaglandin receptors	Thromboxane receptor A_2	Activates platelets via phopholipase A2 and phospholipase C through G_q, G_{i2}, and $G_{12/13}$. Important for autocrine amplification of platelet activation following binding of other receptors
		PGI_2 receptor	Binds endothelial prostacyclin to inhibit platelet activation via G_S signaling and adenylate cyclase
		PGD_2 receptor	Similar in mechanism but distinct from PGI_2 receptor
		PGE_2 receptor	Potentiates platelet response to ADP at low concentrations, but inhibits aggregation at high concentrations
	Lipid receptors	Platelet-activating factor receptor	Activates platelet via G_q and G_i protein signaling
		Lysophosphatidic acid receptor	Causes shape change, degranulation, and aggregation
	Chemokine receptors	CXCR4 CCR4 CCR3 CCR1	May be involved in megakaryocytosis and platelet–leukocyte interactions
	Vasopressin receptor	V_{1a} receptor	Causes rapid but reversible platelet activation via G_{q11} signaling
	Adenosine receptor	A_{2a} receptor	Inhibits vasopressin or PAF-induced platelet activation via G_s signaling
	Epinephrine receptor	β2-Adrenergic receptor	Augments platelet activation caused by other agonists
	Serotonin receptor	$5\text{-}HT_{2A}$ receptor	Causes autocrine platelet activation and degranulation via G-protein and calcium signaling
	Dopamine receptor	D3 D5	Involved in dopamine uptake and may inhibit platelet function
Immunoglobulin superfamily	GPVI	GPVI	Major collagen receptor

leukocyte, as well as transmigration of the leukocyte through the mural thrombus to sites of vascular injury, thus providing a potentially important role for this receptor in inflammation.

GPIb–IX–V also plays a role in tethering of platelets to endothelium via binding of the receptor to P-selectin expressed by endothelial cells (33), and has two binding sites for thrombin, important in the response of platelets to low concentrations (<0.1 U/mL) of thrombin (32, 34), while the PAR family of receptors are more important where higher concentrations are present (see Subheading 3.3). The receptor complex also contributes to the soluble coagulation system through interactions with high-molecular-weight (HMW) kininogen, as well as coagulation factors XII and XI (34, 35).

Despite the advances in understanding of the role of GPIb–IX–V in vWF tethering, maintenance of coagulation, inflammation, and signaling, much remains to be learned about the functions of this unique and complicated receptor complex (25).

3.2 $\alpha_{IIb}\beta_3$

Integrin $\alpha_{IIb}\beta_3$, also known as the GPIIb–IIIa complex, is the most abundant glycoprotein on platelet membranes, and plays an important role in platelet aggregation and signaling as well as interaction with the blood coagulation system and other cell types—such as endothelial cells. $\alpha_{IIb}\beta_3$ binds several adhesive proteins, including fibrinogen (coagulation factor I), prothrombin (coagulation factor II), vWF, fibronectin, neural cell adhesion molecule L1, and vitronectin (36). Much of its binding activity is due to KQAGDV and RGD recognition sequences and binding sites (37).

$\alpha_{IIb}\beta_3$ maintains a low affinity for ligand binding on resting circulating platelets. However conformational changes in $\alpha_{IIb}\beta_3$ as a result of inside-out signaling secondary to ligand binding of agonist receptors (such as ADP, thrombin), as well as clustering of the receptor following release of $\alpha_{IIb}\beta_3$ from the cytoskeleton, lead to a large increase in receptor affinity for its various ligands and increased adhesive capacity (8). Once activated, $\alpha_{IIb}\beta_3$ results in both platelet adhesion to the site of vascular injury and aggregation of platelets causing thrombus propagation. Binding of activated $\alpha_{IIb}\beta_3$ to immobilized fibrinogen and vWF at the site of vascular injury results in spreading of the platelet, firm adhesion of the platelet to the vascular wall, and outside-in signaling leading to amplification of platelet activity, while binding of activated $\alpha_{IIb}\beta_3$ to soluble fibrinogen and vWF promotes cell-to-cell adhesion and platelet aggregation as well as outside-in signaling (36). Therefore $\alpha_{IIb}\beta_3$ is both critical to the adhesive and aggregatory properties of activated platelets as well as essential in the amplification of activation signaling from agonist receptors.

3.3 Thrombin Receptors

Thrombin plays a critical role in the regulation of haemostasis and thrombosis primarily through its proteolytic function within the coagulation cascade. In addition to this action, thrombin also exerts profound effects on a diverse range of cells, including platelets, through cleavage of a number of G-protein-coupled, seven-transmembrane domain, protease-activated receptors (PARs) (38).

PAR1 is the predominant receptor for thrombin-mediated platelet activation and secretion in humans (39, 40). Thrombin interacts with a hirudin-like DKEYPF binding domain on the N-terminus of PAR1, facilitating cleavage at an LDPR/SFLLR sessile bond and generating a new amino terminus, leading to self-activation via a tethered ligand mechanism, resulting in G-protein signaling (40–42). Synthetic peptides containing at least the first five amino acids of the tethered ligand (SFLLR), known as thrombin receptor-activating peptides (TRAP), are able to effect receptor activation without the need for receptor proteolysis, and is commonly employed in laboratory analysis of PAR1 activation without triggering the coagulation system (39, 43). PAR1 is the primary low-dose thrombin receptor on human platelets.

PAR3 is minimally expressed in human platelets. Like PAR1, PAR3 is thought to utilize a hirudin-like domain for thrombin interaction and cleavage at a LPIKTFRGAP sequence generating a tethered ligand (44). However, synthetic peptides of the tethered ligand do not cause PAR3 activation, suggesting that a conformational change in the receptor caused by cleavage is required before the tethered ligand is recognized. PAR3 is the primary low-dose thrombin receptor in mice, but plays little role in humans due to its minimal expression on human platelets.

PAR4, while less abundant than PAR1, is readily expressed on human platelets, although it is much less sensitive to cleavage by thrombin than PAR1 or PAR3 as it lacks the hirudin-like binding sequence of these molecules (45). Instead, thrombin cleaves PAR4 at the Arg-Gly bond in the PAPRGYPGQV sequence, resulting in an exposure of a tethered ligand that binds the PAR4 receptor and activates G-protein signaling. Like PAR1, synthetic peptidomimetics of the tethered ligand can elicit a thrombin-like response from PAR4 without the need for cleavage (45). PAR4 is the principal high-dose thrombin receptor on both mouse and human platelets.

Upon PAR activation, a series of distinct signaling pathways mediated by $G\alpha_s$, $G\alpha_i$, $G\alpha_q$, and $G\alpha_{12/13}$ proteins are initiated (see Subheading 4). These signaling events involve phosphoinositide hydrolysis, protein phosphorylation, increased cytosolic calcium, and suppression of cyclic AMP and ultimately converge in cytoskeletal actin reorganization and integrin activation (10, 46). Shape change resulting in actin reorganization results in the internalization or blebbing off (microparticles) of cleaved thrombin receptors, while cell spreading exposes PAR receptors from the canalicular system to the platelet surface, increasing the potential for further platelet activation by thrombin (47).

The platelet GPIb–IX complex is also a receptor for thrombin (see Subheading 3.1). While the functional relevance of thrombin–GPIb–IX binding on platelet activation is unclear, functional GPIb–IX–V complex is required for optimal thrombin responsiveness in humans, although not necessarily functioning directly in the signal transduction mechanism, and may simply be a result of localization of thrombin to the platelet surface through GPIb–IX–V binding.

3.4 P2Y Nucleotide Receptors

Nucleotide receptors are classified into P1 (A_1 through A_4 adenosine receptors) and P2 (ATP and ADP receptors) (24). The P2 receptors are further categorized as ion-channel linked (P2X) or G-protein linked (P2Y). Two P2Y receptors play a major role in platelet aggregation; these are the G_q-coupled receptor $P2Y_1$ and the G_i-coupled receptor $P2Y_{12}$ (48, 49). Both receptors are bound to and activated by adenosine diphosphate (ADP), while adenosine triphosphate (ATP) acts as an antagonist for both.

$P2Y_1$ signals through phospholipase C and is responsible for the mobilization of intracellular calcium ions, thereby mediating shape change and aggregation (50). $P2Y_{12}$ inhibits adenylate cyclase, thus inhibiting cyclic adenosine monophosphate (cAMP) production, leading to increased platelet activation via dephosphorylation of vasodilator-stimulated phosphoprotein (VASP), which in turn leads to activation of the $\alpha_{IIb}\beta_3$ integrin and decreased inhibition of calcium mobilization and granule release (50).

4 Platelet Signaling

The link between the myriad of surface receptors and their effects on platelet function is network of signaling molecules and regulators including heterotrimeric G-proteins that associate surface receptors and intracellular effectors, Ras proteins that act as GTP-binding switches, and phospholipases that signal via hydrolysis of phosphoinositides and formation of prostanoids, lipid kinases, protein tyrosine kinases, and serine/threonine kinases that regulate enzyme activity (24). In general, this involves activation of phospholipase C and PI 3-kinase-dependent pathways and suppression of cAMP and adenylyl cyclase, which normally act to prevent platelet activation.

In vivo platelet activation is usually initiated by collagen and vWF or, in the case of pathology, thrombin. In collagen-induced platelet activation, collagen and vWF bind to several molecules on the platelet membrane (see Subheading 2) including GPIb–IX–V complex, GPVI, and integrin $\alpha_{IIb}\beta_3$ and $\alpha_2\beta_1$. Collagen causes clustering of GPVI and its constitutively associated Fc receptor γ-chain (51). This leads to phosphorylation of the γ-chain by Src kinases which associate with Syk and phosphorylation and activation of phospholipase $C\gamma_2$ ($PLC\gamma_2$). This results in the production of IP_3—which opens Ca^{2+} channels and thus increases intracellular calcium, and diacylglycerol (DAG) which activates PKC, which phosphorylates serine/threonine to activate $\alpha_{IIb}\beta_3$ to expose fibrinogen-binding sites for aggregation, shape change, and activation. Thus the activation of platelets is a slow process, requiring polymerized collagen and clustering of GPVI. Coincident binding of vWF to $\alpha_{IIb}\beta_3$ to GPIb slows the platelet and localizes it to the endothelium long enough for this process to occur (24).

In contrast, thrombin induces platelet activation via a G-protein-dependent mechanism which results in faster and more intense activation of PLCβ. Thrombin binds to and cleaves the N-terminus of the PAR 1 and 4 in humans. This cleavage exposes a new N-terminus which acts as a tethered ligand (39), signaling via $G_{q\alpha}$, G_{12}, and G_i with downstream activation to a host of intracellular effectors (38, 52). $G_{q\alpha}$ activates PLCβ, resulting in the generation of IP_3 from PIP_2 and release of intracytosolic calcium, and activated PKC from DAG (53, 54). Thus $G_{q\alpha}$ is responsible for integrin activation and fibrinogen binding and increased cytosolic calcium. G_{12} is coupled to guanine nucleotide exchange factors (GEF) which activate Rac and Rho signaling pathways to uncap actin filaments and reorganize the cytoskeleton to produce shape change, degranulation, and spreading (55). G_i inhibits adenylyl cyclase, resulting in diminished cAMP and thus promoting platelet activation (38).

Following initial activation of the platelet, additional circulating platelets are activated and recruited to the thrombus by the local accumulation of molecules that are secreted by the platelets in the primary thrombus, such as ADP or thromboxane A_2 (TxA_2) (Fig. 1). The signaling pathways involved in this extension phase of platelet thrombus formation are predominantly through high-affinity G-protein-coupled receptors similar to thrombin, often with multiple G-proteins activated by the same receptor, and thus rapid amplification of activation can take place. ADP is released by degranulation, while thromboxane is generated by cyclooxygenase from arachidonic acid in response to platelet activation. Both ADP and TxA_2 release result in further platelet activation and recruitment of nearby resting platelets into the growing thrombus in a self-propagating cycle. Binding of the thromboxane prostanoid (TP) receptor leads to shape change via G_q and Rho signaling, and activation of PKC via PLCβ and G_{12}, similar to $P2Y_1$. This stimulated further release of TxA_2 and amplification of the platelet thrombus formation.

Once $\alpha_{IIb}\beta_3$ has been activated by PLC, it binds fibrinogen and platelet aggregation can occur. The close cell-to-cell contact between platelets in aggregation gives rise to another phase of

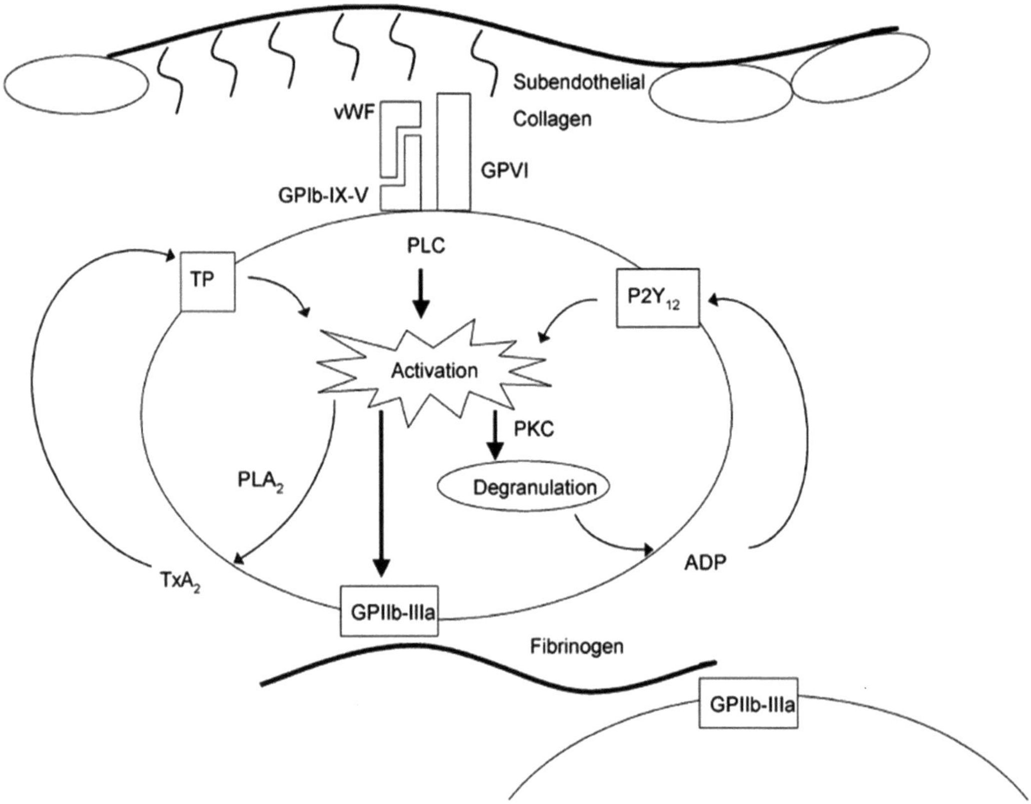

Fig. 1 Platelet activation is normally initiated by exposure of collagen and vWF. This leads to release of ADP through degranulation and synthesis of thromboxane A_2. Both of these bind constitutively expressed receptors on the platelet surface, and represent a self-perpetuating signal amplification loop, and a means of recruiting nearby resting platelets. An activation-dependent conformational change in GPIIb–IIIa allows fibrinogen binding and therefore platelet aggregation

Table 3
G-protein-coupled receptors expressed on human platelets

G-protein	Receptors	Function
G_i	A_{2A}-adrenergic, CXCR4, $P2Y_{12}$, PAR1	Decrease cAMP by inhibiting adenylyl cyclase
		Increase IP_3/DAG via PLC
		Increase 3-PPIs
G_q	PAF, PAR1, PAR4, $P2Y_1$, TPα, TPβ, vasopressin 1	Increase IP_3/DAG via PLC
G_{12}	PAR1, PAR4, $P2Y_1$, TPα, TPβ	Actin assembly and reorganization
G_s	Prostaglandin I receptor	Increases cAMP by adenylyl cyclase

signaling that results in outside-in signaling through integrins and binding of ephrins to Eph kinases (56). Table 3 lists the G-proteins expressed on human platelets, their associated receptors, and function.

5 Platelet Interactions

Platelet physiology cannot be considered in isolation from the other components of blood and the vascular system which interact to contribute to haemostasis and thrombosis. Platelets bind to injured or activated endothelium, while leukocytes bind to activated platelets and the heterotypic thrombus serves as a major procoagulant site (57) and plays an important role in inflammation. These multicellular interactions are mediated by adhesive molecules such as P-selectin from platelet granules, PSGL-1 on leukocytes and endothelium, and GPIb (31).

5.1 Platelet–Leukocyte Interactions

Platelets are a central cellular interface of thrombotic and inflammatory processes (58) and modulate this interface by binding to leukocytes and altering their function (57, 59). Correspondingly, platelets play a pivotal role in recruitment of monocytes and neutrophils to sites of vascular injury, and thus to the atherosclerotic plaque (60). Platelet activation, formation of leukocyte–platelet aggregates (monocyte–platelet aggregates and neutrophil–platelet aggregates), and platelet secretion of inflammatory modulators that affect leukocyte function, such as CD40 ligand (CD40L), are associated with the development of atherosclerosis (61–63), stable coronary artery disease (CAD) (64), unstable angina (65), myocardial infarction (MI) (66), and events following percutaneous coronary intervention (PCI) (66), with a greater magnitude in patients experiencing late clinical events (67).

P-selectin (CD62P) is a component of the α-granule membrane and is not normally expressed on the surface of platelets (59, 68–70). Upon platelet activation α-granule-soluble contents are released and P-selectin is exposed on the platelet surface (59, 69, 70). In vitro, the activation-dependent increase in platelet surface P-selectin is not reversible over time (71, 72). However, in vivo, circulating degranulated platelets rapidly lose their surface P-selectin, yet continue to circulate and function (73).

Surface expression of P-selectin on platelets mediates the initial adhesion of activated platelets to monocytes and neutrophils via PSGL-1, which is constitutively expressed on the surface of these leukocytes (59, 74–76).

Following initial tethering to activated platelets via P-selectin/PSGL-1 interaction, leukocyte activation occurs through signaling via PSGL-1 and platelet-secreted chemokines and lipid mediators (77–82). This response in turn causes activation and upregulation of the Mac-1 integrin ($\alpha_M\beta_2$, CD11b/CD18) on the monocyte surface, allowing firm adhesion to platelets via bridging fibrinogen bound to the activated glycoprotein IIb–IIIa integrin ($\alpha_{IIb}\beta_2$, CD61/CD41) (57, 80), and via direct interaction with GPIbα (30) on the platelet surface. Other adhesion molecules such as

LFA-1 on the monocytes interacting with ICAM-2 on platelets may play a role in stabilizing heterotypic aggregates (83). However, P-selectin/PSGL-1 interaction is first required before these stable secondary adhesions may take place. The exact physiologic significance of leukocyte–platelet aggregation is unknown, but it may represent targeting of both cell types to appropriate inflammatory or haemostatic sites (84).

5.2 Platelet–Endothelial Cell Interaction

Resting platelets under shear roll on activated endothelial cells via interaction of endothelial P-selectin with platelet surface GPIbα or PSGL-1 (33, 85) and vWF interaction with GPIbα (86). This rolling accumulates platelets at the site of injury, and allows for other interactions to take place (85). Following platelet activation, a more stable association between endothelial cells and platelets occurs, mediated by GPIIb–IIIa-bound fibrinogen on platelets binding to ICAM-1 and $\alpha_v\beta_3$ on endothelial cells (87).

5.3 Platelet–Coagulation System Interaction

Platelet adherence and aggregation at the site of vascular injury not only serves to form a platelet-rich haemostatic plug or thrombus but also serves as a site of activation and assembly of the coagulation system, to direct its haemostatic potential to the site of injury and prevent systematic widespread intravascular clot formation. Activated platelets regulate propagation of the coagulation system by releasing granule components that trigger and propagate the coagulation cascade, express specific high-affinity receptors for coagulation components which protect them from inactivation, act as the site for assembly of the tenase and prothrombinase complex formation, and amplify the initial stimulus leading to a rapid and localized thrombin burst (88).

6 Summary

Platelets are specialized, anuclear cells not only of pivotal importance in thrombosis and haemostasis but which also play a role in innate immunity, inflammation, wound healing, haematologic malignancies, and metabolic disorders. Platelets have considerable cross talk with other cells, including other platelets, leukocytes, and endothelial cells. They also interact with the coagulation cascade and the humoral immune system. This is accomplished by a complex array of surface receptors, adhesion proteins, integrins, and glycoproteins coupled to multiple signaling pathways which orchestrate initiation, extension, and propagation of platelet activation both with redundancy and the ability to modulate function. The role of platelets in disease, particularly in atherothrombosis, is increasingly the focus of current research and antiplatelet therapy plays a significant role in the prevention and treatment of atherothrombotic and inflammatory diseases.

References

1. Hartwig JH (2002) Platelet structure. In: Michelson AD (ed) Platelets. Academic, San Diego, CA, pp 37–52
2. Boyles J, Fox JE, Phillips DR, Stenberg PE (1985) Organization of the cytoskeleton in resting, discoid platelets: preservation of actin filaments by a modified fixation that prevents osmium damage. J Cell Biol 101:1463–1472
3. Reed GL (2002) Platelet secretion. In: Michelson AD (ed) Platelets. Academic, San Diego, CA, pp 181–195
4. Hartwig JH, DeSisto M (1991) The cytoskeleton of the resting human blood platelet: structure of the membrane skeleton and its attachment to actin filaments. J Cell Biol 112: 407–425
5. Tablin F, Reeber MJ, Nachmias VT (1988) Platelets contain a 210 K microtubule-associated protein related to a similar protein in HeLa cells. J Cell Sci 90(Pt 2):317–324
6. Kovacsovics TJ, Hartwig JH (1996) Thrombin-induced GPIb-IX centralization on the platelet surface requires actin assembly and myosin II activation. Blood 87:618–629
7. Schwer HD, Lecine P, Tiwari S, Italiano JE Jr, Hartwig JH, Shivdasani RA (2001) A lineage-restricted and divergent beta-tubulin isoform is essential for the biogenesis, structure and function of blood platelets. Curr Biol 11:579–586
8. Shattil SJ, Hoxie JA, Cunningham M, Brass LF (1985) Changes in the platelet membrane glycoprotein IIb.IIIa complex during platelet activation. J Biol Chem 260:11107–11114
9. Berridge MJ (1984) Inositol trisphosphate and diacylglycerol as second messengers. Biochem J 220:345–360
10. Brass LF (1999) More pieces of the platelet activation puzzle slide into place. J Clin Invest 104:1663–1665
11. Hartwig JH (1992) Mechanisms of actin rearrangements mediating platelet activation. J Cell Biol 118:1421–1442
12. Carlier MF, Didry D, Erk I, Lepault J, Van Troys ML, Vandekerckhove J, Perelroizen I, Yin H, Doi Y, Pantaloni D (1996) Tbeta 4 is not a simple G-actin sequestering protein and interacts with F-actin at high concentration. J Biol Chem 271:9231–9239
13. Knezevic I, Leisner TM, Lam SC (1996) Direct binding of the platelet integrin alphaIIbbeta3 (GPIIb-IIIa) to talin. Evidence that interaction is mediated through the cytoplasmic domains of both alphaIIb and beta3. J Biol Chem 271:16416–16421
14. Niewiarowski S, Holt JC, Cook JJ (1994) Biochemistry and physiology of secreted platelet proteins. In: Coleman RW, Hirsh J, Marder VJ, Salzman EW (eds) Haemostasis and thrombosis: basic principles and clinical practice. Lippincott, Philidelphia, PA, pp 546–556
15. Fukami MH (1997) Dense granule factors. In: von Bruchhausen F, Walter U (eds) Platelets and their factors. Springer, New York, pp 419–432
16. Knight DE, Hallam TJ, Scrutton MC (1982) Agonist selectivity and second messenger concentration in Ca2+-mediated secretion. Nature 296:256–257
17. Chang JD, Ware JA (1997) Ca^{2+} and Protein Kinase C in Platelets. In: Bittar EE & Lapretina EG (eds) Advances in Molecular and Cell Biology Vol 18: The Platelet. JAI Press, Greenwich, pp 275–310
18. Shirakawa R, Yoshioka A, Horiuchi H, Nishioka H, Tabuchi A, Kita T (2000) Small GTPase Rab4 regulates Ca2+-induced alpha-granule secretion in platelets. J Biol Chem 275:33844–33849
19. Nieuwland R, Sturk A (2002) Platelet-derived microparticles. In: Michelson AD (ed) Platelets. Academic, San Diego, CA, pp 255–265
20. Wiedmer T, Shattil SJ, Cunningham M, Sims PJ (1990) Role of calcium and calpain in complement-induced vesiculation of the platelet plasma membrane and in the exposure of the platelet factor Va receptor. Biochemistry 29: 623–632
21. Wiedmer T, Sims PJ (1991) Participation of protein kinases in complement C5b-9-induced shedding of platelet plasma membrane vesicles. Blood 78:2880–2886
22. Sims PJ, Faioni EM, Wiedmer T, Shattil SJ (1988) Complement proteins C5b-9 cause release of membrane vesicles from the platelet surface that are enriched in the membrane receptor for coagulation factor Va and express prothrombinase activity. J Biol Chem 263: 18205–18212
23. Sims PJ, Wiedmer T, Esmon CT, Weiss HJ, Shattil SJ (1989) Assembly of the platelet prothrombinase complex is linked to vesiculation of the platelet plasma membrane. Studies in Scott syndrome: an isolated defect in platelet procoagulant activity. J Biol Chem 264:17049–17057
24. Clemetson KJ (2002) Platelet receptors. In: Michelson AD (ed) Platelets. Academic, San Diego, CA, pp 65–84
25. Lopez JA, Berndt MC (2002) The GPIb-IX-V complex. In: Michelson AD (ed) Platelets. Academic, San Diego, CA, pp 85–104
26. Lopez JA (1994) The platelet glycoprotein Ib-IX complex. Blood Coagul Fibrinolysis 5:97–119

27. Fredrickson BJ, Dong JF, McIntire LV, Lopez JA (1998) Shear-dependent rolling on von Willebrand factor of mammalian cells expressing the platelet glycoprotein Ib-IX-V complex. Blood 92:3684–3693
28. Ramakrishnan V, DeGuzman F, Bao M, Hall SW, Leung LL, Phillips DR (2001) A thrombin receptor function for platelet glycoprotein Ib-IX unmasked by cleavage of glycoprotein V. Proc Natl Acad Sci U S A 98:1823–1828
29. Kroll MH, Hellums JD, McIntire LV, Schafer AI, Moake JL (1996) Platelets and shear stress. Blood 88:1525–1541
30. Simon DI, Chen Z, Xu H, Li CQ, Dong J, McIntire LV, Ballantyne CM, Zhang L, Furman MI, Berndt MC, Lopez JA (2000) Platelet glycoprotein ibalpha is a counterreceptor for the leukocyte integrin Mac-1 (CD11b/CD18). J Exp Med 192:193–204
31. McEver RP (2006) P-Selectin/PSGL-1 and other interactions between platelets, leukocytes and endothelium. In: Michelson AD (ed) Platelets. Academic, San Diego, CA, pp 231–250
32. Kansas GS (1996) Selectins and the ligands: current concepts and controversies. Blood 88:3259–3287
33. Romo GM, Dong JF, Schade AJ, Gardiner EE, Kansas GS, Li CQ, McIntire LV, Berndt MC, Lopez JA (1999) The glycoprotein Ib-IX-V complex is a platelet counterreceptor for P-selectin. J Exp Med 190:803–814
34. Berndt MC, Phillips DR (1981) Interaction of thrombin with platelets: purification of the thrombin substrate. Ann N Y Acad Sci 370:87–95
35. Baglia FA, Badellino KO, Li CQ, Lopez JA, Walsh PN (2002) Factor XI binding to the platelet glycoprotein Ib-IX-V complex promotes factor XI activation by thrombin. J Biol Chem 277:1662–1668
36. Hato T, Ginsberg MH, Shattil SJ (2002) Integrin alphallb-beta3. In: Michelson AD (ed) Platelets. Academic, San Diego, CA, pp 105–116
37. Cierniewski CS, Byzova T, Papierak M, Haas TA, Niewiarowska J, Zhang L, Cieslak M, Plow EF (1999) Peptide ligands can bind to distinct sites in integrin alphaIIbbeta3 and elicit different functional responses. J Biol Chem 274:16923–16932
38. Tolentino AR, Bahou WF (2002) Thrombin receptors. In: Michelson AD (ed) Platelets. Academic, San Diego, CA, pp 117–138
39. Vu TK, Hung DT, Wheaton VI, Coughlin SR (1991) Molecular cloning of a functional thrombin receptor reveals a novel proteolytic mechanism of receptor activation. Cell 64:1057–1068
40. Rasmussen UB, Vouret-Craviari V, Jallat S, Schlesinger Y, Pages G, Pavirani A, Lecocq JP, Pouyssegur J, Van Obberghen-Schilling E (1991) cDNA cloning and expression of a hamster alpha-thrombin receptor coupled to Ca2+ mobilization. FEBS Lett 288:123–128
41. Bizios R, Lai L, Fenton JW II, Malik AB (1986) Thrombin-induced chemotaxis and aggregation of neutrophils. J Cell Physiol 128:485–490
42. Liu LW, Vu TK, Esmon CT, Coughlin SR (1991) The region of the thrombin receptor resembling hirudin binds to thrombin and alters enzyme specificity. J Biol Chem 266:16977–16980
43. Vu TK, Wheaton VI, Hung DT, Charo I, Coughlin SR (1991) Domains specifying thrombin-receptor interaction. Nature 353:674–677
44. Ishihara H, Connolly AJ, Zeng D, Kahn ML, Zheng YW, Timmons C, Tram T, Coughlin SR (1997) Protease-activated receptor 3 is a second thrombin receptor in humans. Nature 386:502–506
45. Xu W-F, Anderson H, Whitmore TE, Presnell SR, Yee DP, Ching AC, Gilbert T, Davie EW, Foster DC (1998) Cloning and characterization of the human protease-activated receptor 4. Proc Natl Acad Sci U S A 95:6642–6646
46. Brass LF, Manning DR, Cichowski K, Abrams CS (1997) Signaling through G proteins in platelets: to the integrins and beyond. Thromb Haemost 78:581–589
47. Brass LF (1997) Thrombin receptor antagonists: a work in progress. Coron Artery Dis 8:49–58
48. Ayyanathan K, Webbs TE, Sandhu AK, Athwal RS, Barnard EA, Kunapuli SP (1996) Cloning and chromosomal localization of the human P2Y1 purinoceptor. Biochem Biophys Res Commun 218:783–788
49. Hollopeter G, Jantzen H-M, Vincent D, Li G, England L, Ramakrishnan V, Yang R-B, Nurden P, Nurden A, Julius D, Conley PB (2001) Identification of the platelet ADP receptor targeted by antithrombotic drugs. Nature 409:202–207
50. Jin J, Kunapuli SP (1998) Coactivation of two different G protein-coupled receptors is essential for ADP-induced platelet aggregation. Proc Natl Acad Sci U S A 95:8070–8074
51. Kehrel B, Wierwille S, Clemetson KJ, Anders O, Steiner M, Knight CG, Farndale RW, Okuma M, Barnes MJ (1998) Glycoprotein VI is a major collagen receptor for platelet activation: it recognizes the platelet-activating quaternary structure of collagen, whereas CD36, glycoprotein IIb/IIIa, and von Willebrand factor do not. Blood 91:491–499

52. Woulfe D, Yang J, Prevost N, O'Brien P, Brass LF (2002) Signal transduction during the initiation, extension, and perpetuation of platelet plug formation. In: Michelson AD (ed) Platelets. Academic, San Diego, CA, pp 197–213
53. Hung DT, Wong YH, Vu TK, Coughlin SR (1992) The cloned platelet thrombin receptor couples to at least two distinct effectors to stimulate phosphoinositide hydrolysis and inhibit adenylyl cyclase. J Biol Chem 267: 20831–20834
54. Hung DT, Vu TH, Nelken NA, Coughlin SR (1992) Thrombin-induced events in non-platelet cells are mediated by the unique proteolytic mechanism established for the cloned platelet thrombin receptor. J Cell Biol 116: 827–832
55. Klages B, Brandt U, Simon MI, Schultz G, Offermanns S (1999) Activation of G12/G13 results in shape change and Rho/Rho-kinase-mediated myosin light chain phosphorylation in mouse platelets. J Cell Biol 144:745–754
56. Shattil SJ (1999) Signaling through platelet integrin alpha IIb beta 3: inside-out, outside-in, and sideways. Thromb Haemost 82: 318–325
57. Barnard MR, Linden MD, Frelinger AL III, Li Y, Fox ML, Furman MI, Michelson AD (2005) Effects of platelet binding on whole blood flow cytometry assays of monocyte and neutrophil procoagulant activity. J Thromb Haemost 3:2563–2570
58. Libby P, Simon DI (2001) Inflammation and thrombosis: the clot thickens. Circulation 103:1718–1720
59. McEver RP (2002) P-selectin/PSGL-1 and other interactions between platelets, leukocytes, and endothelium. In: Michelson AD (ed) Platelets. Academic, San Diego, CA, pp 139–155
60. Palabrica T, Lobb R, Furie BC, Aronovitz M, Benjamin C, Hsu YM, Sajer SA, Furie B (1992) Leukocyte accumulation promoting fibrin deposition is mediated in vivo by P-selectin on adherent platelets. Nature 359:848–851
61. Huo Y, Schober A, Forlow SB, Smith DF, Hyman MC, Jung S, Littman DR, Weber C, Ley K (2003) Circulating activated platelets exacerbate atherosclerosis in mice deficient in apolipoprotein E. Nat Med 9:61–67
62. Schonbeck U, Libby P (2001) CD40 signaling and plaque instability. Circ Res 89: 1092–1103
63. Schonbeck U, Libby P (2001) The CD40/CD154 receptor/ligand dyad. Cell Mol Life Sci 58:4–43
64. Furman MI, Benoit SE, Barnard MR, Valeri CR, Borbone ML, Becker RC, Hechtman HB, Michelson AD (1998) Increased platelet reactivity and circulating monocyte-platelet aggregates in patients with stable coronary artery disease. J Am Coll Cardiol 31:352–358
65. Ott I, Neumann FJ, Gawaz M, Scmitt M, Schomig A (1996) Increased neutrophil-platelet adhesion in patients with unstable angina. Circulation 94:1239–1246
66. Michelson AD, Barnard MR, Krueger LA, Valeri CR, Furman MI (2001) Circulating monocyte-platelet aggregates are a more sensitive marker of in vivo platelet activation than platelet surface P-selectin: studies in baboons, human coronary intervention, and human acute myocardial infarction. Circulation 104:1533–1537
67. Mickelson JK, Lakkis NM, Villarreal-Levy G, Hughes BJ, Smith CW (1996) Leukocyte activation with platelet adhesion after coronary angioplasty: a mechanism for recurrent disease? J Am Coll Cardiol 28:345–353
68. Michelson AD, Linden MD, Barnard MR, Furman MI, Frelinger AL (2006) Flow Cytometry. In: Michelson AD (ed) Platelets. Academic Press, San Diego, CA, pp 545–565
69. Hsu-Lin SC, Berman CL, Furie BC, August D, Furie B (1984) A platelet membrane protein expressed during platelet activation and secretion: studies using a monoclonal antibody specific for thrombin-activated platelets. J Biol Chem 259:9121–9126
70. Stenberg PE, McEver RP, Shuman MA, Jacques YV, Bainton DF (1985) A platelet alpha-granule membrane protein (GMP-140) is expressed on the platelet membrane after activation. J Cell Biol 101:880–886
71. Michelson AD, Benoit SE, Kroll MH, Li J, Rohrer MJ, Kestin AS, Barnard MR (1994) The activation-induced decrease in the platelet surface expression of the glycoprotein Ib-IX complex is reversible. Blood 83:3562–3573
72. Ruf A, Patscheke H (1995) Flow cytometric detection of activated platelets: comparison of determining shape change, fibrinogen binding, and P-selectin expression. Semin Thromb Hemost 21:146–151
73. Michelson AD, Barnard MR, Hechtman HB, MacGregor H, Connolly RJ, Loscalzo J, Valeri CR (1996) *In vivo* tracking of platelets: circulating degranulated platelets rapidly lose surface P-selectin but continue to circulate and function. Proc Natl Acad Sci U S A 93: 11877–11882
74. Larsen E, Celi A, Gilbert GE, Furie BC, Erban JK, Bonfanti R, Wagner DD, Furie B (1989)

PADGEM protein: a receptor that mediates the interaction of activated platelets with neutrophils and monocytes. Cell 59:305–312

75. Hamburger SA, McEver RP (1990) GMP-140 mediates adhesion of stimulated platelets to neutrophils. Blood 75:550–554
76. Linden MD, Furman MI (2005) Monocyte-platelet aggregates in patients with ischemic heart disease. In: Morrow DA, Cannon C (eds) Cardiovascular biomarkers: pathophysiology and disease management. Humana, Totowa, NJ, pp 487–493
77. Hidari KI, Weyrich AS, Zimmerman GA, McEver RP (1997) Engagement of P-selectin glycoprotein ligand-1 enhances tyrosine phosphorylation and activates mitogen-activated protein kinases in human neutrophils. J Biol Chem 272:28750–28756
78. Blanks JE, Moll T, Eytner R, Vestweber D (1998) Stimulation of P-selectin glycoprotein ligand-1 on mouse neutrophils activates beta 2-integrin mediated cell attachment to ICAM-1. Eur J Immunol 28:433–443
79. Evangelista V, Manarini S, Sideri R, Rotondo S, Martelli N, Piccoli A, Totani L, Piccardoni P, Vestweber D, de Gaetano G, Cerletti C (1999) Platelet/polymorphonuclear leukocyte interaction: P-selectin triggers protein-tyrosine phosphorylation-dependent CD11b/CD18 adhesion: role of PSGL-1 as a signaling molecule. Blood 93:876–885
80. Weber C, Springer TA (1997) Neutrophil accumulation on activated, surface-adherent platelets in flow is mediated by interaction of Mac-1 with fibrinogen bound to alphaIIbbeta3 and stimulated by platelet-activating factor. J Clin Invest 100:2085–2093
81. Weyrich AS, Elstad MR, McEver RP, McIntyre TM, Moore KL, Morrissey JH, Prescott SM, Zimmerman GA (1996) Activated platelets signal chemokine synthesis by human monocytes. J Clin Invest 97:1525–1534
82. Ostrovsky L, King AJ, Bond S, Mitchell D, Lorant DE, Zimmerman GA, Larsen R, Niu XF, Kubes P (1998) A juxtacrine mechanism for neutrophil adhesion on platelets involves platelet-activating factor and a selectin-dependent activation process. Blood 91:3028–3036
83. Diacovo TG, deFougerolles AR, Bainton DF, Springer TA (1994) A functional integrin ligand on the surface of platelets: intercellular adhesion molecule-2. J Clin Invest 94: 1243–1251
84. Rinder HM, Bonan JL, Rinder CS, Ault KA, Smith BR (1991) Dynamics of leukocyte-platelet adhesion in whole blood. Blood 78:1730–1737
85. Frenette PS, Denis CV, Weiss L, Jurk K, Subbarao S, Kehrel B, Hartwig JH, Vestweber D, Wagner DD (2000) P-Selectin glycoprotein ligand 1 (PSGL-1) is expressed on platelets and can mediate platelet-endothelial interactions in vivo. J Exp Med 191:1413–1422
86. Andre P, Denis CV, Ware J, Saffaripour S, Hynes RO, Ruggeri ZM, Wagner DD (2000) Platelets adhere to and translocate on von Willebrand factor presented by endothelium in stimulated veins. Blood 96:3322–3328
87. Bombeli T, Schwartz BR, Harlan JM (1998) Adhesion of activated platelets to endothelial cells: evidence for a GPIIbIIIa-dependent bridging mechanism and novel roles for endothelial intercellular adhesion molecule 1 (ICAM-1), alphavbeta3 integrin, and GPIbalpha. J Exp Med 187:329–339
88. Bouchard BA, Butenas S, Mann KG, Tracy PB (2002) Interactions between platelets and the coagulation system. In: Michelson AD (ed) Platelets. Academic, San Diego, CA, pp 229–253

Chapter 3

The Role of the Vessel Wall

Nethnapha Paredes and Anthony K.C. Chan

Abstract

The role of the vessel wall is complex and its effects are wide-ranging. The vessel wall, specifically the endothelial monolayer that lines the inner lumen, possesses the ability to influence various physiological states both locally and systemically by controlling vascular tone, basement membrane component synthesis, angiogenesis, haemostatic properties, and immunogenicity. This is an overview of the function and structure of the vessel wall and how disruption and dysfunction in any of these regulatory roles can lead to disease states.

Key words Vessel wall, Vascular tone, Basement membrane, Angiogenesis, Haemostasis, Endothelial cells

1 Introduction

The monolayer of endothelial cells lining the inner lumen of blood vessels is very versatile. It is a selective barrier separating the circulating blood from the underlying tissue, providing a nonthrombogenic surface under physiologic conditions as well as mediating the passage of nutrients, solutes, and hormones from the blood to the interstitium. The endothelium has multifunctional roles in the modulation of vascular tone, blood flow, and permeability. Further, this tissue layer possesses synthesis and metabolic processes that release substances into the bloodstream and basal lamina to maintain and control matrix composition and function. Endothelium also regulates the haemostatic system, angiogenesis, and immune and inflammatory responses by controlling cellular interactions with the vessel wall. Endothelial cell response to physical (shear stress, damage) or chemical (hormones, neurotransmitters, subcellular matrix components, nutrients, oxygen supply, and metabolites) varies depending on the location of these cells in the vascular tree, whether the cells are located in large vessels or capillaries or are arterial or venous in origin. The flexibility of endothelial function and response gives the endothelium the ability to maintain its

Paul Monagle (ed.), *Haemostasis: Methods and Protocols*, Methods in Molecular Biology, vol. 992,
DOI 10.1007/978-1-62703-339-8_3, © Springer Science+Business Media New York 2013

integrity in a dynamic environment. Disruption to any of these systems affecting endothelial structure and function can potentially lead to disease states such as atherosclerosis, haemostatic dysfunction, and altered inflammatory and immune responses.

2 Endothelial Control of Vascular Tone

One function of the endothelium is to regulate vascular tone through the synthesis of vasoactive substances that influence the underlying smooth-muscle cells. The ability to control vascular tone allows endothelial cells to regulate the local environment in response to various stimuli such as shear stress and inflammatory substances, as well as influence cell adhesion, proliferation, and migration. The inability to control vascular tone, as a result of endothelial dysfunction, can potentially lead to pathological states such as heart failure, hypertension, diabetes, and atherosclerosis.

2.1 Vasodilation

Endothelial cells are capable of producing at least three substances that cause relaxation of the underlying vascular smooth muscle. These substances are called endothelium-derived relaxing factors (EDRF) and are discussed below. One of the main factors stimulating the release of EDRF is increase in shear stress (1). Release of EDRF into the endothelial–smooth-muscle cell interstitium results in the upregulation of guanylate cyclase cytosolic enzyme in the smooth-muscle cells, eventually leading to an increase in cyclic 3′,5′-guanosine monophosphate (cyclic GMP) production and resultant relaxation of the vessel wall (2, 3). Several substances are able to stimulate the release of EDRF including circulating hormones (catecholamines, vasopressin), blood vessel wall autacoids (histamine, bradykinin, substance P), platelet products (serotonin, adenosine diphosphate), and coagulation factors (thrombin) (4). Stimulation of endothelial cells to release EDRF will cause, in most cases, a simultaneous release of nitric oxide (NO) and/or endothelial-derived hyperpolarizing factor (EDHF) and/or prostacyclin. Pathological states associated with dysfunctional EDRF release include atherosclerosis (3, 5), hypertension (6, 7), and aging (8, 9).

2.1.1 Endothelium-Derived Nitric Oxide

Endothelial cells possess an enzyme called NO-synthase which is capable of producing NO from a semi-essential amino acid, L-arginine (10). Activation of NO-synthase is dependent on the intracellular calcium ion levels of endothelial cells (11). Once produced, NO is secreted into the vascular lumen and also toward the underlying smooth-muscle cells. In the lumen, NO acts locally to inhibit the adhesion of platelets and leukocytes to the endothelium, and acts synergistically with prostacyclin to inhibit platelet aggregation (11, 12). In the basolateral compartment, NO exerts its influence by stimulating guanylate cyclase in smooth-muscle cells, which in turn, upregulates the formation of cyclic GMP resulting in the relaxation of the smooth-muscle cells (11, 13, 14).

Continuous release of NO maintains basal vessel wall tone. NO production is augmented in the presence of stimuli such as acetylcholine, serotonin, thrombin, shear stress, and oxygen tension (15). Production of NO and its influence on smooth-muscle cells allow the endothelium to regulate blood pressure (16). The ability of NO to relax and dilate vascular vessels has been demonstrated in both animals and humans using NO synthesis inhibitors (6, 7, 16). NO also has the ability to inhibit the growth of vascular smooth-muscles cells (17). One of the hallmark characteristics of endothelial dysfunction is the decrease in the bioavailability of NO, leading to adverse pathological conditions (18).

2.1.2 Prostacyclin

Synthesized from arachidonic acid by endothelial cells, prostacyclin (PGI_2) is a potent, short-lived vasodilator that regulates vascular tone and blood pressure (19, 20). In concert with NO, it is also a potent inhibitor of platelet aggregation (21). Synthesis of prostacyclin is sensitive to a variety of factors that effectively increase cytoplasmic concentrations of calcium, such as thrombin (22), bradykinin (23), histamine (24), and changes in shear stress (25). Many of these agents are produced during onset of coagulation or platelet activation, thus illustrating the importance of prostacyclin in platelet inhibition.

2.1.3 Endothelium-Derived Hyperpolarizing Factor

The degree of influence of EDHF on vasodilation is dependent upon the type and size of the vessel. Unlike NO, which plays a more central role in larger vessels, EDHF is more important in smaller vessels (26). However, its exact chemical nature remains elusive. In several blood vessels, endothelial cell-dependent hyperpolarization is observed in the underlying vascular smooth-muscle cells in the presence of acetylcholine (27, 28). EDHF is thought to be a labile metabolite of arachidonic acid formed through the P-450 pathway (28) and could possibly be a potassium channel opener in smooth-muscle cells. Release of EDHF from the endothelium is dependent on the cytosolic calcium concentration and can be inhibited by calmodulin antagonists (29). Hyperpolarization of the endothelial cells is conducted via the myoendothelial gap junction where the resultant action is EDHF-attributed hyperpolarization and relaxation of the smooth-muscle cells (18).

2.2 Vasoconstriction

Endothelial cells are also able to control vascular tone through the production of diffusible contracting factors that affect the underlying smooth-muscle cells. When endothelial cells are subjected to a specific stimulus, such as neurohumoral mediators, sudden stretch, or A23187 (a Ca^{2+} ionophore), they release vasoconstrictive substances that affect the smooth-muscle cells (30). Factors produced and secreted by endothelial cells which affect the contractility of smooth-muscle cells include vasoconstrictor peptides such as endothelin-1 and angiotensin II, oxygen-derived free radicals that decrease the bioavailability of the vasodilation agent NO, and contracting factors that are metabolites of arachidonic acid.

2.2.1 Endothelin

Endothelin (ET) is a family of contractile peptides, comprised of 21 amino acids, that was initially isolated from the endothelium (ET-1) (31–33). Subsequent studies have revealed that ET-1 is expressed in other nonvascular tissues such as brain, kidney, and lungs (34). ET-2 and ET-3 isomers have been shown to be expressed in the intestine, adrenal gland, and brain (33, 35). ET-1, however, is the only isomer expressed by the endothelium. The ET-1 peptide is continuously released from endothelial cells by the constitutive secretory pathway (36) or from endothelial cell-specific storage granules called Weibel–Palade bodies (37, 38), in response to external stimuli such as thrombin, epinephrine, angiotensin II, growth factors, cytokines, and free radicals (39, 40). In contrast, ET-1 mediators, including NO (41), natriuretic peptide (42, 43), heparin (44, 45), and prostacyclin (46), reduce endogenous ET-1 gene expression from endothelial cells. Another factor influencing the production and release of ET-1 is shear stress (47, 48). An increase in blood flow activates the shear stress receptors of endothelial cells resulting in NO production and release, thereby decreasing ET-1 release and ultimately leading to vasodilation of the vessel wall.

The majority of ET-1 released from endothelial cells (~80 % of the total amount produced) is secreted into the basolateral compartment where it acts in a paracrine manner to elicit a vasoconstrictive response from the smooth-muscle cells (49). Low levels of ET-1 on the arterial lumen side stimulate the release of NO from endothelial cells resulting in relaxation of the smooth-muscle cells. However, higher doses of intravenous ET-1 allow some molecules to diffuse through the endothelial cells and act directly on the smooth-muscle cells. ET-1 acts on the underlying smooth-muscle cells by activating the ET_A receptor to elicit vasoconstriction and ET_B receptors on the endothelium to elicit a relaxing response (50, 51). Additional research has revealed the existence of subsets of ET_B receptors (52–54), ET_{B1} in vascular smooth-muscle cells resulting in vasoconstriction when activated and ET_{B2} in endothelial cells releasing relaxing factors when stimulated. ET has been implicated in several vascular conditions, including hypertension (55, 56), preeclampsia (57, 58), and acute renal failure (59, 60).

Another effect of ET-1 is to promote the proliferation of vascular endothelial cells and smooth-muscle cells, as well as fibroblasts, resulting in the transformation of the structure of the vascular wall (61–63).

2.2.2 Angiotensin II

Acute and chronic maintenance and regulation of blood pressure is through the renin–angiotensin–aldosterone system. In conditions where there are inadequate amounts of salt to maintain volume, renin causes constriction of the vessel wall to maintain blood pressure (64). Renin is an enzyme that converts the protein angiotensinogen to angiotensin I. Angiotensin-converting enzyme (ACE), mainly found at the cell membrane of endothelial cells, converts the less active angiotensin I peptide into the vasoactive angiotensin II. Angiotensin II acts directly on the vascular smooth muscle to cause vasoconstriction. It is also capable of regulating muscle cell growth of the heart and arteries (65, 66). Overactivity of the renin–angiotensin–aldosterone cascade has been linked to hypertension and end-organ damage (67).

2.2.3 Reactive Oxygen Species

Oxygen-derived free radicals, including superoxide anions, are a subgroup of reactive oxygen species (ROS) that contain minimally one unpaired electron (68). Superoxide is produced by vascular cells and is formed from molecular oxygen, affecting vascular tone by direct and indirect effects on the underlying smooth-muscle cells (69, 70). Superoxide anions can be either a vasodilator or vasoconstrictor, leading to the hypothesis that, at least in cerebral arteries, responses to superoxide may be biphasic eliciting vasodilation at lower superoxide concentrations and vasoconstriction at higher concentrations (35, 71, 72). Superoxide also inactivates NO, a potent vasodilatory substance (72). The loss of bioavailability of NO affects vascular tone and results in the constriction of the vessel wall.

3 Biosynthesis of Basement Membrane Components by the Endothelium

The vascular basement membrane (BM) provides structural and functional support to all blood vessels and capillaries. Lining the luminal side of the vascular wall are the endothelial cells, followed by the BM on the basal side of the endothelium, and finally, surrounding the BM are pericytes, specialized smooth-muscle cells controlling the permeability and vascular tone through contractility and apoptosis (73, 74). However, not all vascular BMs are the same. The unique composition is tissue specific and BMs regulate endothelial cell behavior according to the specific environment (75–77).

3.1 Basement Membrane Composition

BMs are always in contact with cells, providing structural support, compartmentalization of tissues, and regulation of cell behavior (75, 78–80). This sheet-like structure (50–100 nm thick) is mainly composed of type IV collagen, laminin, heparan-sulfate proteoglycans (HSPGs), and nidogen/entactin, as well as minor components such as agrin, SPARC/BM-40/osteopontin, fibulins, type XV collagen, and type XVIII collagen (75, 81, 82). Over 50 proteins have been identified as components of the BM, but collagen, especially type IV collagen, is the main component comprising ~50 % of all BM proteins. The specificities of BM components associated with different tissue types are mainly dependent on the composition of type IV collagen isoforms, laminin, and HSPG (76, 77, 83).

Collagen, a class of proteins characterized by a unique sequence of Gly-X-Y motif in which every third amino acid is glycine (84, 85), is one of the primary components of BM, of which collagen type IV is the most abundant. Type IV collagen has the capacity to self-assemble and is highly cross-linked to create a structural network binding other components of the BM (86, 87). Type IV collagen is involved in cell attachment and differentiation, acting primarily through a cell-surface receptor family called integrins (88, 89). Laminins are a family of glycoproteins that are a major non-collagenous structural constituent of the basal lamina (77, 90). It forms an independent network but is associated with type IV collagen through entactin and perlecan. Laminins also bind to integrin receptors on plasma membranes and promote cell attachment, migration, differentiation, and cell growth (35, 90, 91). BM matrix also contains large HSPGs (92), thus creating an anionic defense against the passage of macromolecules (93, 94). Endothelial cells play a role in the structure of BMs by synthesizing BM components, which in turn, they utilize for attachment and migration on these endogenously produced matrix proteins (95–97). Stimulated endothelial cells are also able to remodel the BM through secretion of collagenases that digest collagen types I–V (98–100).

3.2 BM Influence on Angiogenesis

Angiogenesis is the formation of new blood vessels from preexisting vasculature and is crucial to development, reproduction, and repair (101–103). Components of the BM play a vital role in the initiation and resolution of angiogenesis, with mainly matrix metalloproteinases (MMPs) (104, 105) and integrins (106–108) emerging as key mediators. Angiogenesis can be induced by several growth factors, including vascular endothelial growth factor (VEGF), basic fibroblast growth factor (bFGF), platelet-derived growth factor (PDGF), and chemokines (109–114). Initially, BM matrix is degraded by enzymes such as MMPs that are produced by several cells, such as endothelial, stromal, or tumor cells. Matrix degradation allows the endothelial cells to detach and be in contact with several matrix components, such as vitronectin, fibronectin, type I collagen, and thrombin, that provide proliferative cues (115). This degradation of the matrix allows the endothelial cells to migrate and proliferate from their cell-surface anchors (integrins), ultimately resulting in new tube formation and blood flow.

4 Haemostatic Properties of the Endothelium

Maintenance of the fluidity of the blood and regulation of the haemostatic balance are vital roles for the endothelium. The monolayer interface between blood and tissue is the first line of defense against thrombosis, which acts by employing various anticoagulant and antiplatelet mechanisms. Upon vascular injury, endothelial cells ensure clot formation at the site of injury and manage clot evolution and dissolution to restore vascular integrity. Disturbances of the procoagulant or anticoagulant branch of the haemostatic system, whether acquired or genetic, could result in uncontrolled clotting or bleeding.

4.1 Procoagulant Properties

Unperturbed endothelial cells provide an anticoagulant surface but damage or inflammatory challenges can alter this state from an anticoagulant to a procoagulant surface. Tissue factor (TF) is constitutively expressed by adventitial cells surrounding the blood vessels as well as other cell types, including endothelial cells (116–120). TF is a transmembrane glycoprotein that is part of the extrinsic pathway of coagulation and plays a pivotal role in the initiation of the coagulation protease cascade (121, 122). When there is injury to the vessel wall, circulating FVII/FVIIa in plasma is exposed to the extravascular TF. TF serves as a surface receptor for FVIIa. TF/FVIIa reaction, in the presence of calcium, generates FXa, resulting in enhanced thrombin generation (123, 124). Recruitment of platelets to the injury site, and subsequent amplification of thrombin formation by the intrinsic pathway of coagulation (involving FXI, FIX, and FVIII in plasma), results in clot formation and clot stabilization by fibrin deposition.

A large multimeric glycoprotein called von Willebrand factor (vWF) is present in endothelial cells, platelets, and megakaryocytes, as well as in BM matrix of the vessel wall and in circulating plasma. Platelet thrombi, at sites of vascular injury or perturbation, are initially formed when circulating platelets decelerate and adhere to the endothelium through an interaction between platelet glycoprotein (GP) Ib–IX–V complex and vWF immobilized on endothelial cells (125). This association with the endothelium allows the platelets to interact with collagen in the subendothelial matrix, subsequently allowing for platelet activation and firm adherence to the surface (126–128). Activated endothelial cells also release vWF and P-selectin from storage granules (Weibel–Palade bodies), which act as a ligand for the GP Ibα receptor on platelets (129). Thus, releasing vWF may further contribute to platelet activation and enhance platelet–platelet interaction (aggregation) resulting in thrombi formation.

4.2 Anticoagulant Properties

Antithrombin (AT) is a serine protease inhibitor that plays a significant role in the regulation of thrombosis. It is the most abundant endogenous anticoagulant in plasma. The capacity for AT to control thrombosis lies in its ability to bind to a specific pentasaccharide sequence expressed on heparin, glycosaminoglycans (GAGs), and related proteoglycans both within the circulation and on endothelial cell surfaces (130–132). In the presence of heparin or vessel wall-associated GAGs, AT becomes a potent anticoagulant, able to inhibit thrombin as well as other proteases of the coagulation cascade by irreversibly binding the proteases forming an equimolar complex (133–137). AT also has anti-inflammatory properties that are independent of its anticoagulant effects (138–142). Its anti-inflammatory properties seem to be dependent on the interaction of AT with heparin-like GAGs on endothelial cell surfaces (138). AT has been shown to downregulate mRNA expression of lymphocyte growth factors, as well as lymphocyte proliferation and immunoglobulin production (143). The AT inhibitory effect on leukocyte activation may be dependent upon AT interacting with heparin-like GAGs on the endothelial cell surface which leads to the release of prostacyclin, an inhibitor of leukocyte activation (138).

The protein C (PC) pathway is important in regulating FVIIIa and FVa, in the tenase and prothrombinase complexes, respectively, to attenuate the catalytic effects of these complexes on thrombin generation. The major component of this anticoagulant system is PC, a vitamin K-dependent protein that exerts its effects by inhibiting FVIIIa and FVa. The catalytic activation of PC occurs on the endothelial cell surface and is facilitated by the thrombin–thrombomodulin (TM) complex (144). TM is present on all endothelial cells (144–146). Thrombin, when bound to TM, loses its coagulant abilities. Endothelial cells also possess endothelial PC receptor (EPCR) that binds to activated PC to further enhance the stimulation of thrombin–TM-mediated activation of PC (147). Two cofactors, protein S and intact FV, augment the inactivation of FVIIIa and FVa (148). PC plays an important physiologic role in maintaining haemostasis, as evident from genetic defects that increase the patient's risk of venous thrombosis (149, 150).

TF pathway inhibitor (TFPI) is a Kunitz-type proteinase inhibitor primarily expressed by the endothelial cells (151, 152). It is mostly cell-surface bound and can be liberated by heparin and other negatively charged ions (153). Its major role is to regulate the activity of TF-FVIIa by forming a quaternary complex (with TF-FVIIa-FXa) to ultimately inhibit FXa activity, thus diminishing thrombin generation and subsequent clot propagation (153–156).

4.3 Fibrinolytic Properties

The function of the fibrinolytic system is to modify and dissolve the clot. Plasmin is the major enzyme in this system, regulating fibrin degradation. Plasmin is formed from cleavage of plasminogen by plasminogen activators (PAs) that are synthesized and secreted by endothelial cells (157, 158). Thus, plasmin generation primarily takes place on the endothelial cell surface. There are two types of PAs, tissue-type (t-PA) and urokinase-type (u-PA). t-PA is active when bound to fibrin and is mainly involved in fibrin dissolution in the circulation (159). u-PA is able to activate plasminogen in the fluid phase and is involved in pericellular proteolysis (160). Fibrinolysis is controlled by PA inhibitors (PAIs), and this regulation is mediated by the endothelial cells (161).

The thrombin–TM complex, in addition to its role in the PC pathway, can also activate thrombin-activatable fibrinolysis inhibitor (TAFI). TAFI circulates as a proenzyme in plasma but when activated, is able to remove C-terminal lysine and arginine residues from fibrin (162–164). Thus, the essential binding site on fibrin for t-PA, plasminogen, and plasmin is eliminated, leading to a decrease in plasmin formation and eventual inhibition of fibrinolysis. The physiologic importance of TAFI needs further study but elevated TAFI levels have been associated with thrombotic conditions (165).

5 Immunogenicity of the Endothelium

The endothelium is the active interface between circulating blood and the underlying tissue. Its myriad of roles includes anti-inflammatory response to leukocyte adhesion and migration. Dysfunction of the endothelium can result in a specific state of endothelial activation characterized by pro-inflammatory, proliferative, and pro-coagulatory environments favoring the formation of atheromas (166, 167). Activated and damaged endothelial cells have been shown to release intercellular adhesion molecule-1 (ICAM-1), vascular cell adhesion molecule-1 (VCAM-1), vWF, PAI-1, or TM in response to atherosclerotic disease (168). Expression of adhesion molecules by endothelial cells at sites of inflammation facilitates migration of leukocytes to the extravascular space through the endothelial monolayer (169). Atherosclerotic disease has been associated with increased levels of circulating endothelial cells and immunogenic ($CD31^+/CD42^-$) microparticles. Studies have shown that the immunogenicity of endothelial cells is regulated by matrix architecture but further studies are needed to elucidate which components of the extracellular matrix specifically affect endothelial immunogenicity (166, 170).

Endothelial cells are also able to present major histocompatibility complex class II (MHC-II) molecules. Endothelial cell MHC-II up-regulation is evident in human allografts, and may be involved in graft rejection (171). Endothelial cells are able to act as antigen-presenting cells, especially when damaged, through the release of non-HLA antigens resulting in chronic antibody response and may contribute to graft vasculopathy and chronic rejection of solid organ transplant (172).

6 Summary

A vast array of information has been gathered through research on the role of the vessel wall. It is a testament to the complex nature of the endothelium that this thin monolayer of cells is capable of such a myriad of functions which maintain vascular patency in addition to regulating vascular tone, matrix components, haemostasis, angiogenesis, cellular interactions, inflammation, and immune responses. Perturbation of any of these regulatory events can potentially result in disease states. However, our ever-increasing understanding of the basis of how the endothelium functions has allowed for the development of treatments for certain disease states.

Acknowledgments

Anthony Chan is supported by the Bayer Thrombosis and Haemostasis Research Grant.

References

1. Rubanyi GM, Romero JC, Vanhoutte PM (1986) Flow-induced release of endothelium-derived relaxing factor. Am J Physiol 250:H1145–H1149
2. Klinger JR (2007) The nitric oxide/cGMP signaling pathway in pulmonary hypertension. Clin Chest Med 28:143–167
3. Vanhoutte PM (1991) Hypercholesterolaemia, atherosclerosis and release of endothelium-derived relaxing factor by aggregating platelets. Eur Heart J 12:25–32
4. Vanhoutte PM, Boulanger CM, Mombouli JV (1995) Endothelium-derived relaxing factors and converting enzyme inhibition. Am J Cardiol 76:3E–12E
5. Shimokawa H, Vanhoutte PM (1989) Impaired endothelium-dependent relaxation to aggregating platelets and related vasoactive substances in porcine coronary arteries in hypercholesterolemia and atherosclerosis. Circ Res 64:900–914
6. Panza JA, Quyyumi AA, Brush JE Jr, Epstein SE (1990) Abnormal endothelium-dependent vascular relaxation in patients with essential hypertension. N Engl J Med 323:22–27
7. Panza JA, Casino PR, Kilcoyne CM, Quyyumi AA (1993) Role of endothelium-derived nitric oxide in the abnormal endothelium-dependent vascular relaxation of patients with essential hypertension. Circulation 87:1468–1474
8. Shimokawa H, Aarhus LL, Vanhoutte PM (1987) Porcine coronary arteries with regenerated endothelium have a reduced endothelium-dependent responsiveness to aggregating platelets and serotonin. Circ Res 61:256–270
9. Shimokawa H, Vanhoutte PM (1991) Angiographic demonstration of hyperconstriction induced by serotonin and aggregating platelets in porcine coronary arteries with regenerated endothelium. J Am Coll Cardiol 17:1197–1202
10. Palmer RM, Rees DD, Ashton DS, Moncada S (1988) L-arginine is the physiological precursor for the formation of nitric oxide in endothelium-dependent relaxation. Biochem Biophys Res Commun 153:1251–1256
11. Moncada S, Palmer RM, Higgs EA (1991) Nitric oxide: physiology, pathophysiology, and pharmacology. Pharmacol Rev 43:109–142
12. Moncada S, Higgs EA (2006) Nitric oxide and the vascular endothelium. Handb Exp Pharmacol 176:213–254
13. Rapoport RM, Murad E (1983) Endothelium-dependent and nitrovasodilator-induced relaxation of vascular smooth muscle: role of cyclic GMP. J Cyclic Nucleotide Protein Phosphor Res 9:281–296
14. Palmer RM, Ferrige AG, Moncada S (1987) Nitric oxide release accounts for the biological activity of endothelium-derived relaxing factor. Nature 327:524–526
15. Hermann M (2006) Cyclooxygenase-2 and nitric oxide. J Cardiovasc Pharmacol 47: S21–S25

16. Rees DD, Palmer RM, Moncada S (2007) Role of endothelium-derived nitric oxide in the regulation of blood pressure. Proc Natl Acad Sci U S A 86:3375–3378
17. Scott-Burden T, Vanhoutte PM (1994) Regulation of smooth muscle cell growth by endothelium-derived factors. Tex Heart Inst J 21:91–97
18. Desjardins F, Balligand JL (2006) Nitric oxide-dependent endothelial function and cardiovascular disease. Acta Clin Belg 61:326–334
19. Bunting S, Gryglewski R, Moncada S, Vane JR (1976) Arterial walls generate from prostaglandin endoperoxides a substance (prostaglandin X) which relaxes strips of mesenteric and coeliac arteries and inhibits platelet aggregation. Prostaglandins 12:897–913
20. Weksler BB, Marcus AJ, Jaffe EA (1977) Synthesis of prostaglandin I2 (prostacyclin) by cultured human and bovine endothelial cells. Proc Natl Acad Sci U S A 74:3922–3926
21. Radomski MW, Palmer RM, Moncada S (1987) Comparative pharmacology of endothelium-derived relaxing factor, nitric oxide and prostacyclin in platelets. Br J Pharmacol 92:181–187
22. Weksler BB, Ley CW, Jaffe EA (1978) Stimulation of endothelial cell prostacyclin production by thrombin, trypsin, and the ionophore A 23187. J Clin Invest 62:923–930
23. Hong SL (1980) Effect of bradykinin and thrombin on prostacyclin synthesis in endothelial cells from calf and pig aorta and human umbilical cord vein. Thromb Res 18:787–795
24. Baenziger NL, Force LE, Becherer PR (1980) Histamine stimulate prostacyclin synthesis in cultured human umbilical vein endothelial cells. Biochem Biophys Res Commun 92:1435–1440
25. Grabowski EF, Jaffe EA, Weksler BB (1985) Prostacyclin production by cultured endothelial cell monolayers exposed to step increases in shear stress. J Lab Clin Med 105:36–43
26. de Wit C, Wölfle SE (2007) EDHF and gap junctions: important regulators of vascular tone within the microcirculation. Curr Pharm Biotechnol 8:11–25
27. Feletou M, Vanhoutte PM (1988) Endothelium-dependent hyperpolarization of canine coronary smooth muscle. Br J Pharmacol 93:515–524
28. Komori K, Vanhoutte PM (1990) Endothelium-derived hyperpolarizing factor. Blood Vessels 27:238–245
29. Nagao T, Vanhoutte PM (1993) Endothelium-derived hyperpolarizing factor and endothelium-dependent relaxations. Am J Respir Cell Mol Biol 8:1–6
30. Vanhoutte PM, Feletou M, Taddei S (2005) Endothelium-dependent contractions in hypertension. Br J Pharmacol 144:449–458
31. Hickey KA, Rubanyi G, Paul RJ, Highsmith RF (1985) Characterization of a coronary vasoconstrictor produced by cultured endothelial cells. Am J Physiol 248:C550–C556
32. Gillespie MN, Owasoyo JO, McMurtry IF, O'Brien RF (1986) Sustained coronary vasoconstriction provoked by a peptidergic substance released from endothelial cells in culture. J Pharmacol Exp Ther 236:339–343
33. Bloch KD, Eddy RL, Shows TB, Quertermous T (1989) cDNA cloning and chromosomal assignment of the gene encoding endothelin 3. J Biol Chem 264:18156–18161
34. Sakurai T, Yanagisawa M, Inoue A, Ryan US, Kimura S, Mitsui Y, Goto K, Masaki T (1991) cDNA cloning, sequence analysis and tissue distribution of rat preproendothelin-1 mRNA. Biochem Biophys Res Commun 175:44–47
35. Graf J, Ogle RC, Robey FA, Sasaki M, Martin GR, Yamada Y, Kleinman HK (1987) A pentapeptide from the laminin B1 chain mediates cell adhesion and binds the 67,000 laminin receptor. Biochemistry 26:6896–6900
36. Russell FD, Skepper JN, Davenport AP (1998) Evidence using immunoelectron microscopy for regulated and constitutive pathways in the transport and release of endothelin. J Cardiovasc Pharmacol 31:424–430
37. Rondaij MG, Bierings R, Kragt A, van Mourik JA, Voorberg J (2006) Dynamics and plasticity of Weibel-Palade bodies in endothelial cells. Arterioscler Thromb Vasc Biol 26:1002–1007
38. Russell FD, Skepper JN, Davenport AP (1998) Human endothelial cell storage granules: a novel intracellular site for isoforms of the endothelin-converting enzyme. Circ Res 83:314–321
39. Bousette N, Giaid A (2003) Endothelin-1 in atherosclerosis and other vasculopathies. Can J Physiol Pharmacol 81:578–587
40. Marasciulo FL, Montagnani M, Potenza MA (2006) Endothelin-1: the yin and yang on vascular function. Curr Med Chem 13:1655–1665
41. Boulanger C, Lüscher TF (1990) Release of endothelin from the porcine aorta. Inhibition by endothelium-derived nitric oxide. J Clin Invest 85:587–590
42. Kohno M, Yokokawa K, Horio T, Yasunari K, Murakawa K, Takeda T (1992) Atrial and brain natriuretic peptides inhibit the

endothelin-1 secretory response to angiotensin II in porcine aorta. Circ Res 70:241–247

43. Emori T, Hirata Y, Imai T, Eguchi S, Kanno K, Marumo F (1993) Cellular mechanism of natriuretic peptides-induced inhibition of endothelin-1 biosynthesis in rat endothelial cells. Endocrinology 133:2474–2480
44. Imai T, Hirata Y, Emori T, Marumo F (1993) Heparin has an inhibitory effect on endothelin-1 synthesis and release by endothelial cells. Hypertension 21:353–358
45. Yokokawa K, Tahara H, Kohno M, Mandal AK, Yanagisawa M, Takeda T (1993) Heparin regulates endothelin production through endothelium-derived nitric oxide in human endothelial cells. J Clin Invest 92: 2080–2085
46. Prins BA, Hu RM, Nazario B, Pedram A, Frank HJ, Weber MA, Levin ER (1994) Prostaglandin E2 and prostacyclin inhibit the production and secretion of endothelin from cultured endothelial cells. J Biol Chem 269:11938–11944
47. Toda M, Yamamoto K, Shimizu N, Obi S, Kumagaya S, Igarashi T, Kamiya A, Ando J (2008) Differential gene responses in endothelial cells exposed to a combination of shear stress and cyclic stretch. J Biotechnol 133:239–244
48. Busse R, Fleming I (2006) Vascular endothelium and blood flow. Handb Exp Pharmacol (176 Pt 2):43–78
49. Wagner OF, Christ G, Wojta J, Vierhapper H, Parzer S, Nowotny PJ, Schneider B, Waldhäusl W, Binder BR (1992) Polar secretion of endothelin-1 by cultured endothelial cells. J Biol Chem 267:16066–16068
50. Hosoda K, Nakao K, Hiroshi-Arai, Suga S, Ogawa Y, Mukoyama M, Shirakami G, Saito Y, Nakanishi S, Imura H (1991) Cloning and expression of human endothelin-1 receptor cDNA. FEBS Lett 287:23–26
51. Warner TD, Allcock GH, Corder R, Vane JR (1993) Use of the endothelin antagonists BQ-123 and PD 142893 to reveal three endothelin receptors mediating smooth muscle contraction and the release of EDRF. Br J Pharmacol 110:777–782
52. Sumner MJ, Cannon TR, Mundin JW, White DG, Watts IS (1992) Endothelin ETA and ETB receptors mediate vascular smooth muscle contraction. Br J Pharmacol 107:858–860
53. Moreland S, McMullen DM, Delaney CL, Lee VG, Hunt JT (1992) Venous smooth muscle contains vasoconstrictor ETB-like receptors. Biochem Biophys Res Commun 184:100–106
54. Sudjarwo SA, Hori M, Takai M, Urade Y, Okada T, Karaki H (1993) A novel subtype of endothelin B receptor mediating contraction in swine pulmonary vein. Life Sci 53:431–437
55. Schiffrin EL (1995) Endothelin: potential role in hypertension and vascular hypertrophy. Hypertension 25:1135–1143
56. Schiffrin EL, Deng LY, Sventek P, Day R (1997) Enhanced expression of endothelin-1 gene in resistance arteries in severe human essential hypertension. J Hypertens 15:57–63
57. Taylor RN, Varma M, Teng NN, Roberts JM (1990) Women with preeclampsia have higher plasma endothelin levels than women with normal pregnancies. J Clin Endocrinol Metab 71:1675–1677
58. Clark BA, Halvorson L, Sachs B, Epstein FH (1992) Plasma endothelin levels in preeclampsia: elevation and correlation with uric acid levels and renal impairment. Am J Obstet Gynecol 166:962–968
59. Kon V, Sugiura M, Inagami T, Harvie BR, Ichikawa I, Hoover RL (1990) Role of endothelin in cyclosporine-induced glomerular dysfunction. Kidney Int 37:1487–1491
60. Kaddoura S, Curzen NP, Evans TW, Firth JD, Poole-Wilson PA (1996) Tissue expression of endothelin-1 mRNA in endotoxaemia. Biochem Biophys Res Commun 218:641–647
61. Golfman LS, Hata T, Beamish RE, Dhalla NS (1993) Role of endothelin in heart function in health and disease. Can J Cardiol 9: 635–653
62. Hirata Y, Takagi Y, Fukada Y, Marumo F (1989) Endothelin is a potent mitogen for rat vascular smooth muscle cells. Atherosclerosis 78:225–228
63. Bobik A, Grooms A, Millar JA, Mitchell A, Grinpukel S (1990) Growth factor activity of endothelin on vascular smooth muscle. Am J Physiol 258:C408–C415
64. Brown MJ (2007) Renin: friend or foe? Heart 93:1026–1033
65. Weir MR, Dzau VJ (1999) The renin-angiotensin-aldosterone system: a specific target for hypertension management. Am J Hypertens 12:205S–213S
66. Volpe M, Savoia C, De Paolis P, Ostrowska B, Tarasi D, Rubattu S (2002) The renin-angiotensin system as a risk factor and therapeutic target for cardiovascular and renal disease. J Am Soc Nephrol 13:S173–S178
67. Brewster UC, Setaro JF, Perazella MA (2003) The renin-angiotensin-aldosterone system: cardiorenal effects and implications for renal and cardiovascular disease states. Am J Med Sci 326:15–24

68. Faraci FM (2006) Reactive oxygen species: influence on cerebral vascular tone. J Appl Physiol 100:739–743
69. Madamanchi NR, Vendrov A, Runge MS (2005) Oxidative stress and vascular disease. Arterioscler Thromb Vasc Biol 25:29–38
70. Mueller CF, Laude K, McNally JS, Harrison DG (2005) ATVB in focus: redox mechanisms in blood vessels. Arterioscler Thromb Vasc Biol 25:274–278
71. Didion SP, Faraci FM (2002) Effects of NADH and NADPH on superoxide levels and cerebral vascular tone. Am J Physiol Heart Circ Physiol 282:H688–H695
72. Faraci FM, Heistad DD (1998) Regulation of the cerebral circulation: role of endothelium and potassium channels. Physiol Rev 78: 53–97
73. Edelman DA, Jiang Y, Tyburski J, Wilson RF, Steffes C (2006) Pericytes and their role in microvasculature homeostasis. J Surg Res 135:305–311
74. Yamagishi S, Imaizumi T (2005) Pericyte biology and diseases. Int J Tissue React 27:125–135
75. Paulsson M (1992) Basement membrane proteins: structure, assembly, and cellular interactions. Crit Rev Biochem Mol Biol 27:93–127
76. Hudson BG, Reeders ST, Tryggvason K (1993) Type IV collagen: structure, gene organization, and role in human diseases. Molecular basis of Goodpasture and Alport syndromes and diffuse leiomyomatosis. J Biol Chem 268:26033–26036
77. Colognato H, Yurchenco PD (2000) Form and function: the laminin family of heterotrimers. Dev Dyn 218:213–234
78. Vracko R, Benditt EP (1972) Basal lamina: the scaffold for orderly cell replacement. Observations on regeneration of injured skeletal muscle fibers and capillaries. J Cell Biol 55:406–419
79. Vracko R (1974) Basal lamina scaffold-anatomy and significance for maintenance of orderly tissue structure. Am J Pathol 77:314–346
80. Timpl R (1989) Structure and biological activity of basement membrane proteins. Eur J Biochem 180:487–502
81. Schittny JC, Yurchenco PD (1989) Basement membranes: molecular organization and function in development and disease. Curr Opin Cell Biol 1:983–988
82. Yurchenco PD, Schittny JC (1990) Molecular architecture of basement membranes. FASEB J 4:1577–1590
83. Cheng YS, Champliaud MF, Burgeson RE, Marinkovich MP, Yurchenco PD (1997) Self-assembly of laminin isoforms. J Biol Chem 272:31525–31532
84. Prockop DJ, Kivirikko KI (1995) Collagens: molecular biology, diseases, and potentials for therapy. Annu Rev Biochem 64:403–434
85. Kalluri R (2003) Basement membranes: structure, assembly and role in tumour angiogenesis. Nat Rev Cancer 3:422–433
86. Timpl R, Wiedemann H, van Delden V, Furthmayr H, Kühn K (1981) A network model for the organization of type IV collagen molecules in basement membranes. Eur J Biochem 120:203–211
87. Kühn K, Wiedemann H, Timpl R, Risteli J, Dieringer H, Voss T, Glanville RW (1981) Macromolecular structure of basement membrane collagens. FEBS Lett 125:123–128
88. Herbst TJ, McCarthy JB, Tsilibary EC, Furcht LT (1988) Differential effects of laminin, intact type IV collagen, and specific domains of type IV collagen on endothelial cell adhesion and migration. J Cell Biol 106:1365–1373
89. Ruoslahti E, Pierschbacher MD (1987) New perspectives in cell adhesion: RGD and integrins. Science 238:491–497
90. Kleinman HK, Cannon FB, Laurie GW, Hassell JR, Aumailley M, Terranova VP, Martin GR, DuBois-Dalcq M (1985) Biological activities of laminin. J Cell Biochem 27:317–325
91. Graf J, Iwamoto Y, Sasaki M, Martin GR, Kleinman HK, Robey FA, Yamada Y (1987) Identification of an amino acid sequence in laminin mediating cell attachment, chemotaxis, and receptor binding. Cell 48:989–996
92. Hassell JR, Robey FA, Barrach HJ, Wilczek J, Rennard SI, Martin GR (1980) Isolation of a heparan sulfate-containing proteoglycan from basement membrane. Proc Natl Acad Sci U S A 77:4494–4498
93. Kanwar YS, Jakubowski ML, Rosenzweig LJ (1983) Distribution of sulfated glycosaminoglycans in the glomerular basement membrane and mesangial matrix. Eur J Cell Biol 31:290–295
94. Ledbetter SR, Fisher LW, Hassell JR (1987) Domain structure of the basement membrane heparan sulfate proteoglycan. Biochemistry 26:988–995
95. Madri JA, Williams SK (1983) Capillary endothelial cell cultures: phenotypic modulation by matrix components. J Cell Biol 97:153–165
96. Carley WW, Milici AJ, Madri JA (1988) Extracellular matrix specificity for the differentiation of capillary endothelial cells. Exp Cell Res 178:426–434

97. Kramer RH, Bensch KG, Davison PM, Krasek MA (1984) Basal lamina formation by cultured microvascular endothelial cells. J Cell Biol 99:692–698
98. Moscatelli D, Jaffe E, Rifkin DB (1980) Tetradecanoyl phorbol acetate stimulates latent collagenase production by cultured human endothelial cells. Cell 20:343–351
99. Gross JL, Moscatelli D, Jaffe E, Rifkin DB (1982) Plasminogen activator and collagenase production by cultured capillary endothelial cells. J Cell Biol 95:974–981
100. Kalebic T, Garbisa S, Glaser B, Liotta LA (1983) Basement membrane collagen: degradation by migrating endothelial cells. Science 221:281–283
101. Folkman J, Shing Y (1992) Angiogenesis. J Biol Chem 267:10931–10934
102. Carmeliet P, Jain RK (2000) Angiogenesis in cancer and other diseases. Nature 407: 249–257
103. Jain RK, Carmeliet PF (2001) Vessels of death or life. Sci Am 285:38–45
104. Xu J, Rodriguez D, Petitclerc E, Kim JJ, Hangai M, Moon YS, Davis GE, Brooks PC (2001) Proteolytic exposure of a cryptic site within collagen type IV is required for angiogenesis and tumor growth in vivo. J Cell Biol 154:1069–1079
105. Xu J, Rodriguez D, Kim JJ, Brooks PC (2000) Generation of monoclonal antibodies to cryptic collagen sites by using subtractive immunization. Hybridoma 19:375–385
106. Sheppard D (2000) In vivo functions of integrins: lessons from null mutations in mice. Matrix Biol 19:203–209
107. Hynes RO (2008) Integrins: versatility, modulation, and signaling in cell adhesion. Cell 69:11–25
108. Hynes RO (2002) Integrins: bidirectional, allosteric signaling machines. Cell 110: 673–687
109. Kuwano M, Fukushi J, Okamoto M, Nishie A, Goto H, Ishibashi T, Ono M (2001) Angiogenesis factors. Intern Med 40: 565–572
110. Lutsenko SV, Kiselev SM, Severin SE (2003) Molecular mechanisms of tumor angiogenesis. Biochemistry (Mosc) 68:286–300
111. Battegay EJ (1995) Angiogenesis: mechanistic insights, neovascular diseases, and therapeutic prospects. J Mol Med 73: 333–346
112. Suhardja A, Hoffman H (2003) Role of growth factors and their receptors in proliferation of microvascular endothelial cells. Microsc Res Tech 60:70–75
113. Jones AV, Cross NC (2004) Oncogenic derivatives of platelet-derived growth factor receptors. Cell Mol Life Sci 61:2912–2923
114. Bernardini G, Ribatti D, Spinetti G, Morbidelli L, Ziche M, Santoni A, Capogrossi MC, Napolitano M (2003) Analysis of the role of chemokines in angiogenesis. J Immunol Methods 273:83–101
115. Eliceiri BP, Cheresh DA (2001) Adhesion events in angiogenesis. Curr Opin Cell Biol 13:563–568
116. Drake TA, Morrissey JH, Edgington TS (1989) Selective cellular expression of tissue factor in human tissues. Implications for disorders of hemostasis and thrombosis. Am J Pathol 134:1087–1097
117. Fleck RA, Rao LV, Rapoport SI, Varki N (1990) Localization of human tissue factor antigen by immunostaining with monospecific, polyclonal anti-human tissue factor antibody. Thromb Res 59:421–437
118. Flössel C, Luther T, Müller M, Albrecht S, Kasper M (1994) Immunohistochemical detection of tissue factor (TF) on paraffin sections of routinely fixed human tissue. Histochemistry 101:449–453
119. Bouchard BA, Shatos MA, Tracy PB (1997) Human brain pericytes differentially regulate expression of procoagulant enzyme complexes comprising the extrinsic pathway of blood coagulation. Arterioscler Thromb Vasc Biol 17:1–9
120. Schecter AD, Spirn B, Rossikhina M, Giesen PL, Bogdanov V, Fallon JT, Fisher EA, Schnapp LM, Nemerson Y, Taubman MB (2000) Release of active tissue factor by human arterial smooth muscle cells. Circ Res 87:126–132
121. Hoffman M, Monroe DM, Oliver JA, Roberts HR (1995) Factors IXa and Xa play distinct roles in tissue factor-dependent initiation of coagulation. Blood 86:1794–1801
122. Nemerson Y (1988) Tissue factor and hemostasis. Blood 71:1–8
123. Kurachi K, Davie EW (1977) Activation of human factor XI (plasma thromboplastin antecedent) by factor XIIa (activated Hageman factor). Biochemistry 16:5831–5839
124. Nemerson Y (1966) The reaction between bovine brain tissue factor and factors VII and X. Biochemistry 5:601–608
125. Chen J, López JA (2005) Interactions of platelets with subendothelium and endothelium. Microcirculation 12:235–246
126. Coller BS, Beer JH, Scudder LE, Steinberg MH (1989) Collagen-platelet interactions: evidence for a direct interaction of collagen

with platelet GPIa/IIa and an indirect interaction with platelet GPIIb/IIIa mediated by adhesive proteins. Blood 74:182–192

127. Goto S, Tamura N, Handa S, Arai M, Kodama K, Takayama H (2002) Involvement of glycoprotein VI in platelet thrombus formation on both collagen and von Willebrand factor surfaces under flow conditions. Circulation 106:266–272
128. Massberg S, Gawaz M, Grüner S, Schulte V, Konrad I, Zohlnhöfer D, Heinzmann U, Nieswandt B (2003) A crucial role of glycoprotein VI for platelet recruitment to the injured arterial wall in vivo. J Exp Med 197:41–49
129. Wagner DD (1993) The Weibel-Palade body: the storage granule for von Willebrand factor and P-selectin. Thromb Haemost 70:105–110
130. Wu YI, Sheffield WP, Blajchman MA (1994) Defining the heparin-binding domain of antithrombin. Blood Coagul Fibrinolysis 5:83–95
131. Jackson CM (1990) Mechanism of heparin action. Baillieres Clin Haematol 3:483–504
132. Casu B (1990) Heparin structure. Haemostasis 20:62–73
133. Olds RJ, Lane DA, Mille B, Chowdhury V, Thein SL (1994) Antithrombin: the principal inhibitor of thrombin. Semin Thromb Hemost 20:353–372
134. Rosenberg JS, McKenna PW, Rosenberg RD (1975) Inhibition of human factor IXa by human antithrombin. J Biol Chem 250:8883–8888
135. Stead N, Kaplan AP, Rosenberg RD (1976) Inhibition of activated factor XII by antithrombin-heparin cofactor. J Biol Chem 251:6481–6488
136. Damus PS, Hicks M, Rosenberg RD (1973) Anticoagulant action of heparin. Nature 246:355–357
137. Rao LV, Nordfang O, Hoang AD, Pendurthi UR (1995) Mechanism of antithrombin III inhibition of factor VIIa/tissue factor activity on cell surfaces. Comparison with tissue factor pathway inhibitor/factor Xa-induced inhibition of factor VIIa/tissue factor activity. Blood 85:121–129
138. Okajima K, Uchiba M (1998) The anti-inflammatory properties of antithrombin III: new therapeutic implications. Semin Thromb Hemost 24:27–32
139. Dunzendorfer S, Kaneider N, Rabensteiner A, Meierhofer C, Reinisch C, Römisch J, Wiedermann CJ (2001) Cell-surface heparan sulfate proteoglycan-mediated regulation of human neutrophil migration by the serpin antithrombin III. Blood 97:1079–1085
140. Hoffmann JN, Vollmar B, Römisch J, Inthorn D, Schildberg FW, Menger MD (2002) Antithrombin effects on endotoxin-induced microcirculatory disorders are mediated mainly by its interaction with microvascular endothelium. Crit Care Med 30:215–225
141. Souter PJ, Thomas S, Hubbard AR, Poole S, Römisch J, Gray E (2001) Antithrombin inhibits lipopolysaccharide-induced tissue factor and interleukin-6 production by mononuclear cells, human umbilical vein endothelial cells, and whole blood. Crit Care Med 29:134–139
142. Oelschläger C, Römisch J, Staubitz A, Stauss H, Leithäuser B, Tillmanns H, Hölschermann H (2002) Antithrombin III inhibits nuclear factor kappaB activation in human monocytes and vascular endothelial cells. Blood 99:4015–4020
143. Zuo XJ, Nicolaidou E, Okada Y, Toyoda M, Jordan SC (2001) Antithrombin III inhibits lymphocyte proliferation, immunoglobulin production and mRNA expression of lymphocyte growth factors (IL-2, gamma-IFN and IL-4) in vitro. Transpl Immunol 9:1–6
144. Esmon CT (2003) The protein C pathway. Chest 124:26S–32S
145. Weiler H, Isermann BH (2003) Thrombomodulin. J Thromb Haemost 1:1515–1524
146. Van de Wouwer M, Collen D, Conway EM (2004) Thrombomodulin-protein C-EPCR system: integrated to regulate coagulation and inflammation. Arterioscler Thromb Vasc Biol 24:1374–1383
147. Esmon CT (2000) The endothelial cell protein C receptor. Thromb Haemost 83:639–643
148. Nicolaes GA, Dahlbäck B (2002) Factor V and thrombotic disease: description of a janus-faced protein. Arterioscler Thromb Vasc Biol 22:530–538
149. Pescatore SL (2001) Clinical management of protein C deficiency. Expert Opin Pharmacother 2:431–439
150. Nizzi FA Jr, Kaplan HS (1999) Protein C and S deficiency. Semin Thromb Hemost 25:265–272
151. Broze GJ Jr, Warren LA, Novotny WF, Higuchi DA, Girard JJ, Miletich JP (1988) The lipoprotein-associated coagulation inhibitor that inhibits the factor VII-tissue factor complex also inhibits factor Xa: insight into its possible mechanism of action. Blood 71:335–343
152. Piro O, Broze GJ Jr (2004) Role for the Kunitz-3 domain of tissue factor pathway inhibitor-alpha in cell surface binding. Circulation 110:3567–3572

153. Sandset PM (1996) Tissue factor pathway inhibitor (TFPI)—an update. Haemostasis 26:156–165
154. Girard TJ, Warren LA, Novotny WF, Likert KM, Brown SG, Miletich JP, Broze GJ Jr (1989) Functional significance of the Kunitz-type inhibitory domains of lipoprotein-associated coagulation inhibitor. Nature 338:518–520
155. Broze GJ Jr (1995) Tissue factor pathway inhibitor. Thromb Haemost 74:90–93
156. Lindahl AK (1997) Tissue factor pathway inhibitor: from unknown coagulation inhibitor to major antithrombotic principle. Cardiovasc Res 33:286–291
157. Bachmann F (2001) Plasminogen-plasmin enzyme system. In: Colman RW, Hirsh J, Marder VJ, Clowes AW, George JN (eds) Hemostasis and thrombosis: basic principles and clinical practice. Lippincott Williams & Wilkins, Philadelphia, PA, pp 275–320
158. Collen D, Lijnen HR (1991) Basic and clinical aspects of fibrinolysis and thrombolysis. Blood 78:3114–3124
159. Medved L, Tsurupa G, Yakovlev S (2008) Conformational changes upon conversion of fibrinogen into fibrin. The mechanisms of exposure of cryptic sites. Ann N Y Acad Sci 936:185–204
160. Binder BR, Mihaly J, Prager GW (2007) uPAR-uPA-PAI-1 interactions and signaling: a vascular biologist's view. Thromb Haemost 97:336–342
161. Binder BR, Christ G, Gruber F, Grubic N, Hufnagl P, Krebs M, Mihaly J, Prager GW (2002) Plasminogen activator inhibitor 1: physiological and pathophysiological roles. News Physiol Sci 17:56–61
162. Bouma BN, Mosnier LO (2006) Thrombin activatable fibrinolysis inhibitor (TAFI)—how does thrombin regulate fibrinolysis? Ann Med 38:378–388
163. Bouma BN, Meijers JC (2003) Thrombin-activatable fibrinolysis inhibitor (TAFI, plasma procarboxypeptidase B, procarboxypeptidase R, procarboxypeptidase U). J Thromb Haemost 1:1566–1574
164. Bajzar L (2000) Thrombin activatable fibrinolysis inhibitor and an antifibrinolytic pathway. Arterioscler Thromb Vasc Biol 20:2511–2518
165. van Tilburg NH, Rosendaal FR, Bertina RM (2000) Thrombin activatable fibrinolysis inhibitor and the risk for deep vein thrombosis. Blood 95:2855–2859
166. Methe H, Hess S, Edelman ER (2007) Endothelial immunogenicity—a matter of matrix microarchitecture. Thromb Haemost 98:278–282
167. Anderson TJ (2008) Assessment and treatment of endothelial dysfunction in humans. J Am Coll Cardiol 34:631–638
168. Libby P (2002) Inflammation in atherosclerosis. Nature 420:868–874
169. Ross R (1999) Atherosclerosis—an inflammatory disease. N Engl J Med 340: 115–126
170. Methe H, Edelman ER (2006) Tissue engineering of endothelial cells and the immune response. Transplant Proc 38:3293–3299
171. Turesson C (2004) Endothelial expression of MHC class II molecules in autoimmune disease. Curr Pharm Des 10:129–143
172. Rose ML (1997) Role of endothelial cells in allograft rejection. Vasc Med 2:105–114

Part II

General Principles of Haemostatic Testing

Chapter 4

Specimen Requirements for the Haemostasis Laboratory

Linda J. Stang and Lesley G. Mitchell

Abstract

Sample integrity is one of the most important details to consider for the production of quality results in the laboratory. Many factors have the potential to adversely affect the sample: intrinsic patient characteristics (caused by the underlying malady and/or treatment, incorrect patient preparation, etc.), difficult or incorrectly performed collection of sample, correct timing of sample collection relative to drug administration, incorrect processing and transport within the laboratory—just to name a few. This chapter outlines standard common requirements with explanations as a basis for those limitations, and practical laboratory advice to attain and maintain dependable samples.

Key words Blood sampling, Plasma storage, Blood sampling artifacts, Sodium citrate, Vacutainers, Sample stability, Platelet-free plasma, Hemolysis, Lipemia, Interference, Diurnal variation

1 Introduction

The vast majority of coagulation assays are based on the use of anticoagulated plasma from a sodium citrate (blue top) primary collection tube. The mechanism for the anticoagulant effect of sodium citrate is related to the chelation of calcium in the blood sample. As calcium is required for many reactions of the haemostatic system, the blood will not clot in the absence of free calcium. A good portion of coagulation assays, therefore, require re-calcification of the plasma, with other additives, to initiate the clotting process. A few reactions are not calcium dependent; thus calcium chloride is not needed in some reagent systems. For collection tube type, there are some alternatives found in the point-of-care setting. For example—EDTA tubes that do not need to be centrifuged to isolate plasma, but instead use a filter system to remove cellular elements from the sample, resulting in a decreased turn around time for emergency quantitative D-dimers (Biosite Triage meter, San Diego, California). Arterial whole blood from a finger stick for various PT INR point-of-care testing is especially useful for children (and adults) with

Paul Monagle (ed.), *Haemostasis: Methods and Protocols*, Methods in Molecular Biology, vol. 992,
DOI 10.1007/978-1-62703-339-8_4, © Springer Science+Business Media New York 2013

limited venous access who require frequent monitoring after heart valve replacement or prophylaxis for other indications. Other assays with different specimen types include some ELISA-based antiphospholipid antibody assays which may require a serum sample. Also, a specialized collection tube—containing citric acid/sodium citrate, theophylline, adenosine, and dipyridamole—commonly referred to as a CTAD or Diatube H (Becton Dickinson, UK) minimizes the interference from platelet activation that occurs during collection and storage and is used for those markers that are extremely sensitive to platelet activation and granule content release.

General collection of sodium citrate samples will be discussed in this section and where specified, other collection and sample issues are addressed. Specific collection requirements or specimen handling for the various types of assays will be addressed in the sections pertaining to those assays. In general, only commercially available products will be discussed; any specialized in-house requirements are included elsewhere.

Other common collection concerns such as universal precautions, sample labelling, positive patient identification, and common devices or methods for procurement of samples will not be covered here. Only those issues which may have a direct effect on various coagulation assays will be discussed.

2 Patient Preparation, Medication Information, and Timing of Sample Collection

For the most part, no specific patient preparation is required for coagulation assays. One recommendation applicable to optical assays, such as platelet aggregation using platelet-rich plasma, is that the patient should limit themselves to a light breakfast, essentially minimizing any interference from lipemia in the assay. Occasionally, correct timing is essential—for instance, drawing a sample for anti-Xa for low molecular weight heparin analysis 4–6 h after administration of the drug. Specific sections will outline the necessary requirements needed.

For patients having platelet function studies done, such as aggregations or bleeding times, all medications that the patient is currently on should be noted (see Note 1). Many over-the-counter medications contain ASA (acetylsalicylic acid) or NSAIDS (nonsteroidal anti-inflammatories) in combination with other drugs. The patient may not even be aware that a particular medication contains antiplatelet agents and may have ingested the drug for an entirely different indication. The patients should also be asked whether they are using any herbal supplements or alternative medicine products as certain types of these products may affect platelet function.

3 Sodium Citrate Collection Tubes

The current World Health Organization (WHO) and Clinical and Laboratory Standards Institute (CLSI, formerly NCCLS) recommendation for concentration of trisodium citrate (Na citrate) for vacuum blood collection tubes, used for coagulation assays, is 0.109 mol/L (3.2% v/v) (1, 2). A mixture of 1 part citrate to 9 parts blood should be used. The dehydrate form of trisodium citrate is used ($Na^3C^6H^5O^7 \cdot 2H_2O$), and can be buffered or non-buffered.

Historically, coagulation labs have used 3.8% Na citrate for primary collection tubes; the current guidelines recommending the 3.2% concentration were likely adopted after differences were detected between the two concentrations (3). The 3.2% solution is isomolar and does not appear to cause shrinkage of the red cells contained in the sample, in comparison to the 3.8% concentration which causes approximately 6% volume shrinkage of erythrocytes (4). Standardization of the concentration also allows for optimal comparison between both different laboratories within a region for beneficial patient care, and across the realms of laboratory data in published studies. At the time of writing this publication, 3.2% Na citrate tubes are the tube of choice, with 3.8% tubes at about 10% of the market share worldwide, but are no longer available in Canada (personal communication, Becton Dickinson Inc.).

4 Mixing

The Na citrate vacuum collection tubes should be mixed, immediately after collection, by using four complete gentle inversions. Overmixing or harsh mixing may cause hemolysis and/or platelet activation which may affect the results of some assays.

5 Plastic vs. Glass Primary Collection Tubes

Although glass collection tubes may seem contraindicated when working with samples destined for a coagulation laboratory, the commercially available tubes have a siliconized interior surface, which helps prevent activation of factors and platelets. Collection tubes have historically been made of glass, although safety concerns and transport guidelines have motivated tube manufacturers to provide users with a plastic alternative for most collection tube types. Although most published literature has demonstrated that plastic tubes are acceptable for the majority of coagulation assays (5–7), the plastic tubes may not be suitable for collection of samples for specialized platelet assays such as the PFA-100. In this assay, even small platelet clumps can cause an error to be generated as the clumps plug or pass through the tiny aperture (personal communication). As well, some authors have found significant differences in PT INR, between glass and plastic tubes for patients on warfarin (8). Also a worthy note of caution is that results on heparinized patient samples collected in plastic tubes may also be affected, showing a relative decrease in the heparin concentration detected for the comparison of glass to plastic. In Gosselin et al. (5), the means of aPTTs for the patient groups were comparable, but in looking at the range of values, at the top end of the PTT scale, the difference in PTT was 27.1 s, with the plastic tube showing a marked decrease from the glass tube of the same manufacturer. Assumably these differences are due to platelet activation being some degree higher in the plastic vs. the glass collection tubes, causing some small platelet aggregates and release of PF4, which is a potent neutralizer of heparin. This may be in part because some plastic collection tubes are the size of a 4.5 mL draw tube but have an inner sleeve that is long and narrow making complete inversion of the sample difficult due to capillary action; if improper mixing occurs, activation of the sample may occur prior to complete decalcification/anticoagulation. Differences may be tube dependent, and the results of a particular study may not be adaptable to tubes of all manufacturers. Careful evaluation of any tube (with all patient populations, including those on various anticoagulant medications) and its preanalytical variables is needed prior to adopting a new collection tube type. Also, education of the end user as to the correct usage and handling is of paramount importance.

6 Patients with Extreme Hematocrits (>0.55 L/L or <0.20 L/L)

Ideally, the amount of anticoagulant in sodium citrate vacuum collection tubes should be altered for each increment in the range of possible hematocrits. This would keep the plasma to anticoagulant ratio the same for each sample tested in the lab, thus allowing for each sample (plasma) to be diluted identically by the liquid anticoagulant as well as being re-calcified in exactly the same manner during any given assay. Since such a task is impractical and in practice, as long as the amount of calcium added can saturate the anticoagulant, leaving enough calcium for the appropriate reactions to occur, the amount of anticoagulant does not need to be altered, provided that the hematocrit is less than 0.55 L/L. However, for each individual patient with a hematocrit that is above 0.55 L/L, the proper amount of

Table 1
Plasma to anticoagulant ratio for a standard collection tube (all are considered acceptable collections)

HCT (L/L)	Volume of anticoagulant allowed for a 3 mL collection tube (2.7 mL draw) (mL)	Total plasma in tube (mL) (2.7 mL blood × (100 – HCT))	Plasma to anticoagulant ratio
0.55	0.3 (no correction)	1.215	4.05:1
0.20	0.3 (no correction)	2.16	7.20:1
0.12	0.3 (no correction)	2.376	7.92:1

Table 2
Plasma to anticoagulant ratio for a standard tube with one-half of the anticoagulant removed

HCT (L/L)	Volume of anticoagulant remaining (one-half of the total removed from a 2.7 mL draw) (mL)	Total plasma in the tube (mL) (2.7 mL blood × (100 – HCT))	Plasma to anticoagulant ratio
0.78	0.15 (removal of 0.15 mL)	0.594	3.96:1 (lower than acceptable ratio)
0.77	0.15	0.621	4.14:1 (acceptable)
0.76	0.15	0.648	4.32:1 (acceptable)
0.56	0.15	1.188	7.92:1 (acceptable)

anticoagulant should be calculated, according to the following equation (1) (see Note 2):

$$C = \left(1.85\times10^{-3}\right)\left(100-\mathrm{HCT}\right)\left(V_{\mathrm{blood}}\right),$$

where C is the volume of citrate remaining in the tube

HCT is the hematocrit of the patient

V is the volume of blood added (i.e., for a 5 mL tube, use 4.5 mL)

1.85×10^{-3} is the constant

The above guideline also states that in routine practice removal of 0.1 mL of anticoagulant can be used for patients with hematocrit levels between 0.55 and 0.65 L/L. Unfortunately, the reality is that in a large tertiary care hospital, of the samples with a hematocrit higher than 0.55 L/L, approximately 13% of those samples indeed have a hematocrit equal to or higher than 0.65 L/L (unpublished data L.S.).

It should be considered that an acceptable range for plasma/anticoagulant ratio be allowed for the vast difference in hematocrits that fall below 0.55 L/L. A calculation of the allowable amount of plasma volume to citrate anticoagulant (ratio) when considering all the hematocrits below this level causes one to believe that the same overall ratio range should be allowed for hematocrits above 0.55 L/L (see Tables 1 and 2). The three values of Table 1 are hematocrits that are acceptable, with their respective plasma to anticoagulant volume ratios listed. According to literature and published guidelines these samples do not need to have any anticoagulant removed from the primary Na citrate collection tube. Note that the ratio for the sample with the maximum allowable 0.55 L/L hematocrit is 4.05:1; therefore any sample with a ratio less than that should have the anticoagulant adjusted. The four values in Table 2 correspond to hematocrits that are above the 0.55 L/L cutoff and assume that one-half of the total anticoagulant has been withdrawn from the vacuum collection tube, under sterile conditions (see Note 3).

Therefore by removing 0.15 mL of Na citrate anticoagulant from a 2.7 mL draw tube, any patient with a hematocrit up to 0.77 L/L should be accommodated. This is in agreement with previous publications suggesting that 1 part Na citrate anticoagulant be used with 19 parts whole blood to avoid excessive anticoagulation of samples from patients with polycythemia, although the authors used 3.8% Na citrate (4). As there are no current recommendations for altering the anticoagulant when the patient's hematocrit is less that 20 L/L, an excess of plasma to anticoagulant ratio should not be a factor, provided that the anticoagulant is sufficient enough that the sample has not clotted. From the above table of values then, the only sample of concern is that which has a hematocrit of 0.78 L/L (or greater), with its lower plasma volume, producing a ratio of plasma to anticoagulant that is less than the allowed ratio (4.05:1) for the sample with a hematocrit of exactly 0.55 L/L. As well, the likelihood of hematocrits >0.78 L/L is virtually nonexistent, so adjustment of special collection tubes with removal of one-half of the anticoagulant should cover all scenarios of patients with hematocrits higher than 0.55 L/L.

Patients with hematocrits that are lower than 0.20 L/L do not appear to need any adjustment to the citrate volume used for the primary collection tube (1, 9). However data is only available for the more "routine" coagulation assays (i.e., PT, PTT) and is sometimes extrapolated from collections in 3.8% Na citrate (9).

7 Over- or Underfilling of Tubes

The subject of underfilling Na citrate collection tubes has diverse arguments on both sides, at various degrees of fill, using different tube sizes and with both normal subjects and anticoagulated patients. Some authors suggest that underfilling can occur down to 90% fill, with little variation of the PT and PTT on both normal and anticoagulated subjects (10) using 3.2% Na citrate; in this study, underfilling to levels below 90% caused increases in high PTT values, stating however that normal values may be acceptable from underfilled tubes. Others specify that a collection tube for PT can be as low as 60%, with a PTT as low as 70% (11). This is in contrast to the American College of Chest Physicians guideline which recommends that a fill volume of less than 90% to be unacceptable for a PT INR using a 2.7 mL draw pediatric collection tube (12). CLSI guidelines state that underfilling of tubes can lead to inaccurate results and to follow the manufacturer's recommendations (1). However, in another much more general blood collection guideline from the CLSI (H1-A5) a 10% variation in underfilling or overfilling is allowed, and this recommendation has been cited by manufacturers as being an allowable limit (13). One thing to consider is that it may be possible that different sizes, styles (plastic vs. glass), and manufacturer's tubes react differently to underfilling. Also, statistical inaccuracy may not be equivalent to clinical significance and depends on the statistical test used for comparison, and acceptance is subjectively dependent on the interpretation of the user.

The first author (LS) has performed in-house quality assurance studies on glass collection tubes (not published) with the conclusion that a slightly underfilled glass vacuum collection tube does not have a clinically significant effect on routine coagulation results (i.e., PT, PTT, Fibrinogen), provided that the tube is filled to at least 80% of its total volume (i.e., 5.0 mL, 3.0 mL, or 2.0 mL). If sufficient plasma volume for end testing is a concern, a minimum volume of 90% could be used, especially for the smaller tube sizes. The experiments described here were done using underfilled tubes that had been underfilled to various degrees at the time of sample collection. Manipulation of the sample to mimic underfilling, for instance by adding more anticoagulant was not performed; post-draw manipulation of samples has been viewed by some authors as adding another variable to an already complex situation that may not be reflective of actual lab practice.

The recommendation of this publication is that any allowance of underfilling of Na citrate tubes should be verified with the lab's own reagent/instrument combination, as well as the exact tube type, style, and size needed, prior to implementation of altering the allowable acceptance rules within the laboratory (see Note 4).

Overfilling of a tube can be an issue when the sample is collected via syringe, usually from an access line. The tube cap is removed and whole blood is then added to the tube without accurate measurement. Vacuum collection tubes are designed such that if a substantial amount of overfilling occurs, the cap will not be able to be properly seated and will pop off because of the air pressure in the small remaining airspace. For a glass 4.5 mL draw collection tube (Becton Dickinson), an extra 200 μL is all that can be added, which equates to only 4% of the total volume; an extra 300 μL does not allow adequate airspace for the lid to be secured, and it will continually pop off. Overfilling a tube results in larger plasma to anticoagulant ratio and is essentially the equivalent of a sample with a low hematocrit, for which there is currently no recommendation of citrate adjustment.

8 Collections Other than Standard Venous Collections

Collection through vascular access devices in the clinical reality is sometimes unavoidable. However, there are certain precautions that should be followed.

A line that has been flushed with heparin should be avoided if at all possible; the concentration of heparin in the line can be much greater than a prophylactic or therapeutic dosage; therefore even a small amount of contamination would produce a large error in the coagulation results. For sample collection from a line, it is necessary to first flush the line with 5 mL of sterile saline solution and then discard 5 mL of blood or 5–6 volumes of the dead space of the device or tubing (1).

If a butterfly needle or similar apparatus is used, and coagulation testing is the only blood work being drawn, a discard tube (nonadditive or Na citrate tube) should be used first, followed by the number of tubes required. Essentially this discard tube will withdraw the air from the tubing in the butterfly device; this tube does not need to be fully filled, as long as all the air has been removed from the tubing in the collection device.

If collection is performed using a syringe, the sample must be added to the vacuum collection tube with 1 min of the actual draw from the patient (1). As well, a small volume syringe is recommended. Generally a syringe capacity of <20 mL is used with some type of transfer device to improve safety.

In the point-of-care setting, capillary samples are suitable for some analyzers, the most common being PT INR analysis. For other routine collections from a capillary sample, it is usually crucial to wipe away the first drop obtained which contains the tissue factor released by the initial lancet puncture. However, some manufacturers of PT INR point-of-care equipment actually recommend using the first "hanging" drop of blood for the assay. It is important to follow the specific manufacturer's directions, as reference ranges have been determined in the same manner. Loading the cartridge quickly (manufacturer will recommend a maximum time) is also important, as obviously, the sample contains no anticoagulant.

9 Processing and Stability of the Sample Within the Laboratory

Prior to centrifugation, the sample should be visually examined for proper fill volume. Large clots can also be detected with a gentle inversion. After centrifugation, each sample should be visually inspected for presence of hemolysis in the plasma layer, as well as a high hematocrit. Unacceptable specimens should have all tests cancelled and recollection requested. Samples with hemolysis and high hematocrit are discussed in detail in other sections. Other problem samples include, but are not limited to the following: clotted samples, incorrect anticoagulant, or incorrect plasma to Na citrate anticoagulant ratio (see Note 5).

Samples should be centrifuged as soon as possible after collection. This is especially true of PTT samples drawn on patients on therapeutic heparin, which should be centrifuged within 1 h of collection (11). These samples should also be assayed as quickly as possible. Although CLSI published guidelines state 4 h stability for PTT, the heparin is neutralized quickly by the platelet factor 4 released from the platelets as the sample ages; heparin neutralization can be anywhere from 10 to 70%, 5 h after the sampling time point (14). PTT reagent manufacturer's have variation in their respective package inserts regarding acceptable stability times for testing patients on heparin and can be as low as 2 h. Each lab should set its own defined limits for heparinized patients, after proper investigation using the appropriate tube type, as well as the other inherent pre-analytical and analytical variables. For those samples from patients not on heparin, with PTT ordered, stability is generally 4 h, centrifuged or uncentrifuged.

Optimally, samples should be centrifuged to obtain a platelet count (on the plasma) of $<10 \times 10^9$/L. There are various recommendations for centrifuge speed and time (i.e., $1{,}500 \times g$ for 15 min, $1{,}700 \times g$ for 10 min, $3{,}000 \times g$ for 10 min) that differ between the various published guidelines, manufacturer's product inserts, etc. The common denominator of all the recommendations is to ensure a plasma platelet count of $<10 \times 10^9$/L, prior to freezing the samples for subsequent testing. For samples with platelet counts higher than this, when the platelets undergo a freeze-thaw cycle which essentially causes them to lyse, the remaining platelets will release platelet factor 4 and various phospholipids, neutralizing heparin and antiphospholipid antibodies, respectively. There is evidence that fresh plasma samples with platelet counts of up to 200×10^9/L do not have significantly different results for routine coagulation assays (15, 16), but in practice, this is actually a normal count and would likely only occur if the sample is unspun or poorly enough spun to leave remaining red cells and platelets in the plasma. Also, to have different plasma sample types within the laboratory (some with platelet counts of <10 and some up to 200×10^9/L) may cause errors when samples are inadvertently frozen which contain too many remaining platelets. Samples for lupus anticoagulant, inhibitor screens, and heparin monitoring (as well as the aPTTs for these same patients) may be affected by platelets present in the samples; these assays are often frozen and run in batches. Platelet counts of $<10 \times 10^9$/L are recommended for lupus anticoagulant testing and for some activated protein C resistance testing (17, 18). Centrifuges are generally tested twice annually to ensure that they are capable of producing samples with platelet counts $<10 \times 10^9$/L and should be retested after any major maintenance has taken place.

For immediate testing of the sample, the plasma may remain on the cells after centrifugation. If the samples are batch run, the plasma should be removed after centrifugation, using only plastic tubes and transfer pipettes to avoid contact activation of the coagulation factors. As a general rule for the majority of coagulation assays, at room temperature storage with the plasma sample remaining on the cells, stability is 4 h. This can be prolonged up to 24 h at room temperature for a PT INR. Prolonged storage at 4°C is generally not recommended and may result in cold activation of factor 7, which can affect the PT INR. Overall sample stability on some patients (i.e., with DIC, or on fibrinolytic drugs) may be shorter than listed; however the samples will usually be ordered on a STAT basis, due to the patient acuity.

For samples frozen at −20 to −24°C, a non-frost-free freezer should be used, as a frost-free cycle may cause partial thawing of the sample. Samples stored at −24°C (or lower) are good for 3 months, whereas samples stored below −74°C are good for approximately 18 months (1). The specific chapters will contain more detailed information of stability maximums at various temperatures for each assay that may deviate from the above recommendations.

Frozen samples should be snap thawed in a 37°C water bath for 5–10 min (dependent on sample volume) to ensure the sample is completely thawed as well as bringing back into solution any of the cryoprecipitate that may have formed. Following adequate mixing, these samples should be assayed as soon as possible. Certain tests, such as PTT, may be affected by freezing and this should be taken into consideration when verifying results or comparing reagents or analyzers. It is prudent to compare "like" samples—i.e., frozen to frozen, fresh to fresh for the most accurate evaluations—and is an especially important consideration in reference range determinations.

10 Preparation of Platelet-Free Plasma

Preparation of platelet-free plasma is necessary prior to sample freezing for those assays which will be affected by any platelet component that will be released as a cause of the platelet lysis that occurs during a freeze-thaw cycle. These assays include anti-Xa in which the heparin or low molecular weight heparin will be neutralized by the resulting platelet factor 4 that is now in solution. Also affected are lupus anticoagulant assays, which can exhibit some neutralization of antibodies in the patient sample from the various phospholipids that are released from the cell membrane during the freeze-thaw.

There are two different methods of platelet-free preparation. The first one is to double spin the sample. Essentially, after the first centrifugation, the plasma is removed to a secondary plastic tube and then recentrifuged using a high-speed centrifuge at approximately 13,000 × *g* for 5 min. For those sites that do not have a high-speed centrifuge, the option is to repeat the original spin, at the same speed and time. The plasma is then removed to the appropriate plastic tube for freezing, avoiding the tiny cell button which has formed in the bottom of the tube.

The second method is discussed here (with some reservation) and again involves removal of the plasma after the first centrifugation, followed by a filtering step. The plasma is drawn into a 1 mL syringe and dispensed through a 0.22 μm filter into a second plastic tube. Each method should produce adequate platelet-free plasma.

It is important to note that the filtering method can also remove fibrinogen and some high molecular weight multimers (19). The loss of fibrinogen appears to reach a saturation point, thus is likely caused by direct binding of the fibrinogen to the filter material. Loss of high molecular weight multimers, however, occurs to the same degree for each of multiple sample passes through the filter, implying that the loss is due to either the adhesive properties of the vWF or the molecular size or structure being impenetrable to the pore diameter. As a result of this loss of components post filtering, it is vitally important that filtered platelet-free samples are only tested for anti-Xa and lupus anticoagulant assays. If these samples are inadvertently assayed for von Willebrands workup, they may appear to mimic type II disease. Patient fibrinogen levels would be lowered as well; PTT and factor VIII levels also appear to be affected.

11 Transport

Transport of samples must follow local regulations. As a general guideline, plastic tubes can be shipped in a biohazardous zipper closure bag with enough adsorbent material to accommodate the amount of total liquid present. To minimize breakage, glass collection tubes are usually individually sleeved in a continuous strip of "bubble wrap" designed to hold individual tubes, and then placed in the appropriate zipper closure bag with adsorbent material. Since most samples being shipped are destined for reference laboratories, the likelihood is that these samples are frozen to prolong stability, and should be shipped on dry ice, using the appropriate dangerous goods transport rules specific to the region.

There are many unforeseen complications that can arise from collection/processing in one location and analysis/reporting from a second location. This could include test name confusion, basic sample type errors or artifact from freeze/thaw, all of which can be difficult errors to detect (see Notes 6–9).

12 Heparin Removal

For samples contaminated with heparin that are difficult to redraw, there are various commercial products for heparin removal. The sample can be incubated (room temperature) with either a lyophilized enzyme or a heparin adsorbent material, the latter which requires a centrifugation step prior to assay of the sample. For some random-access analyzers, the lyophilized enzyme preparation has shown carryover to the next sample, which will have an effect on the amount of heparin assayed in this second sample. It is important to adopt a thorough sample needle washing step after the sample with heparin removal has been aspirated to avoid heparin neutralization, and thus errors, in subsequent samples (see Note 10). Of interest, it is also important to note that reagents containing heparin neutralizers should be evaluated for carryover in random-access analyzers as well. This is especially important if the reagent and analyzer are from two distinct manufacturers, as this combination may never have been evaluated in the past (see Note 11).

The lab must also ensure that the patient is not on therapeutic heparin, prior to sending results to the end user. The use of heparin removal products must be carefully explained to the physicians and patient care personnel; as well, explanatory comments should accompany the results. It would be prudent to send results of both values—the pre- and post-heparin removal—to help avoid confusion and assist the caregiver to understand the significance of the difference between the two values.

13 Hemolysis

Samples with visible hemolysis likely indicate a difficult venipuncture, which in turn may have produced clotting factor activation, which could have an effect on clot-based assays. As well, results from optical endpoint detection analyzers may be affected by various levels of hemolysis. For very mild hemolysis, the laboratory may choose to send the results obtained, along with a comment specifying that slight hemolysis was noted and may affect the results, leaving recollection up to the discretion of the ordering physician. For samples with more than slight hemolysis due to collection technique, tests should be cancelled and the specimen recollected.

For some patient groups, the hemolysis present is an in vivo phenomenon, caused by stress on the red cells from ECMO (extra corporeal membrane oxygenation), cardiopulmonary bypass, hemolytic disease states, etc. Obviously, in these cases a recollection of sample is not going to be helpful, although a suitable comment should be sent out with the patient's results, which will help the laboratory staff track the sample appearance over time and may prevent further rejection of samples for which recollection is of no benefit.

Chromogenic assays (such as anti-Xa for unfractionated or low molecular weight heparin) generally do not show interference from slightly hemolyzed samples, as the quantitation is calculated from a rate vs. time reaction. However some optical detection methods have a maximum OD value that can be read. For patients on

ECMO, whose in vivo hemolysis can sometimes be quite profound, if the "background" OD reading is such that in addition to the reaction reading, the maximum value is superseded somewhere during the time the reaction is monitored, then an error is generated, and no value is attainable. For these samples, a 1 in 2 dilution in normal pooled plasma (not containing heparin) will usually dilute out the hemolysis enough so that the maximum OD reading is not reached and therefore a result is generated, which then needs to be multiplied by the appropriate corrector factor of the dilution performed. It is important to remember that the pooled normal plasma contains antithrombin 3, as well as all other factors in normal amounts. If using an anti-Xa assay that does not contain antithrombin, thus relying on the patient's own antithrombin to exhibit a more physiological value, this may not be a plausible solution. This may be of clinical significance, especially for the pediatric population, who can occasionally have lower antithrombin values. It is also important to remember that if a dilution is done on a sample the lower limit of detection be taken into consideration when calculating the result to be given out. For instance, if an assay cannot accurately detect anti-Xa levels below 0.10 U/mL and a one-half dilution is made on the patient sample, then the lower limit of detection should be resulted as <0.20 U/mL.

Hemolysis may also be related to the size of needle gauge used for the venipuncture, with the theory being that smaller gauge needles may have a greater propensity to produce hemolyzed samples. For this reason, generally 25 gauge needles (or smaller diameter) are discouraged for use in blood collection.

14 Lipemia and Icterus

Samples with extreme lipemia or icteric qualities are usually only a concern with optical endpoint detection systems. For laboratories with these analyzer types, the degree of interference should be documented at the time of instrument evaluation and appropriate measures in place to be able to generate results on these rare samples. Usually slight lipemia or icterus does not interfere with results, although this should be verified for the specific analyzer in use by each lab (see Note 12).

Although rare, for samples with gross lipemia, centrifugation may produce an unusually large layer of lipids, which sits atop the plasma layer. Automated analyzers are usually designed so that the sampling needle descends until the liquid is detected and then the sample is aspirated. For these particular samples, the sampling needle of the analyzer may actually aspirate the defined lipid layer, causing an inadequate volume of actual plasma to be sampled, leading to incorrect results being generated. When assaying this type of sample, a good practice is to withdraw the plasma layer, including the lipemic layer, to a secondary plastic tube and remix the sample prior to testing. This would represent the physiologic nature of in vivo plasma for this particular patient. Alternatively, if using an optical endpoint detection analyzer, this may not be suitable, as the sample may produce an error, due to the gross lipemia present.

15 Interference from Anticoagulants

Although detection and quantitation or ensuring adequate effect of anticoagulants is usually desired within the coagulation lab, some assays show effects/direct interference from these compounds which is undesirable. For instance protein C and S are vitamin K dependent, and therefore are decreased in patients on vitamin K antagonists, and should be tested if possible prior to or when the patient has discontinued use of this medication. Heparin neutralizers (i.e., protamine sulfate, polybrene) are incorporated into many of the coagulation reagents; however heparin will still interfere with assays such as PTT-based factor assays. Direct thrombin inhibitors will interfere with almost all assays that have thrombin present, either as a reagent or generated from within the patient sample, which encompasses a large proportion of coagulation tests. Assays with very large amounts of thrombin may not show interference, as they are able to neutralize the direct thrombin inhibitors and have ample left over for the reaction to occur. Interference may be dependent on the type and amount of thrombin in an individual assay, and the pertinent lab assays should be tested to verify that the various drugs (argatroban, lepirudin, etc.) from this class do not interfere. The other downfall of the direct thrombin inhibitors for the laboratory is that we currently have no way to remove them from the sample for interference-free testing, as can be done with a sample containing heparin. For suspicious coagulation results, always review the medication history at the time of collection, which may help elucidate the cause.

16 CTAD Collection Tube

The CTAD evacuated blood collection tube is commercially available (Becton Dickinson, Franklin Lakes, NJ) and contains Na citrate, citric acid, and various inhibitors of platelet aggregation and release reaction: theophylline, adenosine, and dipyridamole. Also called Diatube H, this tube can be used for assays of PAI-1, β-thromboglobulin, or platelet factor 4, among others. It also decreases the progressive neutralization of heparin from platelet factor 4 release (which occurs over time) in a sample drawn from a therapeutically heparinized patient. Preservation of this sample type extends to at least 4 h before centrifugation is necessary. This tube can also be used for the more common special coagulation assays such as protein C or S and factor assays. One of the drawbacks of using this tube type is that the dipyridamole is light sensitive and can inactivate to unacceptable levels after only 48 h of exposure to light (either natural or artificial) (20). This property is likely one of the issues preventing this tube from being used as a standard routine coagulation collection tube, although it does have its place in the aforementioned ultrasensitive assays.

17 Diurnal Variation

Although circadian variation is not considered to be of paramount importance in coagulation assays, it is important to note that some assays are affected (21). Platelet function appears to be most robust in the morning, as is factor VIII, factor VIIa, protein C and S, β-thromboglobulin, and F1 + 2.

Overall, fibrinolysis tends to be lowest in the early morning: tPA and PAP (plasmin-α2-antiplasmin complexes) exhibiting trough levels, and PAI-1 at its peak. Plasminogen appears unchanged.

Factor V activity, von Willebrands antigen, and factor VII antigen appear to remain unchanged during the course of the day. There is conflicting evidence surrounding the variation seen with antithrombin, which may peak in the afternoon, or remain unchanged.

These differences are especially important in the realm of research studies. The diurnal variation will influence the results, prompting the investigator to assume that a significant change has occurred between two time points. In reality, those naturally occurring differences are inherent issues in the study design.

18 Guideline Table

The following summary (Table 3) is a general guideline for sample collection, volume, and special handling for the most common coagulation assays. It is expected that there will be variations between laboratories to accommodate various analyzers and commercial kits, etc. Sample stability is 4 h unless otherwise specified for a particular assay. As a general rule, three aliquots of 0.5 mL each can be attained from a single 4.5 mL draw primary collection tube. Similar assays and assays that are often ordered together are grouped together to minimize the size of the table.

There are numerous variables affecting the quality of a patient sample, which in turn affect the results that are generated from that sample. It does not matter how extremely precise and accurate the methodology and equipment in a laboratory is if the sample entering the system is not optimal because of the aforementioned variables. No matter what the perceived efficiency of the reagent/instrument system, results and patient treatment may be negatively affected by a less than perfect sample.

Table 3
Guideline for sample collection, volume, and special handling for the most common coagulation assays

Test description	Specimen type/transport	Special handling/recommendations
PT	3.2% Na citrate tube	Sample stable 24 h
PTT	3.2% Na citrate tube	Patient on heparin—stable 4 h or *less* Sample should be centrifuged within 1 h of collection
Fibrinogen	3.2% Na citrate tube	Sample stable 8 h
D-dimer—quantitative	3.2% Na citrate tube	Sample stable 8 h
Antiphospholipid antibodies	Gold top or other serum separator tube	2 × 0.5 mL serum (mark serum on label)
Activated protein C resistance (clot based)	3.2% Na citrate tube	2 × 0.5 mL plasma
Factor V Leiden mutation and/or prothrombin 20210 (or factor II) mutation	1–4 mL mauve top tube (preferably at 4°C)	MUST be sterile, dedicated sample Sample stable 24–48 h
– Factor assays—II, V, VII, VIII, IX, X, XI, XII – Ristocetin cofactor – von Willebrand factor	3.2% Na citrate tube (prolonged storage on ice may activate FVII)	2 × 0.5 mL plasma/test
Factor VIII inhibitor	3.2% Na citrate tube	2 × 1.0 mL plasma
Factor XIII	3.2% Na citrate tube	2 × 1.0 mL plasma
Heparin-induced thrombocytopenia assay	Gold top or other serum separator tube	2 × 1.2 mL serum
Lupus anticoagulant *or* dilute Russell's Viper Venom Time	2–(3.2%) Na citrate tube	3 × 1.0 mL plasma Make platelet free by double-spin method or filtering
Anti-Xa assay: – Low molecular weight heparin – Orgaran – Unfractionated Heparin	3.2% Na citrate tube—transport at room temperature LMWH, Orgaran—collect 4–6 h post dose	2 × 0.5 mL plasma/test Make platelet free by double-spin method or filtering Mark PFP on label
– Antithrombin – Protein C – Protein S	3.2% Na citrate tubes	2 × 0.5 mL plasma/test
PT inhibitor screen	2–(3.2%) Na citrate tubes	2 × 2.0 mL plasma
PTT inhibitor screen	3–(3.2%) Na citrate tubes	2 × 3.0 mL plasma Make platelet free by double-spin method *only* Mark PFP on label

(continued)

Table 3 (continued)

Test description	Specimen type/transport	Special handling/recommendations
Plasminogen	3.2% Na citrate tube	2 × 0.5 mL plasma/test
Thrombin time	3.2% Na citrate tube	2 × 0.5 mL plasma/test
Reptilase time	3.2% Na citrate tube	2 × 0.5 mL plasma/test
Euglobulin lysis time (ELT)	3.2% Na citrate tube on ice	Sample should be collected with no venous stasis Assay should be done within 30 min of collection
Platelet aggregation (platelet-rich plasma method)	5–4.5 mL (3.2%) Na citrate tube	Centrifuge at 150 × *g* for 15 min with no brake Remove platelet-rich plasma (PRP) Centrifuge remainder at 3,000 × *g* for 10 min Remove platelet-free plasma (PFP) for blanking Platelets are viable for 4 h

19 Notes

1. To aid in the investigation of platelet function studies, all drugs that a patient is currently on should be documented. The pharmacy department can be a valuable resource for literature regarding those medications available on the institution's formulary as well as what is available in a specific country. Providing the front-line staff with an alphabetical list which contains both generic and trade names of each drug of interest is useful—patients and staff may only know the drug by either the generic or the trade name. The alphabetical list helps to avoid confusion, making it simple to find the drug no matter what name is given.

2. When patients with hematocrits higher than 0.55 L/L are first identified, it is usually via their first venipuncture, with a "regular" collection using a Na citrate tube that has not had the citrate amount adjusted properly. For resulting PT INR and PTT on those samples, if the results are normal, they can be sent with a comment stating that future collections need to be drawn using the special collection tube. If the excess anticoagulant were to affect the result, there would be a false prolongation; the calcium would be chelated by the anticoagulant, resulting in a slower rate of clot formation. There may also be a slight dilutional effect, which may prolong the results. Therefore, if the initial results (collected in a regular collection

tube) are prolonged, these tests should be cancelled and the special collection tube with the appropriate amount of anticoagulant used for the recollection.

3. For withdrawal of anticoagulant from vacuum collection tubes, for patients with high hematocrits, a 1 mL syringe with a small bore needle (i.e., 25 gauge) can be inserted into a sterilized tube top to remove some of the anticoagulant. If done carefully, the vacuum will still remain, allowing the tube to be used in the usual manner. During the withdrawal, pay close attention to any sound that may indicate loss of the vacuum; discard any suspect tubes. Sometimes a more successful removal is achieved if a 2.7 mL pediatric draw tube is used. With some of the 4.5 mL draw tubes, the type of cap used can have a propensity to lose the vacuum when the needle is inserted or withdrawn. It is important to sterilize the top of the tube with an alcohol swab prior to anticoagulant removal. Depending on the type of syringe used, the volume in the hub of the syringe may need to be measured prior to special tube preparation, or too much anticoagulant may be removed from the tube; alternatively, the syringe hub can be "primed" with Na citrate from another Na citrate tube. This altered tube should be assigned a shorter expiry than the unaltered tube of the same type. As a general rule, tubes may be made up monthly or using a similarly short interval, which may depend on the total usage.

4. An easy way to have a minimum volume acceptability standard within the lab for quick decision making is to add water and food colorant in the amount of the smallest acceptable volume, taking into consideration the amount of liquid anticoagulant already in the tube (i.e., 0.5 mL for a 5 mL tube, 0.3 mL for a 3 mL tube). Evaporation from the tube will occur over time, so a line drawn on the tube at the time of preparation will assist the front-line user in determining if a given tube is acceptable, or if a recollection should be performed for accurate results.

5. In most laboratories, coagulation assays on sodium citrate collection tubes that require repeat are checked for the presence of a clot. This is usually done with two wooden applicator sticks, rimming the tube. When checking the sample for a clot using this method, if subsequent testing may be needed, it is important to first remove some of the plasma from the sample. When the primary collection tube has been centrifuged, then checked for a clot, subsequently recentrifuged, and retested, heparin levels can drop dramatically from the original value. Also, samples for stat analysis are sometimes checked for a clot prior to centrifugation, to improve turnaround times; however, this will result in falsely low heparin levels. The likely cause is platelet activation with release of platelet factor 4, which neutralizes the heparin.

6. The variations in sample type that come into a reference coagulation lab can be a source of error. Generally the samples are frozen at peripheral sites and sent to the central reference center. Depending on the LIS (lab information system) used, a single accession number may be generated for all tests on a patient at a given time point. This would potentially mean that plasma, platelet-free plasma, and serum from the same patient may all come into the lab with the same collection date and time and the same lab assigned accession number. Normal (or even high) results, for certain clot-based assays that usually require citrated plasma, can even be attained when serum is accidentally used for the assay. The results are dependent on whether consumption of the particular analyte occurs during clotting in the serum collection tube. As an example, Factor VII levels are actually higher on serum than plasma owing to the conversion of FVII to FVIIa during the clotting of the sample, and the fact that consumption of the FVII does not occur during the clotting process. In an effort to discriminate questionable serum samples, perform a fibrinogen, PT, and PTT. A serum sample should give above maximum times for the PT and PTT, and a very low fibrinogen. Platelet-free samples prepared using a filter will be lower in fibrinogen, FVIII, and the higher molecular weight multimers of von Willebrand factor than standard plasma samples, as outlined in the preparation of platelet-free plasma section.

   In an effort to overcome the potential mix-ups, peripheral laboratories should be instructed to document on individual sample aliquots the specifics other than the norm, such as "PFP" (platelet-free plasma) and "serum."

7. On rare occasions, frozen samples that have been made platelet free by the filtering or double-spin method still exhibit a large loss of anti-Xa activity in comparison to the fresh sample. This experience is drawn from a specific pediatric patient, awaiting cardiac bypass surgery. The post-freeze-thaw values had lost approximately one half (0.30 U/mL) of the anti-Xa activity, when compared to the fresh sample from the same time point (unpublished data). The reason for the loss is not easily definable, but could be due to platelet microparticles that were not removed by the platelet-free processing of the sample prior to freezing. If anti-Xa values on a particular patient do not seem to correlate with the dosage of heparin being given and the other laboratory data, it may be prudent to verify if a difference exists between values pre- and post-freeze-thaw cycle.

8. Different assays within the coagulation laboratory (and some in other labs) have names that are very similar. Education of ordering physicians who do not order these assays with some frequency will help to ensure the correct assays are being requested.

The most common error is ordering a "factor V" in place of a "factor V Leiden." Another set of assays which is commonly exchanged is "factor X" and "anti-Xa." The third most common mistake, which is not likely to be picked up (as one of the assays is generally done outside the coagulation lab), is that of a "C-reactive protein" requested in place of a "protein C." Education of front-line staff is also important to recognize combinations of requests on the same patient that may appear in error. For instance, a factor V ordered with a typical hypercoagulable workup of protein C and protein S would need some investigation, and would likely conclude with a factor V Leiden being exchanged for the original order of factor V.

9. There is potential for specimen mix-up to occur when large central laboratories receive frozen patient samples from small referral sites. Collections for factor V Leiden genotype are usually collected at the same time as the clot-based test for activated protein C resistance. The error occurs when the EDTA plasma is frozen, instead of this tube being submitted as whole blood for the genotype. When the sample arrives at the central laboratory, the data entry personnel assume it is frozen citrated plasma. This sample will generally give very long clotting times for the activated protein C resistance clot-based assays. As well, EDTA plasma, when tested for standard coagulation screening tests (PTT, PT INR, and fibrinogen), gives plausible coagulation results—usually the PTT is only slightly increased and the other assays can appear normal. Therefore, the usual method which differentiates plasma from serum is of no use. One way to elucidate the nature of the sample is to run a potassium, calcium, and sodium on the sample. Characteristically, a pattern of results will aide in differentiation of the respective tubes (Table 4). The range of results was determined from five samples of each type, on a Beckman Synchron LX 20 chemistry analyzer.

10. It is especially important to verify that no carryover of heparin adsorbent (contained in reagents) occurs when using analyzer/reagent combinations that are marketed by two different companies. Generally the carryover of heparin adsorbent has been investigated for an assay kit on a particular analyzer from the same company; however not all products on the market would have been investigated for each available analyzer. If unacceptable carryover is detected, a suitable washing step, such as loading a wash solution as a patient sample, or even repeating of the anti-Xa unfractionated heparin controls may be necessary to verify results of subsequent samples.

11. When using a heparin removal product, there are certain limits to the amount of heparin that can be adequately removed. Some commercial products allow for a sample to be treated twice—after the first removal process, a second removal step

Table 4
Electrolyte results associated with different anticoagulant tubes used in haemostatic testing

	Sodium level (mmol/L)	Potassium level (mmol/L)	Calcium level (mmol/L)
EDTA plasma	131.6–134.5	18.79–20.89	<0.50
Na Citrate plasma	148.9–156.6	3.11–4.63	1.27–1.42

can sometimes be done for those samples that contain an amount of heparin exceeding the capability of the system. Always follow the manufacturer's product insert.

12. Assays such as automated quantitative D-dimer usually have interference from at least the most markedly lipemic samples. However the inserts to these products usually give the interference information in a way that is not particularly useful for day-to-day decision making within the laboratory. For example, the insert for Diagnostica Stago quantitative D-dimer states that if the patient sample is diluted 1/6 with buffer only, and this mixture reads an OD higher than 0.35 at same wavelength at which the assay is read, then interference could occur. It is unreasonable to expect front-line staff to use these instructions for their decision making. As well, most laboratories do not have access to manual spectrophotometers, in order to determine this each time a lipemic sample is encountered.

This can be circumvented by interference testing as follows. Load only buffer in place of reagent on the analyzer and then allow samples to be picked up. The required one-sixth dilution is made by the analyzer (STAR, Diagnostica Stago) in buffer only, and when the OD readings begin, viewing of the graphics allows the user to verify if the maximum OD has been exceeded. The OD must be viewed while the analyzer is reading—because there is no reagent in the cuvette, the analyzer will throw an error, causing the initial OD reading to be lost. Spiking samples with Intralipid over a large range of OD values will alert the user to the amount of lipemia that will interfere. These spiked samples can then be run on either a chemistry analyzer that produces a lipemic index value or on a hematology analyzer in much the same manner as a lipemic blank would be run for interference in the hemoglobin value of a patient. Then an alert value (in either lipemic index or hemoglobin blank values) can be written in the standard operating procedure. Samples which generate numbers above either cutoff alert the technologist that the result may be incorrect, and an appropriate comment can be added to the result.

This technique could be modified and applied to virtually any laboratory assay that may have interference from lipemia, giving a more defined piece of information that can be used on day-to-day basis.

Acknowledgments

In memory of my father, who stressed to his children the value of education and kind deeds, and from whom I learnt that a good day's work can feed both your family and your mind. L. Stang.

Funding support was from the Canadian Institute of Health Research (L Mitchell Grant#114981).

References

1. Clinical and Laboratory Standards Institute (CLSI) (2008) Collection, transport and processing of blood specimens for testing plasma-based coagulation assays. Approved Guideline, 5th edn. NCCLS document H21-A5
2. World Health Organization (2002) Use of anticoagulants in diagnostic laboratory investigations. Document WHO/DIL/LAB/99.1 Rev 2, Geneva, 15 Jan 2002
3. Adcock DM, Kressin DC, Marlar RA (1997) Effect of 3.2% vs. 3.8% sodium citrate concentration on routine coagulation testing. Am J Clin Pathol 107(1):105–110
4. Koepke JA, Rodgers JL, Olivier MJ (1975) Pre-instrumental variables in coagulation testing. Am J Clin Pathol 64(5):591–596
5. Gosselin RC, Janatpour K, Larkin EC, Lee YP, Owings JT (2004) Comparison of samples obtained from 3.2% sodium citrate glass and two 3.2% sodium citrate plastic blood collection tubes used in coagulation testing. Am J Clin Pathol 122:843–848
6. Biron-Andreani C, Mallol C, Seguret F, Schved JF (2000) Plastic versus siliconized glass tubes: evaluation in current laboratory practice. Thromb Haemost 83:800–801
7. Kratz A, Stanganeli N, Van Cott EM (2006) A comparison of glass and plastic blood collection tubes for routine and specialized coagulation assays: a comprehensive study. Arch Pathol Lab Med 130(11):1600
8. Fiebig EW, Etzell JE, Ng VL (2005) Clinically relevant differences in prothrombin time and INR values related to blood sample collection in plastic vs. glass tubes. Am J Clin Pathol 124(6):902–909
9. Siegel JE, Swami VK, Glenn P, Peterson P (1998) Effect (or lack of it) of severe anemia on PT and APTT results. Am J Clin Pathol 110(1):106–110
10. Reneke J, Etzell J, Leslie S, Ng VL, Gottfried EL (1998) Prolonged prothrombin time and activated partial thromboplastin time due to underfilled specimen tubes with 109 mmol/L (3.2%) citrate anticoagulant. Am J Clin Pathol 109:754–757
11. Adcock DM, Kressin DC, Marlar RA (1998) Minimum specimen volume requirements for routine coagulation testing: dependence on citrate concentration. Am J Clin Pathol 109(5):595–599
12. Chuang J, Sadler MA, Witt DM (2004) Impact of evacuated collection tube fill volume and mixing on routine coagulation testing using 2.5-mL (pediatric) tubes. Chest 126: 1262–1266
13. NCCLS (2003) Tubes and additives for venous blood specimen collection. Approved Standard, 5th edn. NCCLS document H1-A5, vol 23, no 33. Dec 2003
14. Contant G, Gouault-Heilmann M, Martinoli JL (1983) Heparin inactivation during blood storage: its prevention by blood collection in citric acid, theophylline, adenosine, dipyridamole—DTAD mixture. Thromb Res 31:365–374
15. Carroll WE, Wollitzer AO, Harris L et al (2001) The significance of platelet counts in coagulation studies. J Med 32:83–96
16. Barnes PW, Eby CS, Lukoszyk M (2002) Residual platelet counts in plasma prepared for routine coagulation on testing with the Beckman Coulter power processor. Lab Hematol 8:205–209
17. Brien WF, Schaus MR, Cooper KE, O'Keefe BT, Inwood M (1993) Lupus anticoagulant testing: effect of the platelet count on the activated partial thromboplastin time. Br J Biomed Sci 50(2):114–116
18. Tripodi A, Velsecchi C, Chantarangkul V, Vattaglioli T, Mannucci PM (2003)

Standardization of activated protein C resistance testing: effects of residual platelets in frozen plasmas assessed by commercial and home-made methods. Br J Haematol 120:825–828
19. Favaloro EJ, Mohammed A, Coombs R, Mehrabani PA (1995) Filtered plasma as a potential cause of clinical misdiagnosis: inappropriate testing in a haematology laboratory. Br J Biomed Sci 52:243–248
20. Diatube H product insert (1995) Becton Dickinson Franklin Lakes NJ, 061196 Nov 1995
21. Blomback M, Konkle BA, Manco-Johnson MJ, Bremme K, Hellgren M, Kaaja R, on behalf of the ISTH SSC subcommittee on Women's Health Issues (2007) Preanalytical conditions that affect coagulation testing, including hormonal status and therapy. J Thromb Haemost 5:855–888

Chapter 5

Methods of Coagulation

Gemma Crighton

Abstract

The investigation of haemostasis is aimed to replicate normal blood coagulation in the laboratory. There are a number of different methods employed including clot-based coagulation tests, chromogenic assays, immunological tests, and aggregation studies. Today automated machines are designed to be able to perform a number of different methodologies.

To guarantee the results produced by a laboratory are reliable and accurate, laboratories need to follow international standards and guidelines and use established methodologies. The laboratory needs a quality management plan, to perform internal quality control and participate in an external quality assurance program.

Key words Clot-based coagulation tests, Chromogenic assays, Immunological tests, Aggregation studies, Quality management, Standardization

1 Introduction

The study of coagulation began in the 1700s with observation of the time taken for blood to clot after being removed from an animal. With advances in technology, clotting has been examined under the microscope, in capillary tubes and later in test tubes (1). The coagulation laboratory has changed dramatically over the last 30 years, and so has coagulation methodology. It has seen a move from manual tests, to semi-automated tests and currently to fully automated machines. These can perform and analyze at the same time clot-based tests apostrophe chromogenic and immunological assays (2, 3). Fully automated systems when compared with manual methods are efficient in terms of time and labor, as well as being economical in sample and reagent use (1, 3). Automated methods have improved test precision, with variation coefficients of <5% compared with 20% for manual techniques (4).

Coagulation analysis aims to simulate in the laboratory what happens in vivo. In vitro tests may be misrepresentative of what actually happens in the body and even be inaccurate. The bleeding

Paul Monagle (ed.), *Haemostasis: Methods and Protocols*, Methods in Molecular Biology, vol. 992,
DOI 10.1007/978-1-62703-339-8_5, © Springer Science+Business Media New York 2013

time is the only in vivo test of coagulation. Historically the bleeding time was used as a means to screen for bleeding risk prior to major surgery (5) and involved a blood pressure cuff being placed on the arm and two incisions being made in the forearm. The time taken for the blood to clot was timed and the bleeding time recorded; an average bleeding time was 5 min (6). Bleeding time is hard to standardize and has not been shown to predict surgical bleeding (5). It may be painful leave scars and hence the bleeding time is not performed routinely today.

2 The Manual Tilt-Tube Method

The manual tilt-tube test is the gold standard method for the determination of prothrombin time using international reference preparations of thromboplastin (7) and is the reference method for assessing new coagulation tests (8, 9). Laboratories should be able to perform manual methods in the case of equipment failure and in the event of inconsistent results. Lipemia and hyperbilirubinemia are thought to impede automated analyzer clot detection systems and manual methods may be employed for testing such samples. When doing manual tests, they should be performed in duplicate and the clotting times within 10%; otherwise they should be repeated (4). Ideally an experienced technician with consistent technique is required in order to obtain reliable results and dependable endpoint recognition. A test tube containing the sample and reagents is tilted every 5 seconds in a water bath at 37 °C under constant examination for clot sensing its formation. At the first detectable evidence of macroscopic fibrin strands or web, the clotting time is recorded in seconds (4).

3 Clot-Based Coagulation Tests

Clot-based tests are functional assays, aiming to replicate the extrinsic and intrinsic coagulation pathways in the test tube and give an overall assessment of coagulation function. They measure the exact time the plasma takes to clot and are measured in seconds. They are often used as screening tests to investigate patients with possible bleeding disorders and to monitor anticoagulant treatments. Automated clot-based tests rely on the ability of a machine detect fibrin clot formation by either observing or sensing its formation (1). The main techniques utilized are mechanical clot detection, viscosity-based detection systems, optical clot detection, and nephelometry (4).

The principle behind mechanical clot detection systems is that as the clotting reaction occurs fibrin forms and this can be sensed. As the fibrin strands fix to a stainless steel ball in a test cuvette, they displace the ball from its initial position. This movement is detected by a magnetic sensor which causes a change in electric current and the clotting time is recorded (1). The viscosity-based method is based on electromechanical detection of increasing viscosity of the plasma when fibrin forms. A steel ball sits in a cuvette, to which an electromagnetic field is applied and the steel ball swings like a pendulum inside the cuvette. When clot formation occurs, there is increased viscidness of the sample and the ball's swinging slows. This change in swing is detected and is used to measure the clotting time (4). The advantage of these electromechanical methods is that small reagent and patient volumes are needed and they are able to test lipemic and icteric samples. The downside is that endpoint detection in the setting of low fibrinogen levels can be difficult and the machine provides no information about the dynamics of clot formation (3).

Optical based clot detection systems are founded on visually detecting clot formation by increased scattered light and decreased transmitted light. When coagulation occurs and fibrin strands form within the test cuvette, there is increased turbidity of the plasma sample. Less light is transmitted through the cuvette and this causes a change in light absorbance per minute (ΔOD/min). The principle of nephelometry is measuring the amount of light scattered at an angle, often perpendicular to the incident beam by a detector. As fibrin forms there is increased light scattering, which is recorded. Clotting waveforms can be plotted and give information about the dynamics of clot formation. Photo-optical methods are more sensitive at detecting the initial point of fibrin formation, compared to the manual tilt-tube technique, as photo-optical methods are based on changes in optical intensity rather than waiting for macroscopic fibrin strands to form (10). Advantages of photo-optical techniques are that they are able to plot clot formation. Their drawback is that interference from lipemia, hemolysis, and hyperbilirubinemia can affect some optical clot detection systems. When mechanical clot detection systems have been compared with photo-optical methods for basic coagulation studies (PT, APTT, and fibrinogen) there is high correlation with r squared values ≥ 0.96 for all tests (8).

One of the main advantages of clot-based tests is that they are physiological tests that try to best replicate the coagulation system in the body in vitro. Because their basis is clot formation, they give some assessment of overall functioning (8). However they are only screening tests and they only provide information about one endpoint, clot formation. The clot-based prothrombin time (PT) and activated partial thromboplastin time (APPT) have been adapted to perform one-stage factor assays. These are simple to perform and accurate, but they do have limitations. Fibrin clot formation is the endpoint of the PT- or APTT-based test and this may be a number of steps away from the factor being assessed (8). Recombinant FVIII can interfere with clot-based versus chromogenic assays, and product-specific recombinant FVIII reference standard may need to be used (11). The one-stage FVIII assay depends on the APTT reagent and this can be affected by lupus anticoagulants, heparin, low molecular weight heparin, and lepirudin (12). Some cases of mild hemophilia and some genetic mutations in the factor VIII gene can produce incongruent results, when matched against the 2-stage chromogenic assay (13).

4 Chromogenic Assays

Chromogenic assays use color-producing chemical substances or chromophores, of which *para*-nitroaniline (*p*NA) is commonly used. The chromophore is attached to a synthetic peptide, which has an amino acid sequence that mimics the active site of the specific coagulation protein of interest. In the inactivated state the peptide is colorless, and only absorbs light near the ultraviolet region. When the synthetic peptide reacts with the appropriate enzyme, *p*NA is released and has a yellow color that can be measured photometrically and quantified by its absorbance at 405 nm. The intensity of the color is directly proportional to the enzyme activity being tested (14, 15). Fluorogenic techniques are based on similar principles and commonly use 5-amino isophthalic acid dimethyl ester (AIE), which is measured by a fluorometer, by its emission at 340–425 nm. Chromogenic assays were first applied to coagulation in 1972, in determining thrombin levels (16). Since the discovery of coagulation enzymology, chromogenic substrates have been adapted for the investigation of coagulation factors, their inhibitors, fibrinolysis, and haemostasis (14). The advantages of chromogenic assays are that they are simple, reliable, and precise. The degree of color change can be measured accurately by optical absorption and they can quantify high and low factor levels (15). Chromogenic assays are easily automated and therefore batches of samples can be run, allowing rapid turnaround times and labor efficiency (14, 17). Disadvantages of chromogenic assays are that reagents and instruments are costly and a large number of tests need to be performed for them to be cost efficient. The tests may be limited by the coagulation machines wavelength, although newer machines are able to run more than one wavelength and detect more than one endpoint (4). Care needs to be taken with sample integrity before running a chromogenic test, as contaminating substances such as hemoglobin, cellular debris, and bilirubin may interfere with spectrophotometric readings (15). Discrepant results have occurred with chromogenic PT (which is not routinely done) in patients with congenital dysfibrinogenemia or hypofibrinogenemia (15, 18). A patient's bleeding phenotype in congenital FX and FII deficiencies may correlate better with a clotting assay, rather than a chromogenic test (19, 20).

5 Immunological Tests

Immunological tests are based on the principle that antibodies are highly specific for their corresponding antigen and this has been applied to the field of coagulation. A variety of methods have been employed including immunodiffusion, immunoelectrophoresis, radioimmunometric assays, latex agglutination test, and enzyme-linked immunosorbent assays. Immunodiffusion is based on antigens reacting with their specific antibodies, to form complexes, which at the ideal concentrations will eventuate in precipitation (21). Radial immunodiffusion is a type of simple immunodiffusion, where antibodies are integrated into agar solution before a gel is made and are evenly distributed through the gel. Wells are cut into the gel; antigen is added to the wells and allowed to diffuse. When the concentration of the diffusing antigen becomes equal to the antibody in the gel, precipitation occurs. By taking predetermined antigen concentrations and running them, it is possible to create a calibration graph. Radial immunodiffusion has been accurately and reliably used for fibrinogen measurement (22).

Immunoelectrophoresis also known as the electroimmunoassay method is based on an electric field being applied to an agarose gel plate with antibodies distributed through it. Antigens are applied to the gel plate and precipitation cones or spikes form. These can be assessed in terms of length and surface area; the surface area is proportional to the amount of antigen (23). Immunoelectrophoresis has been used to distinguish between von Willebrand disease (vWD) type 1, type 2A, and type 2B based on multimeric analysis. Electrophoresis clearly separates bands of high, intermediate, and low molecular weight multimers. A normal pattern will have many large multimers and a visible triplet pattern of low molecular multimers (23). Type 1 vWD results in an overall decrease in the pattern of multimers, but in normal triplet pattern and in type 3 vWD there is virtually no von Willebrand factor (vWF) detected. In type 2A vWD, there is a lack of high and intermediate multimers and an abnormal triplet pattern in low molecular multimers. In type 2B there is loss of large multimers, but preserved triplet pattern (23, 24).

ELISA or enzyme-linked immunosorbent “sandwich” assays or capture assays can be used to quantitate or semi-quantitate antigen concentration. A solid structure, commonly a polystyrene microtiter plate, is coated with antibodies against the antigen of interest. After washing away any excess antibodies, the antigen is added and binds the adsorbed antibodies. Next an enzyme-labeled antibody is added, which binds the antigen. Any excess antibody is removed by washing (25, 26). After incubation, a chromogenic substrate for the enzyme is added, which produces a colored product. The intensity of the color produced is proportional to the amount of conjugated enzyme and hence proportional to the amount of bound antigen molecule. The antigen can be detected either directly by a labeled primary antibody or indirectly by a labeled secondary antibody (26). ELISAs have been applied to all areas of hematology and have been used to quantify factor IX, factor X, protein C assays, and fibrinogen degradation products (27, 28). Today they are routinely used for quantitative assessment of von Willebrand factor antigen (vWF:Ag) and von Willebrand factor collagen binding assay (vWF:CoBA). They have been key in research and in our understanding of how proteins work including lupus anticoagulants and anti-cardiolipin antibodies (29). ELISAs are used to detect very small amounts of coagulation protein (in the nanogram region); they are sensitive and have good reproducibility and low variation coefficients (5–10%) (27).

In latex agglutination testing, latex particles are covered in antibodies specific for the antigen under investigation. When the plasma sample containing the antigen of interest is combined with the latex mixture, agglutination of the latex particles occurs as the antigen and antibodies form complexes. The increased agglutination or turbidity was initially determined visually, whereas today it is detected using spectrophotometers or nephelometers as absorbed or scattered light. The amount of antigen is proportional to the amount of latex agglutination (30). Clinical applications to coagulation include the D-dimer test and vWF:Ag immunoturbidimetric assay (31). Compared with ELISA techniques, latex agglutination tests are simpler and quicker to perform and can be performed as individual tests rather than in batches. However latex agglutination tests are not as sensitive as ELISA tests (26, 28). Cloudy plasma can lead to underestimation of agglutination.

Rheumatoid factor and paraproteins can cross-react and potentiate agglutination, leading to overestimation of the amount of antigen (32).

Advantages of immunological assays are that they are sensitive, relatively simple with rapid turnaround times, and hence are labor and time efficient. Today many kit sets have been produced, which are able to be automated and run in batches. Immunoassays are able to detect very small amounts of antigen in the nanogram range, whereas immunodiffusion or immunonephelometry methods rely on medium-high concentration >10 μg/mL (27). The shortcoming of immunological testing is that it is not able to provide information about the functional capability of a protein of interest but only quantifies how much of the antigen is detected. The polyclonal antibodies used can detect whole proteins, and have high sensitivities, but lower specificities; monoclonal antibody on the other hand can detect a single epitope or protein and are very specific (21). ELISAs are costly in their initial setup; however once set up the ongoing labor costs are low.

6 Aggregation Studies

The von Willebrand factor:ristocetin cofactor (vWF:RCoF) assay is based on ristocetin-induced platelet agglutination and gives a functional measure of vWF activity in the body. Ristocetin is an antibiotic that stimulates platelet agglutination through interactions with the glycoprotein (GP1b) platelet receptor. The original studies used fresh, washed platelets, and showed that these did not aggregate in the presence of ristocetin, unless plasma was present (33). Today commercially frozen or formaldehyde-fixed platelets are used and the speed and amount of platelet aggregation are measured (25). The advantages of this test are that it is a functional assay and it is specific and provides some indication of what is happening in vivo. However the assay takes time to perform and there is considerable inter-assay and inter-laboratory variability (variation coefficients of 10–20%) (27).

The turbidimetric technique for measurement of platelet aggregometry uses changes in optical density and was described by Born in 1962. It uses platelet-rich plasma, which is cloudy at baseline, and as the platelets aggregate there is reduced turbidity and increased light penetration (34). As light transmission increases, optical density or absorbance of the platelet-rich plasma decreases. The turbidity is measured constantly by recoding the light transmission and obtaining an "aggregation trace." Standardization for the procedure includes the preparation of the patient and control samples, controlling for platelet count, temperature, and time period. The patient and the healthy control should have avoided any medications or foods that could interfere with platelet aggregation for the preceding 10 days. Platelet-rich plasma is diluted with the platelet-poor plasma to obtain a platelet count of $200–300 \times 10^9$ L for the patient and the control. The aggregometer should be pre-warmed to 37° and the samples should be kept at room temperature, as cooling them leads to platelet activation (35). Platelets aggregate in reaction to the addition of an agonist. Typical agonists used include adenosine-5-diphosphate (ADP), collagen, Ristocetin Sulfate, epinephrine, and arachidonic acid (28). The important features to observe are the shape of the trace, looking at the angle and height of aggregation, ADP primary and secondary wave aggregation, and the lag phase with collagen. Of note, normal platelet-rich plasma does not aggregate with concentrations of ristocetin that are <1.0 mg/mL. External factors need to be controlled that may affect optical quality including air bubbles, debris, red cells, white cells, cryoglobulins, and lipemia (36).

7 Standardization

Important clinical decisions are made on the basis of blood tests and the results of the blood tests therefore must be accurate and precise. Laboratory errors are usually a result of system and procedure problems, rather than the fault of individual people. Standardization can help set in place protocols and quality management systems to prevent errors and provide high-quality laboratory practice. Standards are the minimum requirement for a procedure, method, staffing resource, or a laboratory facility that are required before a laboratory can attain accreditation whereas guidelines are consensus recommendation for best laboratory practice (37). A number of organizations exist worldwide which contribute to the standardization of methods and practices in hematology. In the United Kingdom, the British Committee for Standards in Haematology (BCSH) publishes guidelines for books and journals. In America, the Clinical and Laboratory Standards Institute (CLSI) formerly the National Committee for Clinical Laboratory Standards (NCCLS) produce a number of standards and guidelines to develop best practice in clinical and laboratory medicine. There are two quality systems and international standard setting bodies in widespread use throughout the world: the International Organization for Standardization (ISO) and CLSI. ISO produced the document ISO 15 189: 2003, *Medical laboratories—Particular requirements for quality and competence*. This is a key document in laboratory standardization and outlines the quality management system requirements particular to medical laboratories (37). Clinical coagulation laboratories should comply with international standards and guidelines and follow the recommendations of the International Society on Thrombosis and Haemostasis.

The World Health Organization is the main authority in the production of material standards and reference preparations. The WHO has a critical role in laboratory medicine in the development of WHO International Biological Reference Preparations, which serve as reference materials of defined biological activity, reported in an internationally decided measurement unit. Reference laboratories and manufacturers use WHO International Standards for blood coagulation factors and inhibitors to calibrate their secondary plasma coagulation standards (38). The Scientific and Standardization Committee of the International Society on Thrombosis and Haemostasis produces coagulation standards with assigned values of the coagulation-related analytes by assay relative to its relevance to the WHO International Standards (39). Reference preparations or standards are used to calibrate analytic instruments and to assign quantitative values to calibrators.

8 Quality Management

Quality management is an essential component of laboratory medicine. Blood results issued by the laboratory need to be accurate, reliable, and reproducible and to ensure this quality management is key. There are a number of facets to quality assurance and these include having an up-to-date quality policy and manual, quality control, quality assessment (internal and external), and internal audit (40). Internal quality control is the constant evaluation of the reliability of the day-to-day results being issued by the laboratory and their precision (41). It encompasses performing duplicate assays, using commercially produced control preparations to run routine tests and comparing these with expected values, day-to-day evaluation of laboratory results, checking mean values obtained for population data, delta check, correlation with blood films, and accurate record keeping (42). Partaking in external quality assessment is a mandatory requirement for laboratories. At regular intervals throughout the year, samples will be sent to laboratories for assessment and interpretation. An external body scrutinizes the performance of the results produced and compares them to those obtained by other laboratories. The laboratory should be enrolled in an appropriate quality assessment scheme for every test the laboratory performs, if there is one available (37). The main objective of external quality control is to help facilitate high-quality laboratory performance (41).

Total quality management includes the control of pre-analytical variables as these can have significant impact on the accuracy of coagulation results and obtained (43). In order to try and produce results that replicate what is happening in vivo, care must be taken in the collection and handling of the sample (42). The pre-analytic stage starts from the point of blood collection and encompasses patient variables, positive patient verification and sample labeling, phlebotomy techniques, blood volumes attained, anticoagulant used, and specimen handling and storage (1, 43). Attempts need to be made to control for these pre-analytical variables and laboratories should comply with international quality documents, in order to maintain the accuracy of the blood test results produced.

Finally, it is important to understand the coagulation tests may be normal; they are only attempts to replicate what happens in the body and are only as good as their laboratory. They are numbers and they do not necessarily ensure that a patient will not bleed; they need to be taken in the context of the clinical and family history.

References

1. McGlinchey K (2010) Coagulation automation. ADVANCE for Administrators of the Laboratory 19:26
2. Flanders MM, Crist R, Safapour S, Rodgers GM (2002) Evaluation and performance characteristics of the STA-R coagulation analyzer. Clin Chem 48:1622–1624
3. Milos M, Herak D, Kuric L, Horvat I, Zadro R (2007) Evaluation and performance characteristics of the coagulation system: ACL TOP analyzer—HemosIL reagents. Int J Lab Hematol 31:26–35
4. Kitchen S, McCraw A, on behalf of the WFH Laboratory Sciences Committee (2010) Diagnosis of haemophilia and other bleeding disorders: a laboratory manual, 2nd edn. World Federation of Hemophilia, Montreal, QC
5. Lind SE (1991) The bleeding time does not predict surgical bleeding. Blood 77: 2547–2552
6. Mielke CH Jr, Kaneshiro MM, Maher IA, Weiner JM, Rapaport SI (1969) The standardized normal Ivy bleeding time and its prolongation by aspirin. Blood 34:204–215
7. World Health Organisation (1997) Recommended methodology for using WHO International Preparations for thromboplastin, WHO, 1121 Geneva 27, Switzerland
8. Bai B, Christie DJ, Gorman RT, Wu JR (2008) Comparison of optical and mechanical clot detection for routine coagulation testing in a large volume clinical laboratory. Blood Coagul Fibrinolysis 19:569–576
9. D'Angelo A, Seveso MP, D'Angelo SV, Gilardoni F, Macagni A, Manotti C, Bonini P (1989) Comparison of two automated coagulometers and the manual tilt-tube method for the determination of prothrombin time. Am J Clin Pathol 92:321–328
10. Johnstone IB (1984) The activated partial thromboplastin time of diluted plasma: variability due to the method of fibrin detection. Can J Comp Med 48:198–201
11. Lippi G, Franchini M, Favaloro EJ (2009) One-stage clotting versus chromogenic assays for assessing recombinant factor VIII: two faces of a haemostasis coin. Blood Coagul Fibrinolysis 20:1–3
12. Chandler WL, Ferrell C, Lee J, Tun T, Kha H (2003) Comparison of three methods for measuring factor VIII levels in plasma. Am J Clin Pathol 120:34–39
13. Keeling DM, Sukhu K, Kemball-Cook G, Waseem N, Bagnall R, Lloyd JV (1999) Diagnostic importance of the two-stage factor VIII:C assay demonstrated by a case of mild haemophilia associated with His 1954–> Leu substitution in the factor VIII A3 domain. Br J Haematol 105:1123–1126
14. Fareed J, Messmore HL, Walenga JM, Bermes EW Jr (1983) Diagnostic efficacy of newer synthetic-substrates methods for assessing coagulation variables: a critical overview. Clin Chem 29:225–236
15. Hutton RA (1987) Chromogenic substrates in haemostasis. Blood Rev 1:201–206
16. Svendsen L, Blomback B, Blomback M, Olson PI (1972) Synthetic chromogenic substrates for determination of trypsin, thrombin and thrombin-like enzymes. Thromb Res 1:267–278
17. Francis JL (1979) A new chromogenic assay for the specific determination of prothrombin. J Clin Pathol 32:651–654
18. Tripodi A, Mannucci PM (1984) Clinical evaluation of a fully automated chromogenic method for prothrombin time compared with a conventional coagulation method. Clin Chem 30:1392–1395
19. Girolami A, Vettore S (2009) Discrepancies between clotting and chromogenic assays in congenital coagulation disorders: the hemostatic coin has only one face, chromogenic substrates many. Blood Coagul Fibrinolysis 20:484–485
20. Peyvandi F, Menegatti M, Santagostino E, Akhavan S, Uprichard J, Perry DJ, Perkins SJ, Mannucci PM (2002) Gene mutations and three-dimensional structural analysis in 13 families with severe factor X deficiency. Br J Haematol 117:685–692
21. Walker JM (ed) (1996) The protein protocols handbook. Humana, Totowa, NJ
22. Palareti G, Maccaferri M, Manotti C, Tripodi A, Chantarangkul V, Rodeghiero F, Ruggeri M, Mannucci PM (1991) Fibrinogen assays: a collaborative study of six different methods. C.I.S.M.E.L. Comitato Italiano per la Standardizzazione dei Metodi in Ematologia e Laboratorio. Clin Chem 37:714–719
23. Verbruggen (1975) Quantitative immunoelectrophoretic methods: a literature survey. Clin Chem 21:5–43
24. Ruggeri ZM, Zimmerman TS (1981) The complex multimeric composition of factor VIII/von Willebrand factor. Blood 57:1140–1143
25. Engvall E (2010) The ELISA, enzyme-linked immunosorbent assay. Clin Chem 56:319–320
26. Voller A, Bartlett A, Bidwell DE (1978) Enzyme immunoassays with special reference to ELISA techniques. J Clin Pathol 31:507–520
27. Amiral J, Adalbert B, Adam M (1984) Application of enzyme immunoassays to coagulation testing. Clin Chem 30:1512–1516

28. van der Graaf F, van den Borne H, van der Kolk M, de Wild PJ, Janssen GW, van Uum SH (2000) Exclusion of deep venous thrombosis with D-dimer testing—comparison of 13 D-dimer methods in 99 outpatients suspected of deep venous thrombosis using venography as reference standard. Thromb Haemost 83:191–198
29. Pengo V, Thiagarajan P, Shapiro SS, Heine MJ (1987) Immunological specificity and mechanism of action of IgG lupus anticoagulants. Blood 70:69–76
30. Gella FS, Gener J, Latex J (1991) Agglutination procedures in immunodiagnosis. Pure Appl Chem 63:1131–1134
31. Ewenstein BM (2001) Use of ristocetin cofactor activity in the management of von Willebrand disease. Haemophilia 7(Suppl 1): 10–15
32. Lewis SM, Bain BJ, Bates I (eds) (2006) Dacie and Lewis practical haematology, 10th edn. Churchill Livingstone Elsevier, Philadelphia, PA
33. Weiss HJ, Hoyer LW, Rickles FR, Varma A, Rogers J (1973) Quantitative assay of a plasma factor deficient in von Willebrand's disease that is necessary for platelet aggregation. Relationship to factor VIII procoagulant activity and antigen content. J Clin Invest 52: 2708–2716
34. Born GV, Cross MJ (1963) The aggregation of blood platelets. J Physiol 168:178–195
35. Yardumian DA, Mackie IJ, Machin SJ (1986) Laboratory investigation of platelet function: a review of methodology. J Clin Pathol 39: 701–712
36. British Committee for Standards in Haematology (1988) Guidelines on platelet function testing. The British Society for Haematology BCSH Haemostasis and Thrombosis Task Force, 1988/12/01 ed, p 1322–1330, J Clin Pathol
37. National Pathology Accreditation Advisory Council (2009) Requirements for participation in external quality assessment, Commonwealth of Australia
38. World Health Organisation (2011) International reference materials. www.who.int/bloodproducts/ref_materials/en/
39. Hubbard AR, Kitchen S, Beeharry M, Bevan SA, Bowyer A, on behalf of the SSC Working Group on Coagulation Standards of the ISTH. (2011) Long-term stability of the Scientific and Standardization Committee Secondary Coagulation Standard (SSC Lot no. 3). J Thromb Haemost 9:2146–2148
40. Clinical Laboratory Standards Institute (2011) Working together to improve the quality of medical care–the Global Application of CLSI Documents, Lab Medicine, p 440–441
41. Lewis SM (1988) The WHO international external quality assessment scheme for haematology. Bull World Health Organ 66:283–290
42. Lewis SM (1996) Quality control: good laboratory practice—an overview of quality assurance. In: XXVIth World Congress of the International Society of Haematology. ICSH, Singapore
43. Garvey MB, Black JM (1972) The detection of fibrinogen-fibrin degradation products by means of a new antibody-coated latex particle. J Clin Pathol 25:680–682

Chapter 6

Reference Ranges of Coagulation Tests

Oliver Speer, Markus Schmugge, Claudia Metzger, and Manuela Albisetti

Abstract

Reference ranges are a set of values that correctly include most of the subjects with characteristics similar to the reference group and exclude the others. When accurate, reference ranges aid physicians to interpret results of clinical measurements and thus establish diagnosis. However, obtaining accurate reference ranges is a very demanding procedure. This chapter provides basic definitions and theories as well as a step-by-step procedure for the analysis of reference values and determination of reference ranges of coagulation, focusing on quantitative clinical laboratory assays. Preanalytical and analytical factors as well as dependence on the age influencing reference values for coagulation assays and their transference are discussed.

Key words Reference ranges, Reference value, Coagulation assays, Age dependence of coagulation assays, Parametric, Nonparametric

1 Introduction

"Practical medicine is basically founded on comparison." A.J. Schneider states in 1960 in his publication "Some thoughts on normal, or standard, values in clinical medicine" (1): "If medicine is to be scientific, we must not only understand the structural, functional and chemical relations operating in individuals, but we must also understand the basis of our comparisons." Today, almost 50 years later, in the age of evidence-based medicine, and in contrast with the enormous developments in the field of medicine, a sound basis for these comparisons is often lacking in the clinical laboratory. Nevertheless, according to Horn and Pesce, comparison of laboratory results using reference ranges is the most widely used medical decision-making tool, even if its practical usefulness is lower than its theoretical power (2). This is due to the fact that obtaining a "good" reference range is a very demanding activity, in terms of time, money, and knowledge. But what does a "good" reference range mean? To answer this question the Scientific Committee of the International Federation of Clinical Chemistry

Paul Monagle (ed.), *Haemostasis: Methods and Protocols*, Methods in Molecular Biology, vol. 992,
DOI 10.1007/978-1-62703-339-8_6, © Springer Science+Business Media New York 2013

(IFCC) created an expert panel in 1970 that developed a nomenclature and guidelines for the production of reference ranges (3–8). In 1977, the International Committee for Standardization in Hematology (ICSH) established a corresponding expert panel. This group adopted recommendations from other scientific organizations for hematology (9–19). The Clinical and Laboratory Standards Institute also published recently a guideline for the definition and determination of reference ranges in the clinical laboratory (20).

Although these recommendations have been widely adopted, the concepts of reference values and reference ranges are constantly evolving due to changing technologies, changing populations, and increasing knowledge of old and new diseases (21). Very detailed critics and discussions about new developments, additions, and expansions of the theories of reference ranges are now available (22–47), and the reader may also be referred to Subheading 5.

This chapter will review the still valid guidelines from the IFCC and ICSH for the determination of reference ranges of coagulation and provide information on factors that may influence both the procedure and interpretation of these ranges.

2 Definitions

Reference ranges are a set of values that, when applied to the population serviced by the laboratory, correctly includes most of the subjects with characteristics similar to the reference group and excludes the others. In Fig. 1 the most important terms (according to IFCC) for determining reference values are set in relations to each other and are defined as follows:

1. The reference individual is an individual with a defined state of health selected for comparison.
2. The reference population consists of all possible reference individuals and is a hypothetical entity.
3. The reference sample group is an adequate number of randomly drawn reference individuals representing the reference population.
4. The reference value is obtained by measuring a certain quantity on a reference individual.
5. The reference distribution is the statistical distribution of reference values.
6. The reference limits are derived from the reference distribution.
7. The reference range lies between the upper and lower reference limit including both limits.

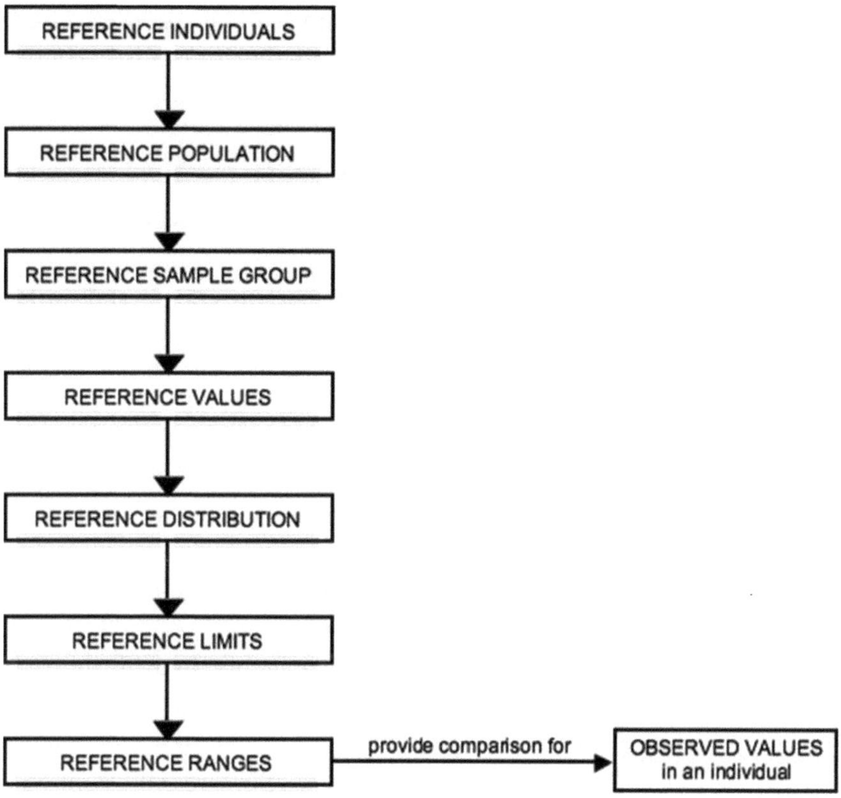

Fig. 1 Concept of reference values and the relationship of recommended terminology. Adapted from "approved recommendation on the theory of reference values" (3)

Usually we consider "health-related" reference ranges to mean that the subjects with values within the range have a lower probability of being affected by a specific disease, while those outside the interval have a higher statistical probability of having the disease or, at least, that the observed value is not normal for a healthy person. The percentage of unhealthy people included in the reference range or, vice versa, the percentage of healthy subjects outside the range defines the "goodness" of the interval.

3 Method

To assess reference ranges for a coagulation test, blood samples from at least 120 healthy males and females of all age categories are required (20). The interpretation and definition is funded according to the statistical data. In case that there is time or physiological fluctuations to the determining factor, reference range from a plasma pool should be determined and/or ascertained. The procedures for determining health-associated reference values or ranges derived from a reference sample group without disorders of coagulation and in general of good health are the primary focus of this chapter. However other types of reference values, e.g., for other physiological or pathological conditions, could also be established in the same manner.

3.1 Protocol Outline

1. Establish an appropriate list of biological variations and analytical interferences from the literature.
2. Establish selection and exclusion criteria and an appropriate questionnaire designed to reveal these criteria in the potential reference individual.
3. Decide on an appropriate number of reference individuals in consideration of desired confidence limits.
4. Obtain the approval from the local ethical committee for the study protocol, questionnaire, and consent forms.
5. Obtain the appropriate written consent form for participation in the reference study and have the individual complete the questionnaire.
6. Categorize the potential reference individuals based on the questionnaire findings and results of other appropriate health assessments.
7. Exclude individuals from the reference sample group based on the exclusion criteria or other conditions indicating a possible coagulation disorder.
8. Prepare the selected individuals for specimen collection consistent with the routine practice for patients.
9. Collect and handle the biological specimen consistent with routine practice for patient specimen, and thus keep at the same preanalytical conditions.
10. Analyze the specimens according to the respective analytical methodology under well-defined conditions and consistent with the routine practice for patient specimens, and thus keep at the same analytical conditions.
11. Inspect the value data by preparing histograms to evaluate the distribution of data. Identify possible errors and outliers.
12. Analyze the reference values. Select a method to estimate the reference limits and the reference range. If appropriate include partitioning into subclasses for separate reference ranges, i.e., female vs. male, or different age-related groups.
13. Document all steps and procedures.

The previous sequence is consistent with a prospective approach of selecting reference individuals and determining reference values. When examining individuals that are expected to be healthy for the reference group, questionnaire completion and specimen collection are practically performed at the same time. In case of exclusion of a reference individual the analytical measurement of this individual should be cancelled if possible.

A retrospective approach may be useful or necessary for coagulation tests, which are new or poorly studied, and for which there is little information in the literature. Because the factors defining criteria for inclusion and exclusion of reference individuals or for partitioning of the reference sample group may not be known initially, these decisions are taken after sampling and analyzing. This approach includes a collection of data already obtained on medically examined individuals. For the retrospective approach, the same considerations for inclusion or exclusion of reference individuals should be taken.

3.2 Selection and Exclusion Criteria

Health is a relative condition lacking a quantitative definition. However according to the WHO health is a state of complete physical, mental, and social well-being, not merely the absence of disease or infirmity (48). Establishing criteria to exclude the non-healthy individual from the reference sample group is the first step in selecting reference individuals. While each institution or investigator may have own criteria, the latter should be defined before starting the reference range study. The designation of good health for a candidate reference individual may involve a variety of examinations, such as history taking, physical examination, and certain clinical laboratory tests. Criteria used for any reference range study have to be documented in the study protocol, and are important for both the acceptance by an ethical committee and by peer-investigators to evaluate the status of the reference sample group.

Exclusion criteria are details about the candidate reference individual that, if present, serve to keep that person from being included in the reference sample group. Examples are oral anticoagulation, other drugs interfering with coagulation, recent transfusion, known genetic factors as inherited disease, or recent illness. These examples are far from being exhaustive and should only stimulate thinking about criteria for the study under design.

Partitioning criteria are characteristics of the individuals in the reference sample group that may divide the reference sample group into significant subclasses (4). The most common criteria are sex and age. But also blood group or the ethnic background might be important.

3.3 Sample Questionnaire and Written Consent

As previously described, questionnaires are mainly suitable for the prospective approach of collecting reference individuals and their specific reference values. A questionnaire should primarily give information on age and sex but also on other features and disease states possibly affecting haemostasis like blood groups, pregnancy, ethnic background, renal failure, liver diseases, and intake of pharmacological active substances like anticoagulation drugs, contraceptive, tobacco, and alcohol. Disease states and drug intake may constitute exclusion criteria.

The written informed consent is a mandatory prerequisite which has to be obtained from each reference individual. The consent form should give information about the respective reference value project in an easily understandable fashion. Further, the consent form has to state clearly that medical personnel are allowed to obtain blood samples, and to use the laboratory data and questionnaire information for the determination of reference ranges. Examples of questionnaires can be retrieved from Internet sources, which are listed below.

3.4 Analysis of Reference Values

The reference range is defined as the interval between and including the upper and lower reference limit, which are estimated to enclose a specified percentage (usually 95%) of the values for a population from which reference subjects have been drawn. For most analyses, the lower and upper reference limits are assumed to demarcate the estimated 2.5th and 97.5th percentiles of the underlying distribution of values, respectively. In some cases, only one reference limit is of medical importance, usually an upper limit, i.e., the 97.5th percentile. It should be noted that the 2.5th and 97.5th percentile are not estimable unless the 0.025 and 0.975 fractiles are well above $1/n$, whereas n denotes the sample size. Thus, the determination of the 0.025 and 0.975 fractiles requires at least 40 values. As a standard for general practice a minimum of 120 reference individuals is recommended (7, 20). This number assumes that no observations were deleted from the reference set. If aberrant or outlying observations are deleted, additional individuals should be included in the study until at least 120 acceptable reference values are obtained. Moreover, if separate intervals are needed for different subclasses (e.g., sex or age classes) each subclasses interval should be based on the recommended 120 observations. Independently on the number of values obtained, the data should be analyzed by the nonparametric method and reported by percentiles appropriate to the number of values obtained. Analysis by the nonparametric method makes no assumption on the type of distribution (i.e., Gaussian distribution), and is based on the ranks of the observation.

3.4.1 Procedure for the Nonparametric Method

Sort the n reference values according to increasing numerical values and assign rank numbers such that the lowest value has rank no. 1 and the highest value has rank no. n: $x_1 \le x_2 \le \ldots \le x_n$. Consecutive rank numbers should also be assigned to two or more values that are equal ("ties"). Ties may often be avoided by using more digits in the reference values than are commonly used for reporting of patient results. Compute the rank number of the 0.025 fractile as $0.025 \times (n+1)$ and that of the 0.975 fractile as $0.975 \times (n+1)$. Set the lower reference limit equal to the reference value corresponding to the rank number of the 0.025 fractile if this number is an integer. Otherwise the reference limits should be determined by interpolation between two reference values. The upper reference limit is similarly determined by the rank number of the 0.975 fractile (7).

3.4.2 Procedure for the Parametric Method

The parametric method assumes that the observed values, or some mathematical transformation of those values, follow a Gaussian distribution curve. Because the reference values of many analyses do not follow the Gaussian distribution, use of the parametric method requires transformation of values to some other measurement scale, which will "normalize" them. This requires selecting the most suitable transformation (i.e., log, power, or some other transformation from the original scale) and then testing whether the reference values on this new scale indeed reflect a Gaussian distribution. In general the upper reference limit is defined as the arithmetic mean plus the double standard deviation, the lower limit as the arithmetic mean minus the double standard deviation (7).

4 Factors Affecting Procedure and Interpretation

4.1 Pre-analytical and Analytical Considerations

Analytical results from reference populations must reflect all of the pre-analytical and analytical variables that can influence the results. Therefore all pre-analytical factors such as sample collection, processing, analytical method, and instrumentation as shown in Table 1 must be defined and consistently applied both for testing the reference sample group as well as the patient population.

The laboratory should document the outline of collection, handling, and storage of specimens. Care should be taken to specify the appropriate blood collection method, which might interfere, i.e., with platelet activation. Further, it will be necessary to define whether the sample should be arterial, venous, and capillary and which anticoagulant is acceptable. The conditions

Table 1
Preanalytical factors potentially influencing reference values

Subject	Specimen collection	Specimen handling
• Fasting vs. nonfasting • Drug regimen • Sampling time in relation to biological rhythms • Physical activity • Rest or stress before collection	• Body posture • Specimen type (i.e., serum, EDTA, citrate) • Collection site • Site preparation • Blood flow • Equipment • Technique	• Transport • Standing time • Clotting • Separation of serum/plasma • Storage • Preparation for analysis

for standardized specimen collection by venipuncture and skin puncture are described elsewhere (5, 49, 50).

The handling of some specimen may require procurement at a specific temperature (e.g., room temperature to maintain platelet activity measurement, 37°C to measure factor activity). In addition preservation of some specimen will require snap freezing and storage at −20°C or −80°C. It is essential to establish any special condition, document, and strictly adhere to them. In general, specimens should be processed promptly after collection. Measurements of factor activities in plasma require for example immediate removal of platelets and red cells from the plasma.

4.2 Age

Pioneer works by M. Andrew et al. in the late 1980s and subsequent studies by other investigators have shown that the haemostatic system in children is a dynamic process with specific age-dependent features (51–53). While all components of the coagulation and fibrinolytic system are present at birth, their concentration and turnover rate differ substantially from adults.

In the coagulation system of children, plasma concentrations of the vitamin K-dependent factors (F) and contact factors are decreased while other factors such as fibrinogen, FV, FVIII, and FXIII are similar or increased in newborns as compared to adults. Plasma concentrations of the inhibitors antithrombin, heparin cofactor II, protein C, and protein S are decreased at birth up to 50% of adult values. By contrast, the plasma concentration of α_2-M in newborns is increased approximately twice compared to adult values. After birth, plasma concentration of antithrombin increased to adult values by approximately 3–6 months of age, while plasma concentration of α_2-M remains increased throughout childhood (51, 52, 54). In the fibrinolytic system of children, plasma concentrations of plasminogen and α_2-AP are decreased up to 80% of adult values until the age of 6 months. Plasma concentrations of tPA are decreased and of PAI-1 increased throughout childhood (55).

While being physiologic, differences of the haemostatic system between children and adults may lead to misclassification of children as having coagulation defects when reference ranges of coagulation established for adults are used to evaluate children. Therefore, accurate interpretation of coagulation tests in children can only be performed using age-dependent reference ranges.

4.3 Transference

Because the determination of reliable reference ranges can be laborious and costly, it would be useful to be able to transfer reference ranges from one laboratory to another by some process of validation that is less costly and more convenient. As more and more tests and methods are introduced in many laboratories in parallel, it is unrealistic to expect that each laboratory develops its own reference ranges. Consequently, clinical laboratories rely on manufacturers of diagnostic tests to generate and provide appropriate reference value data that can be transferred. The transference of reference values can be a complex issue and might be impossible if manufacturers do not provide pediatric reference ranges.

The reference values reflect and depend on the inaccuracy and interference of the analytical system as well as the use of calibrators or standards and reported unit. These facts render reference values reagent and analyzer specific. If the analytical system including reagents and analyzer is comparable, reference values can be transferred within the laboratory and also from one laboratory to another. If however comparability is not given, new reference values have to be obtained.

5 Internet Sources

Different organizations involved in standardization:

International Federation of Clinical Chemistry and Laboratory Medicine http://www.ifcc.org/

Clinical and Laboratory Standards Institute (the former National Committee on Clinical Laboratory Standards NCCLS) http://www.clsi.org/

The British Society for Haematology, member of the International Committee for Standardization in Hematology (ICSH) http://www.b-s-h.org.uk/; unfortunately the ICSH has no own home page.

http://www.westgard.com/guest27.htm

This home page reviews a Clinical Chemistry and Laboratory Medicine special issue on Reference Values (Volume 42, Number 7, 2004), and thereby gives a good overview about new developments and critics of the theories about reference values published by the IFCC (3–8).

Examples of questionnaires and consent sheets can be found at the following links:

http://patienteducation.stanford.edu/research/diabquest.pdf

http://www.tinnitusresearch.org/en/consensus/consensusdocuments/en/TINNITUS_SAMPLE_CASE_HISTORY_QUESTIONNAIRE.pdf

http://pages.unibas.ch/itpbasel/

References

1. Schneider AJ (1960) Some thoughts on normal, or standard, values in clinical medicine. Pediatrics 26:973–984
2. Horn PS, Pesce AJ, Copeland BE (1998) A robust approach to reference interval estimation and evaluation. Clin Chem 44:622–631
3. Solberg HE (1987) International Federation of Clinical Chemistry (IFCC), Scientific Committee, Clinical Section, Expert Panel on Theory of Reference Values, and International Committee for Standardization in Haematology (ICSH), Standing Committee on Reference Values. Approved Recommendation (1986) on the theory of reference values. Part 1. The concept of reference values. J Clin Chem Clin Biochem 25:337–342
4. PetitClerc C, Wilding P (1984) International Federation of Clinical Chemistry (IFCC), Scientific Committee, Clinical Section. The theory of reference values. Part 2. Selection of individuals for the production of reference values. J Clin Chem Clin Biochem 22:203–208
5. Solberg HE, PetitClerc C (1988) International Federation of Clinical Chemistry (IFCC), Scientific Committee, Clinical Section, Expert Panel on Theory of Reference Values. Approved recommendation (1988) on the theory of reference values. Part 3. Preparation of individuals and collection of specimens for the production of reference values. J Clin Chem Clin Biochem 26:593–598
6. Solberg HE, Stamm D (1991) International Federation of Clinical Chemistry IFCC. IFCC recommendation—theory of reference values. Part 4. Control of analytical variation in the production, transfer and application of reverence values. Clin Chim Acta 202:S5–S11
7. Solberg HE (1987) International Federation of Clinical Chemistry (IFCC), Scientific Committee, Clinical Section, Expert Panel on Theory of Reference Values, and International Committee for Standardization in Haematology (ICSH), Standing Committee on Reference Values. Approved Recommendation (1986) on the theory of reference values. Part 5. Statistical treatment of collected reference values. Determination of reference limits. Clin Chim Acta 170:S13–S32
8. Solberg HE (1987) International Federation of Clinical Chemistry (IFCC), Scientific Committee, Clinical Section, Expert Panel on Theory of Reference Values, and International Committee for Standardization in Haematology (ICSH), Standing Committee on Reference Values. Approved Recommendation (1986) on the theory of reference values. Part 6. Presentation of observed values related to reference values. Clin Chim Acta 170:S33–S42
9. (1981) The theory of reference values: international committee for standardization in haematology (ICSH). Clin Lab Haematol 3:369–373
10. (1982) Standardization of blood specimen collection procedure for reference values. International Committee for Standardization in Haematology (ICSH). Clin Lab Haematol 4:83–86
11. (1984) Recommendation for a selected method for the measurement of plasma viscosity. International Committee for Standardization in Haematology. J Clin Pathol 37:1147–1152
12. (1988) The assignment of values to fresh blood used for calibrating automated blood cell counters. International Committee for Standardization in Haematology; Expert Panel on Cytometry. Clin Lab Haematol 10:203–212
13. (1989) Recommended methods for an additional red cell enzyme (pyrimidine 5 -nucleotidase) assay and the determination of red cell adenosine-5 -triphosphate, 2,3-diphosphoglycerate and reduced glutathione. International Committee for Standardization in Haematology. Clin Lab Haematol 11:131–138
14. (1990) ICSH recommendations for the analysis of red cell, white cell and platelet size distribution curves. Methods for fitting a single reference distribution and assessing its goodness of fit. International Committee for Standardization in Haematology. ICSH Expert Panel on Cytometry. Clin Lab Haematol 12: 417–431
15. (1993) ICSH recommendations for measurement of erythrocyte sedimentation rate. International Council for Standardization in Haematology (Expert Panel on Blood Rheology). J Clin Pathol 46:198–203
16. (1993) Recommendations of the International Council for Standardization in Haematology for ethylenediaminetetraacetic acid anticoagulation of blood for blood cell counting and sizing. International Council for Standardization in Haematology: Expert Panel on Cytometry. Am J Clin Pathol 100:371–372
17. (1994) Reference method for the enumeration of erythrocytes and leucocytes. International Council for Standardization in Haematology; prepared by the Expert Panel on Cytometry. Clin Lab Haematol 16:131–138
18. (1994) Guidelines for the evaluation of blood cell analysers including those used for differential leucocyte and reticulocyte counting and cell marker applications. International Council for Standardization in Haematology: prepared by the ICSH Expert Panel on Cytometry. Clin Lab Haematol 16:157–174

19. (1998) Proposed reference method for reticulocyte counting based on the determination of the reticulocyte to red cell ratio. The Expert Panel on Cytometry of the International Council for Standardization in Haematology. Clin Lab Haematol 20:77–79
20. NCCLS (2000) How to define and determine reference intervals in the clinical laboratory. Approved Guideline, 2nd edn. NCCLS Document C28-A2, Wayne
21. Henny J, Petitclerc C, Fuentes-Arderiu X, Petersen PH, Queralto JM, Schiele F, Siest G (2000) Need for revisiting the concept of reference values. Clin Chem Lab Med 38:589–595
22. Goldschmidt HM (2004) The NEXUS vision: an alternative to the reference value concept. Clin Chem Lab Med 42:868–873
23. Henny J, Hyltoft Petersen P (2004) Reference values: from philosophy to a tool for laboratory medicine. Clin Chem Lab Med 42:686–691
24. Grasbeck R (2004) The evolution of the reference value concept. Clin Chem Lab Med 42:692–697
25. Petitclerc C (2004) Normality: the unreachable star? Clin Chem Lab Med 42:698–701
26. Ritchie RF, Palomaki G (2004) Selecting clinically relevant populations for reference intervals. Clin Chem Lab Med 42:702–709
27. Solberg HE (2004) The IFCC recommendation on estimation of reference intervals. The RefVal program. Clin Chem Lab Med 42:710–714
28. Hyltoft Petersen P, Blaabjerg O, Andersen M, Jorgensen LG, Schousboe K, Jensen E (2004) Graphical interpretation of confidence curves in rankit plots. Clin Chem Lab Med 42:715–724
29. Lahti A (2004) Partitioning biochemical reference data into subgroups: comparison of existing methods. Clin Chem Lab Med 42:725–733
30. Virtanen A, Kairisto V, Uusipaikka E (2004) Parametric methods for estimating covariate-dependent reference limits. Clin Chem Lab Med 42:734–738
31. Boyd JC (2004) Reference regions of two or more dimensions. Clin Chem Lab Med 42:739–746
32. Jorgensen LG, Brandslund I, Hyltoft Petersen P (2004) Should we maintain the 95 percent reference intervals in the era of wellness testing? A concept paper. Clin Chem Lab Med 42:747–751
33. Klee GG (2004) Clinical interpretation of reference intervals and reference limits. A plea for assay harmonization. Clin Chem Lab Med 42:752–757
34. Fraser CG (2004) Inherent biological variation and reference values. Clin Chem Lab Med 42:758–764
35. Queralto JM (2004) Intraindividual reference values. Clin Chem Lab Med 42:765–777
36. Fuentes-Arderiu X, Mas-Serra R, Aluma-Trullas A, Marti-Marcet MI, Dot-Bach D (2004) Guideline for the production of multicentre physiological reference values using the same measurement system. A proposal of the Catalan Association for Clinical Laboratory Sciences. Clin Chem Lab Med 42:778–782
37. Rustad P, Felding P, Lahti A (2004) Proposal for guidelines to establish common biological reference intervals in large geographical areas for biochemical quantities measured frequently in serum and plasma. Clin Chem Lab Med 42:783–791
38. Johnson AM, Hyltoft Petersen P, Whicher JT, Carlstrom A, MacLennan S (2004) Reference intervals for serum proteins: similarities and differences between adult Caucasian and Asian Indian males in Yorkshire, UK. Clin Chem Lab Med 42:792–799
39. Ichihara K, Itoh Y, Min WK, Yap SF, Lam CW, Kong XT, Chou CT, Nakamura H (2004) Diagnostic and epidemiological implications of regional differences in serum concentrations of proteins observed in six Asian cities. Clin Chem Lab Med 42:800–809
40. Siest G (2004) Study of reference values and biological variation: a necessity and a model for Preventive Medicine Centers. Clin Chem Lab Med 42:810–816
41. Jorgensen LG, Brandslund I, Hyltoft Petersen P, Stahl M, de Fine Olivarius N (2004) Creation of a low-risk reference group and reference interval of fasting venous plasma glucose. Clin Chem Lab Med 42:817–823
42. Jensen E, Hyltoft Petersen P, Blaabjerg O, Hansen PS, Brix TH, Kyvik KO, Hegedus L (2004) Establishment of a serum thyroid stimulating hormone (TSH) reference interval in healthy adults. The importance of environmental factors, including thyroid antibodies. Clin Chem Lab Med 42:824–832
43. Dhondt JL (2004) Difficulties in establishing reference intervals for special fluids: the example of 5-hydroxyindoleacetic acid and homovanillic acid in cerebrospinal fluid. Clin Chem Lab Med 42:833–841
44. Thienpont LM, Van Uytfanghe K, Rodriguez Cabaleiro D (2004) Metrological traceability of calibration in the estimation and use of common medical decision-making criteria. Clin Chem Lab Med 42:842–850
45. Klein G, Junge W (2004) Creation of the necessary analytical quality for generating and using reference intervals. Clin Chem Lab Med 42:851–857
46. Ricos C, Domenech MV, Perich C (2004) Analytical quality specifications for common reference intervals. Clin Chem Lab Med 42:858–862

47. Westgard JO (2004) Design of internal quality control for reference value studies. Clin Chem Lab Med 42:863–867
48. WHO (2006) Constitution of the World Health Organization. Basic Documents, 45th edn, 1
49. NCCLS (2004) Procedures and devices for the collection of diagnostic capillary blood specimens. Approved Standard, 5th edn. NCCLS Document H04-A5, Wayne
50. NCCLS (2007) Procedures for the collection of diagnostic blood specimens by venipuncture. Approved Standard, 6th edn. NCCLS Document H03-A6, Wayne
51. Andrew M, Paes B, Milner R, Johnston M, Mitchell L, Tollefsen DM, Powers P (1987) Development of the human coagulation system in the full-term infant. Blood 70:165–172
52. Andrew M, Vegh P, Johnston M, Bowker J, Ofosu F, Mitchell L (1992) Maturation of the hemostatic system during childhood. Blood 80:1998–2005
53. Hathaway W, Corrigan J (1991) Report of Scientific and Standardization Subcommittee on Neonatal Hemostasis. Normal coagulation data for fetuses and newborn infants. Thromb Haemost 65:323–325
54. Schmidt B, Mitchell L, Ofosu FA, Andrew M (1989) Alpha-2-macroglobulin is an important progressive inhibitor of thrombin in neonatal and infant plasma. Thromb Haemost 62:1074–1077
55. Albisetti M (2003) The fibrinolytic system in children. Semin Thromb Hemost 29: 339–348

Chapter 7

Lupus Anticoagulant Testing

Karen Moffat, Anne Raby, and Mark Crowther

Abstract

Antiphospholipid antibodies are a heterogenous group of autoantibodies directed against glycoproteins in concert with anionic phospholipids. In clinical laboratory practice, antiphospholipid antibody evaluations usually consist of a combination of the following: anticardiolipin antibody assay, anti-beta 2 glycoprotein I assay, and at least two lupus anticoagulant assays with an appropriate confirmatory test. Lupus anticoagulants produce their laboratory effect by prolonging recalcification times in assays within which phospholipid content is limited. Although many assays are available, all are based on the fundamental principle of demonstrating normalization of prolonged recalcification times with the addition of exogenous phospholipid. The antibody specificity of an individual lupus anticoagulant is difficult or impossible to determine; however a small proportion do demonstrate avidity for selected proteins such as prothrombin or beta 2 glycoprotein I. The mechanism by which these antibodies cause their clinical manifestations remains unknown; however their relationship to increased risk of thrombosis, pregnancy loss, and autoimmune thrombocytopenia is undoubted. There is no correlation between the "strength" of lupus anticoagulants and the level of thrombotic risk; thus it is important to identify both "weak" and "strong" lupus anticoagulants.

Key words Antiphospholipid antibodies, Lupus anticoagulants, Anticardiolipin antibody, Anti-beta 2 glycoprotein I

1 Introduction and Background

Antiphospholipid antibodies are a heterogenous group of autoantibodies directed against glycoproteins in concert with anionic phospholipids. Antiphospholipid antibodies were initially described as a result of their ability to produce false-positive serologic assays for syphilis. The high prevalence of antiphospholipid antibodies in patients with systemic lupus erythematosus and the association of antiphospholipid antibodies with a false-positive VDRL remain the explanation for the inclusion of a false-positive VDRL in diagnostic criteria for systemic lupus erythematosus (1, 2).

In clinical laboratory practice, antiphospholipid antibody evaluations usually consist of a combination of the following:

Paul Monagle (ed.), *Haemostasis: Methods and Protocols*, Methods in Molecular Biology, vol. 992,
DOI 10.1007/978-1-62703-339-8_7,

anticardiolipin antibody assay, anti-beta 2 glycoprotein I assay, and at least two lupus anticoagulant assays with an appropriate confirmatory test. Frequently uninformed clinicians will ask for "antiphospholipid antibody testing"; as there is no such single test the laboratory should develop policies and procedures to determine which assays will be performed should this request be received. In general, these tests will be ordered for patients with systemic autoimmune conditions or as part of an assessment to determine if selected clinical problems are due to an antiphospholipid antibody (1).

The lupus anticoagulant was first described in the 1950s as a cause of a bleeding diathesis in patients with systemic lupus erythematosus who presented with prolonged calcium-dependent clotting times (2). As a result of their clinical presentation the term "lupus anticoagulant" was coined. This name has subsequently proven unfortunate given the observation that many patients with these abnormalities do not have lupus and the principal clinical manifestation is a pro-coagulant, rather than anticoagulant, effect. In fact, the bleeding diathesis in the originally described patients was likely due to a rare effect wherein the lupus anticoagulant had specificity for prothrombin producing an acquired form of hemophilia.

The "anticoagulant" term reflects the prolongation of phospholipid-dependent clotting assays, which is due to the lupus anticoagulant's specificity for phospholipids. Lupus anticoagulants produce their laboratory effect by prolonging recalcification times in assays within which phospholipid content is limited. Although many assays are available, all are based on this fundamental principle. The presence of a lupus anticoagulant can be confirmed by demonstrating normalization of recalcification times with the addition of exogenous phospholipid.

The antibody specificity of an individual lupus anticoagulant is difficult or impossible to determine; however a small proportion do demonstrate avidity for selected proteins such as prothrombin or beta 2 glycoprotein I (3). The small subgroup of antibodies that bind with prothrombin may reduce its circulating half-life resulting in an acquired form of hemophilia with an associated bleeding risk. In addition to rare presentations with acquired hemophilia, patients with lupus anticoagulants appear to be at increased risk of clinically important thrombocytopenia, venous and arterial thromboembolism, and pregnancy loss (4). Specific discussion of treatment recommendations for these disorders is beyond the scope of this text: briefly, thrombocytopenia usually responds to immunosuppressive therapy and/or splenectomy, thromboembolism may be prevented or treated using "usual anticoagulants," and recurrent pregnancy loss may be addressed through vigorous and careful antenatal care perhaps coupled with prophylactic dose anticoagulation. The mechanism by which these antibodies cause their clinical manifestations remains unknown.

There is no correlation between the "strength" of lupus anticoagulants and the level of thrombotic risk; thus it is important to identify both "weak" and "strong" lupus anticoagulants.

2 Monitoring of Anticoagulants in Lupus Anticoagulant Patients

Some lupus anticoagulants produce baseline prolongation of the prothrombin time, making laboratory monitoring of oral anticoagulant therapy difficult. Such antibodies are, in general, uncommon and the prolongation is largely limited to selected reagents. If a patient is identified to have baseline prolongation, the prothrombin time reagent should be switched. If an unaffected reagent cannot be found monitoring of the oral anticoagulants with functional coagulation factor levels might be considered. Although reported, there is little evidence that lupus anticoagulants cause "INR instability"; if this is suspected compliance of the patient should be evaluated and corrected.

3 Standardization

Because of the heterogeneity of lupus anticoagulants there is no one diagnostic assay for detecting the lupus anticoagulant since some tests are more sensitive than others. Given epitope variation, expert panels such as the International Society on Thrombosis and Haemostasis (ISTH) have developed recommendations for standardized patient testing of lupus anticoagulants (5, 6). In general, such panels recommend a battery of screening tests with a "positive" being abnormalities on any one constituent test with a positive confirmatory assay.

The fundamental requirements of the laboratory evaluation of a lupus anticoagulant include:

1. Prolongation of one or more phospholipid-dependent clotting assays
2. Evidence that the above prolongation is due to an inhibitor as demonstrated by mixing studies
3. Confirmation of the phospholipid-dependent nature of the inhibitor
4. Lack of specific inhibition of any one coagulation factor

4 Interpretation of Results

Interpreting qualitative results is challenging for a physician because of the variation of test nomenclature, heterogeneity of lupus anticoagulant, and the absence of one main diagnostic assay.

Lupus anticoagulants are generally reported as positive or negative. False-positive results may be obtained in some patients receiving therapeutic dose anticoagulation, particularly with warfarin. Prolongation of the screening assay with a failure to correct the confirmatory assay may be due to other nonspecific inhibitors of coagulation, specific inhibitors of coagulation, and/or deficiencies of individual coagulation factors. Generally speaking, clinically important lupus anticoagulants will be persistently positive in the laboratory tests. Clinical importance is generally assigned to an antibody that is present on two occasions separated by a minimum of 12 weeks (7).

5 Quality Control

A positive and negative lupus anticoagulant control should be included with each run of patient samples. Controls should be retested with a reagent change or major instrument adjustment. Strong positive, weak positive, and negative lupus anticoagulant controls are available through commercial manufacturers and are preferred to the traditional plasma samples of local lupus anticoagulant-positive patients (7).

6 External Quality Assessment and Impact of Anticoagulant Therapy on the Testing for Lupus Anticoagulants

External quality assessment (EQA) is an important component of the clinical laboratory's overall quality assurance management program. Distribution of thrombophilia investigation surveys has improved inter- and intra-laboratory reliability for these assays (8). EQA provides the opportunity for programs to monitor if laboratories are conforming to the 1995 ISTH recommendations by performing two or more lupus anticoagulant tests based on different testing principles and at least one test confirming phospholipid dependence.

EQA samples may be obtained from known lupus anticoagulant-positive patients and the frozen plasmas distributed to participants on dry ice. Other types of samples are prepared using normal pooled plasma spiked with monoclonal antibodies against beta 2 glycoprotein I, prothrombin, or affinity-purified IgG from a positive lupus patient. Artificially prepared plasmas may not perform in the same way as clinical lupus anticoagulant samples (9).

Plasma samples from patients known to have a lupus anticoagulant and undergoing treatment with warfarin produce varied Russell viper venom time results (RVVT). Dependent on the RVVT reagent kit, a wide spread of results were reported both within and between methods, producing positive and negative results. In addition, other tests are prolonged due to warfarin making it difficult to interpret screening, mixing studies, and confirmatory testing as most lupus anticoagulant tests have not been validated when a patient is receiving oral anticoagulants (10). For this reason, it is recommended by the authors that a free text comment be included on a laboratory's report, for example, "Testing was performed for a lupus anticoagulant by an APTT-based assay and a dilute RVVT test, with a confirmatory reagent. The dilute RVVT-based test for lupus anticoagulant is positive. If warfarin therapy is a potential cause of this abnormality, it may be worthwhile to repeat the testing, off warfarin therapy."

7 Reference Intervals

It is recommended that each laboratory determine a reference interval specific for their reagent and instrument combination using accepted laboratory principles, such as those promulgated by the Clinical and Laboratory Standards Institute (CLSI), formerly NCCLS (11, 12). Reference intervals should be verified with a change in reagent lot number, instrument, collection system, or at least once per year.

Better precision can be achieved when laboratories determine their own cutoff levels for positive results. An appropriate way to establish the cutoff level for lupus anticoagulant test such as dilute RVVT or APTT using a lupus-sensitive reagent is to determine the geometric mean ±2 standard deviation (SD) of 40 healthy individuals (7).

8 Blood Collection

Blood samples for lupus anticoagulant testing should be collected into buffered 3.2% (0.109 M) trisodium citrate (3). Collection of the blood sample using a vacuum draw system is acceptable. Venous sample collection is recommended (13).

9 Stability

Plasma samples should be centrifuged as soon as possible after collection to prevent in vitro absorption of the antibody to the cell phospholipid surface resulting in the neutralization of the lupus anticoagulant and false-negative laboratory test results. Separation of the plasma from the cells should occur within 4 h of sample collection.

10 Processing

Plasma samples should be centrifuged at room temperature. The centrifugation force and time used to separate the plasma and the cells must produce plasma with a platelet count of $<10 \times 10^9$/L (12). Current recommendations state that this may be obtained using 1,500 RCF (g-force) for a minimum of 15 min. When a sample is frozen and thawed, residual platelets will release phospholipids causing neutralization of the lupus anticoagulant. Therefore, prior to analysis or freezing, recentrifugation or filtration should be performed when the platelet count is $>10 \times 10^9$/L. It should be noted that filtration may cause loss of such high-molecular-weight coagulation proteins as von Willebrand factor, and consequently factor VIII causing an artificial prolongation of the APTT (6, 10). Samples that have visible hemolysis should not be used because of possible clotting factor activation and end point measurement interference (13).

11 Storage

Samples for lupus anticoagulant should be stored in an ultralow freezer at −70°C. When testing is to be performed within 4 h of sample collection plasma may be stored at 4°C. Samples are stable at −70°C for at least 6 months. A frost-free freezer should not be used as the freeze thaw cycle allows the temperature of the sample to increase and then drop when the sample refreezes (13).

12 Thawing

Samples should be thawed in a circulating water bath at 37°C (±1°C); thawing should be assessed frequently beginning at 5 min. Samples must be removed from the water bath as soon as the last ice crystals have melted. Invert gently to ensure homogeneity of sample prior to use. If there is flocculation possibly due to cryoprecipitate continue to thaw the sample at 37°C for 3 additional minutes. Test immediately (14).

13 Reagents and Reagent Preparation

Reagents should be prepared as per manufacturer's recommendations. Reagents should be at room temperature prior to use. If the reagent is to be reconstituted, purified water with a pH 5.3–7.2 (distilled, deionized, or type 1 reagent grade) should be used (15).

14 Principal

Lupus anticoagulant testing requires demonstration of a prolongation of recalcification times in phospholipid-dependent coagulation assays. The presence of the antibody can be confirmed by correction of the prolonged clotting times through the addition of excess phospholipid.

15 Methods

As no single assay detects a lupus anticoagulant laboratories should heed consensus recommendations to run a minimum of two screening tests that use different test principles (2). Common screening tests include the following: lupus-sensitive activated partial thromboplastin time (APTT), dilute Russell viper venom time (dRVVT), dilute prothrombin time (dPT), and the kaolin clotting time (KCT). These assays are clot based and are easily adapted to automated coagulation instrumentation. The assays have low concentrations of phospholipid and in the presence of a lupus anticoagulant the time in seconds is prolonged.

The general approach to testing for a lupus anticoagulant is to perform several phospholipid-limited recalcification clotting times and, if prolongation is detected, perform mixing studies (to rule out a specific inhibitor of factor deficiency and demonstrate the inhibitory effect on normal plasma) followed by confirmatory assays for the lupus anticoagulant. Confirmatory tests include confirmation of phospholipid dependency which may include dRVVT confirm test and platelet neutralization procedures. Figures 1 and 2 show algorithms commonly used within laboratories to delineate their testing pathways.

15.1 Lupus-Sensitive APTT Reagents

All lupus anticoagulant sensitive reagents contain a low concentration of phospholipid—often referred to as being phospholipid limited. In APTT-based assays, activation of the contact factors of coagulation occurs on negatively charged surfaces, such as silica or ellagic acid. Platelet poor plasma is incubated with the reagent for a predetermined time. Calcium is added and the clotting time in seconds is determined. The lupus anticoagulant antibody binds to the phospholipid contained in the reagent causing a prolongation in the clot times. Used on its own this test does not confirm the presence of a lupus anticoagulant since other conditions may also cause prolonged clotting times, as in the presence of direct thrombin inhibitors such as dabigatran (10).

15.2 Dilute Russell Viper Venom Time

The dRVVT activates factor X to factor Xa directly in the presence of a low concentration of phospholipid. The dRVVT reagent is

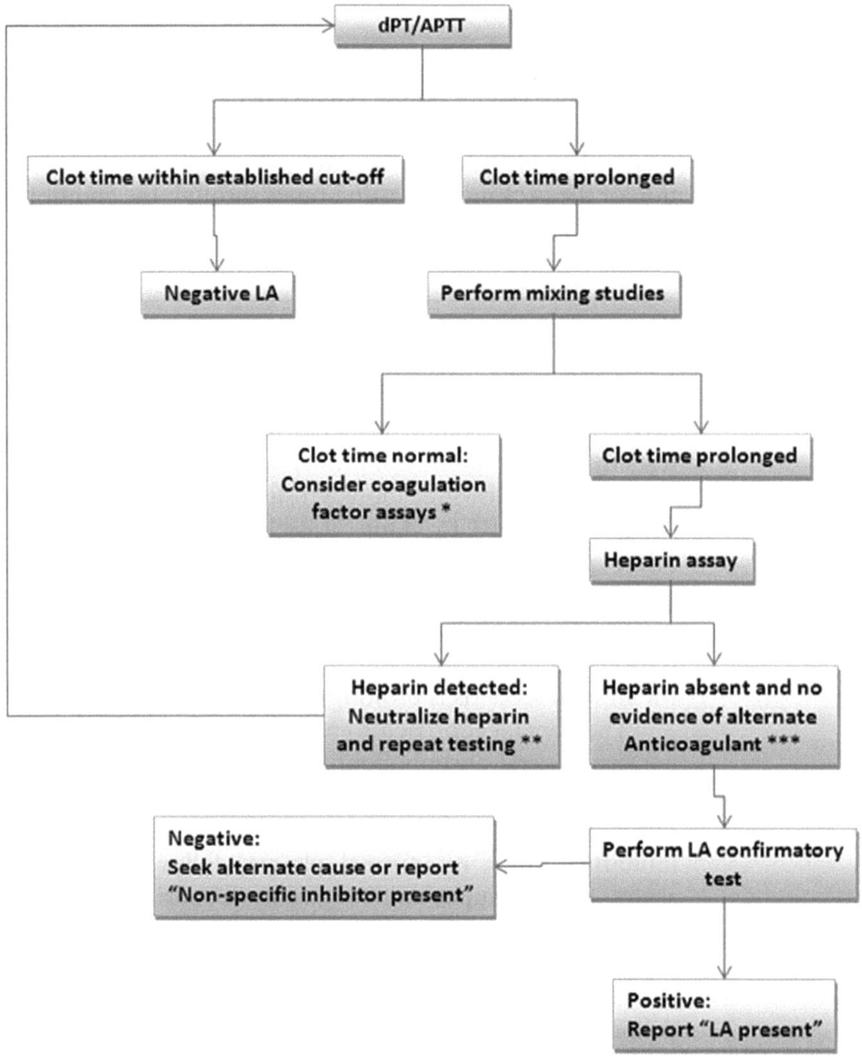

Fig. 1 Suggested algorithm for the laboratory testing in the investigation of lupus anticoagulant (LA) using a dPT reagent and/or a lupus-sensitive APTT reagent. APTT-based assays include lupus-sensitive APTT reagent and/or a kaolin clotting time. Caution: No one laboratory test is diagnostic for LA. (*Asterisk*) Report should include a comment advising the clinician of the possibility of a single or multiple factor deficiency. (*Double asterisk*) Report should include a comment advising the clinician that the testing was performed on a neutralized sample. (*Triple asterisk*) The effect of novel anticoagulants such as direct thrombin inhibitors (e.g., dabigatran) or Xa inhibitors (e.g., apixaban) on LA assays are unknown. As a result, caution should be used when reporting investigation results in the presence of these anticoagulants

added to the plasma and the clotting time in seconds is determined. Most commercial dRVVT reagents neutralize unfractionated heparin (up to 1 unit/mL) and low molecular weight heparin within the therapeutic range (10). Commercial manufacturers often have a confirmation reagent with a higher concentration of phospholipid available to run in parallel with the dRVVT. The calculated

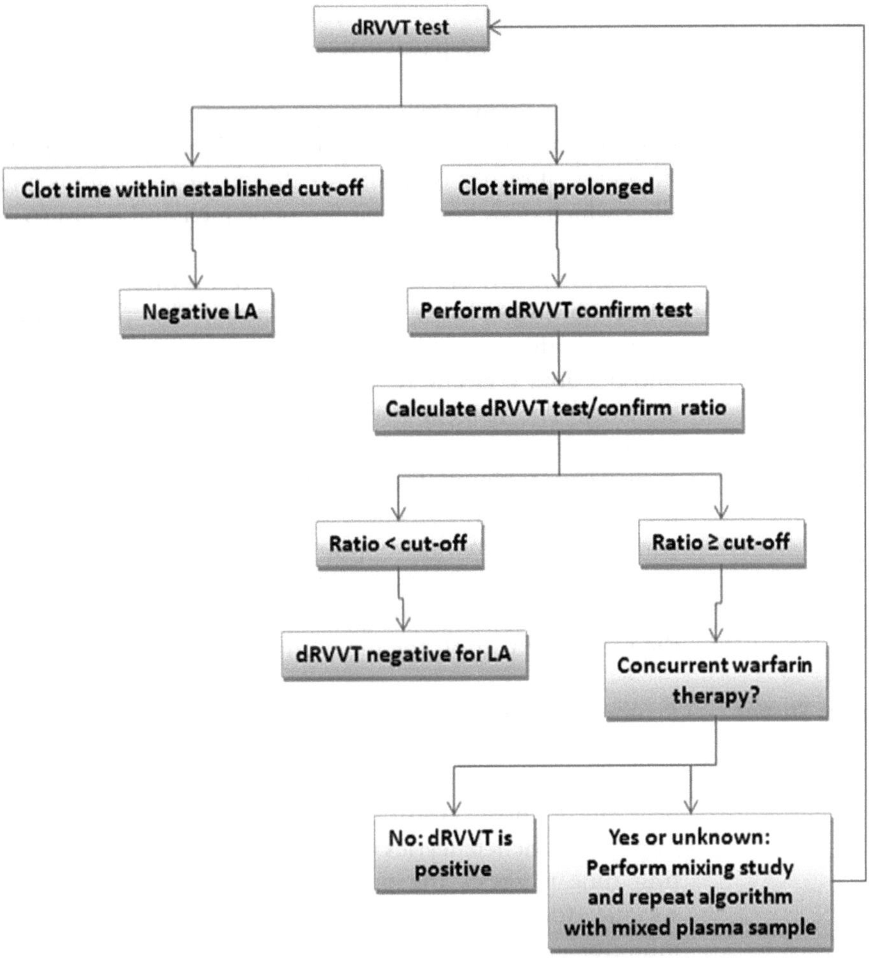

Fig. 2 Suggested algorithm for the laboratory testing in the investigation of lupus anticoagulant (LA) using a dilute Russell viper venom time (dRVVT) assay. Caution: No one laboratory test is diagnostic for LA. Most commercial dRVVT test and confirm reagents contain a heparin neutralizer. If warfarin use is suspected or confirmed a comment should be included on patient's report indicating that warfarin may interfere with the assay

ratio of the dRVVT test/dRVVT confirm of the patient sample is compared to a specified cutoff ratio to determine the presence of a lupus anticoagulant. If the ratio is greater than the established cutoff then the lupus anticoagulant is confirmed—caution is needed in the interpretation of these assays, as noted, because of the potential for oral anticoagulants to produce a "falsely positive" test.

15.3 Kaolin Clotting Time

Kaolin is a negatively charged particulate that activates the contact factors for the ultimate generation of thrombin and the conversion of fibrinogen to fibrin. Kaolin is added to the plasma sample which activates the contact factors. Calcium is added and the time for clot formation is determined. This test is considered a sensitive screening test because of its low content of phospholipids. However, it is problematic as the particulate substance can cause difficulty with optical clot detection and may also form sediment within the coagulation instrument dispensing system and cuvettes. In addition, the long clotting times in healthy individuals and patients make reproducibility of results difficult. An alternative to kaolin is micronized silica which does not exhibit the same technical issues (6).

15.4 Dilute Prothrombin Time

The dilute prothrombin time (dPT) test is often referred to as the dilute thromboplastin inhibition test. The prothrombin time reagent is diluted, often as high as a 1/500 dilution to obtain a phospholipid concentration that allows detection of lupus anticoagulants. The reagent is comprised of a relipidated recombinant human tissue factor which in the presence of calcium activates the tissue factor pathway. The assay is similar to the dilute RVVT in that there is a screening and confirmatory test. The dPT screening assay contains lower amounts of phospholipid and the confirmatory test contains higher amounts of phospholipid. The ratio is derived from the dilute divided by the confirmatory. If the ratio is greater than the established cutoff the lupus anticoagulant is confirmed (10).

15.5 Mixing Studies

Prolongation of the clotting time in any of the above assays should be investigated with mixing studies. Generally a 1:1 mix with pooled platelet poor normal plasma followed by repeat testing is performed—normalization of the clotting time suggests one or more factor deficiency(ies) (6). Persistent prolongation of the clotting time suggests the presence of an inhibitor which is either specific (for example heparin or an acquired coagulation factor inhibitor) or nonspecific (for example a lupus anticoagulant). Nonspecific inhibitors should be investigated using confirmatory tests. Examples of confirmatory tests include the DRVVT confirm and the platelet neutralization procedure. Factor assays may be considered if the 1:1 mixing study demonstrates correction of the clotting time. However such reflexive testing is both expensive and may be unneeded—for example in patients tested inadvertently while receiving oral vitamin K antagonists. The authors suggest that rather than reflectively testing all samples with evidence of a coagulation factor deficiency, a statement be attached to the results alerting clinicians that the 1:1 mixing study is corrected, thereby suggesting a factor deficiency, and factor assays should be ordered, if clinically indicated.

15.6 Platelet Neutralization Procedure

The PNP is often used to confirm the presence of a lupus anticoagulant. The correction or neutralization of the lupus-sensitive APTT in seconds of the patient's platelet poor plasma after the addition of a platelet membrane preparation is determined and confirms the presence of a lupus anticoagulant. Both platelet membrane preparations and commercial kits are available commercially (10).

16 Sources of Error

False-negative lupus anticoagulant testing may be caused by:

1. Pre-analytic factors leading to either delays in processing or platelet activation—both of these effects can cause platelet-derived phospholipid to neutralize the lupus anticoagulant. Of note, weak lupus anticoagulants may be lost during the freezing and thawing performed when the platelet count is $>10\times10^9$/L.
2. Ineffective centrifugation leading to excess platelet-derived phospholipid in the test system.

False-positive lupus anticoagulant testing may be caused by:

1. Prolongation of the clotting time in clot-based lupus-sensitive assays such as APTT, dPT, KCT, and dRVVT due to factor deficiencies or specific factor inhibitors
2. Prolongation of the clotting time by oral anticoagulant therapy.

References

1. Abo SM, DeBari VA (2007) Review: laboratory evaluation of the antiphospholipid syndrome. Ann Clin Lab Sci 37:3–14
2. Triplett DA (2002) Antiphospholipid antibodies. Arch Pathol Lab Med 126:1424–1429
3. Pengo V, Biasiolo A, Gresele P, Marongiu F, Erba N, Veschi F, Ghirarduzzi A, De Candia E, Montaruli B, Testa S, Barcellona D, Tripodi A, on behalf of Participating Centres of Italian Federation of Thrombosis Centres (FCSA) (2007) Survey of lupus anticoagulant diagnosis by central evaluation of plasma samples. J Thromb Haemost 5:925–30
4. Lim W, Crowther MA, Eikleboom JW (2006) Management of antiphospholipid antibody syndrome: a systematic review. JAMA 295:1050–1057
5. Brandt JT, Triplett DA, Alving B, Scharrer I (1995) Criteria for the diagnosis of lupus anticoagulants: an update. On behalf of the Subcommittee on lupus anticoagulant/antiphospholipid antibody of the Scientific and Standardisation Committee of the ISTH. Thromb Haemost 74:1185–90
6. Tripodi A (2007) Laboratory testing for lupus anticoagulants: a review of issues affecting results. Clin Chem 53:1629–1635
7. Miyakis S, Lockshin MD, Atsumi T, Branch DW, Brey RL, Cervera R, Derksen RHWM, de Groot PG, Koike T, Meroni PL, Reber G, Shoenfeld Y, Tincani A, Vlachoyiannopoulos PG, Krills SA (2006) International consensus statement on an update of the classification criteria for definite antiphospholipid syndrome (APS). J Thrombo Haemost 4:295–306
8. Jennings I, Greaves M, Mackie IJ, Kitchen S, Woods TAL, Preston FE (2002) Lupus anticoagulant testing: improvements in performance in a UK NEQAS proficiency testing exercise after dissemination of national guidelines on laboratory methods. Br J Haematol 119: 364–369
9. Jennings I, Mackie I, Arnout J, Preston FE, on behalf of the UK National External Quality Assessment Scheme for Blood Coagulation (2004) Lupus anticoagulant testing using plasma spiked with monoclonal antibodies: performance in the UK NEQAS proficiency testing programme. J Thromb Haemost 2:2178–84
10. Teruya J, West AG, Suell MN (2007) Lupus anticoagulant assays: questions answered and to be answered. Arch Pathol Lab Med 131:885–889
11. Pierangeli S, Harris EN (2005) Review: clinical laboratory testing for the antiphospholipid syndrome. Clinica Chimica Acta 357:17–33
12. Clinical and Laboratory Standards Institute/NCCLS (June 2000) How to define and determine reference intervals in the clinical laboratory; approved guideline. 2nd edn. CLSI/NCCLS document C28-A2. Clinical and Laboratory Standards Institute, Wayne (PA).
13. Clinical and Laboratory Standards Institute/NCCLS (June 2003) Collection, transport,

and processing of blood specimens for testing plasma-based coagulation assays; approved guideline. 4th edn. CLSI/NCCLS document H21-A4. Clinical and Laboratory Standards Institute, Wayne (PA).
14. Clinical and Laboratory Standards Institute/ NCCLS (June 1997) Determination of factor coagulant activities; approved guideline. CLSI/ NCCLS document H48-A. Clinical and Laboratory Standards Institute, Wayne (PA).
15. Clinical and Laboratory Standards Institute/ NCCLS (June 2006) Preparation and testing of reagent water in the clinical laboratory; approved guideline. 4th edn. CLSI/NCCLS document C3–A4. Clinical and Laboratory Standards Institute, Wayne (PA).

Part III

Examples of Global Tests of Haemostasis

Chapter 8

Activated Partial Thromboplastin Time

Vera Ignjatovic

Abstract

Activated partial thromboplastin time (APTT) is a commonly used coagulation assay that is easy to perform, is affordable, and is therefore performed in most coagulation laboratories, both clinical and research, worldwide. The APTT is based on the principle that in citrated plasma, the addition of a platelet substitute, factor XII activator, and $CaCl_2$ allows for formation of a stable clot. The time required for the formation of a stable clot is recorded in seconds and represents the actual APTT result.

Key words APTT, aPTT, PTT, Clotting test, Heparin monitoring

1 Introduction

Activated partial thromboplastin time (APTT) is one of the most commonly used coagulation assays, which measures the clotting time from the time of activation of factor XII to the formation of a stable fibrin clot. This assay has been used since 1953 (1), and was modified significantly in 1961 (2), closely resembling the assay that is used currently. Since that time, the APTT has become time- and cost-efficient and simple to perform using automated coagulation analyzers. Clinically, the APTT is often performed in conjunction with prothrombin time (PT) and the fibrinogen assay, with these tests known as the "coagulation screen." This standard set of assays represents the starting point for clinicians when diagnosing a bleeding and/or a clotting disorder and is also useful for pre-surgical assessment of patients, to rule out coagulation defects (3–5).

The APTT test specifically involves re-calcification of plasma once the sample has been incubated with a platelet substitute and a factor XII activator. This test can therefore be used to detect the deficiency of the following factors: high molecular weight kininogen (HMWK); prekallikrein; factors XII, XI, IX (hemophilia), VIII (hemophilia), X, and V; prothrombin; and fibrinogen. In addition, this assay is widely used for monitoring anticoagulant therapy (unfractionated heparin, argatroban, hirudin) as well as for detection

Paul Monagle (ed.), *Haemostasis: Methods and Protocols*, Methods in Molecular Biology, vol. 992,
DOI 10.1007/978-1-62703-339-8_8, © Springer Science+Business Media New York 2013

of lupus anticoagulants (6). Recent studies have demonstrated an association between shortened APTT and the risk of venous thromboembolism (VTE) (7), allowing for an additional use of this assay, that for prediction of VTE (8).

1.1 Principle

Activation of the coagulation system in a plasma sample in the presence of a platelet substitute (silica), activator of factor XII, and $CaCl_2$ leads to the formation of a stable clot. The time from activation to formation of a stable clot is recorded in seconds, and represents the APTT. The absence of the tissue factor from this reaction mixture has lead to the use of the term "partial."

1.2 Standardization

Despite the fact that the APTT assay itself is easy to perform, to date efforts to standardize it have not been possible. The variables that need to be considered include the phospholipid content and its source, type of activator (nature and amount), length of incubation, the buffers used, as well as the method used to measure clot formation (9, 10). This is further complicated by the fact that there are more than 300 different APTT methods in use (11). In addition, when the same reagents are used on different coagulation analyzers, different results are obtained. Despite the fact that most of the APTTs are performed on automated analyzers, to date, attempts to standardize all aspects of the APTT assay have to date been unsuccessful.

The main differences in the reagents used for the APTT assay include the origin of the phospholipids component, as well as the lipid composition. The result of this variation is that some reagents are more/less sensitive to particular factor deficiencies. The phospholipid content of the APTT reagent is very important in how sensitive the assay is to the presence of lupus anticoagulants. Synthetic phospholipids have previously been shown to reduce batch-to-batch variation, compared to the reagents derived from rabbit brain and soybean (12).

In the situation where APTT is used to monitor unfractionated heparin (UFH) therapy, the use of this assay is complicated by the fact that different reagents have different sensitivity to UFH (13, 14). In addition, some reagents are designed to be insensitive to UFH (up to 1 IU/ml). This is useful in situations where the effect of UFH is not important and makes the assay quicker, with no need for addition of a heparin inactivator (i.e., heparinase).

The latest approach to the design of APTT reagents includes the use of completely synthetic polymer activators, such as the Cephascreen reagent designed by Diagnostica Stago. This reagent is based on a polyphenolic activator, and comes in a ready to use form, reducing the possibility of errors during the preparation of the reagent.

An ideal APTT reagent should be sensitive to therapeutic doses of UFH, be able to detect lupus anticoagulants, and identify mild to moderate factor deficiency.

1.3 Clinical Applications

The clinical application of APTT is mostly directed towards detecting the deficiencies of factors VIII and IX and the presence of inhibitors and screening patients prior to surgery and is also used as a screening test for detection of lupus anticoagulants. Despite this, the factor deficiencies to a level of up to 45% can still lead to an APTT result within reference ranges (15).

The APTT is widely used in monitoring of UFH (16), despite the fact that numerous studies have shown poor correlation between the APTT and the anti-Xa assay (17–19). Due to the variability of the APTT reagents, as well as the methods used for testing, it is recommended that each laboratory determines their own APTT ranges corresponding to therapeutic levels of UFH (0.35–0.70 IU/ml by anti-Xa assay) (16). In children, the correlation between the APTT and the anti-Xa assay is poor and could be attributed to the age-related differences in the hemostatic system (developmental haemostasis) (20–22). A recent study has confirmed poor correlation between the APTT and the anti-Xa assay in children and suggested that this correlation improves in patients with elevated factor VIII levels (23).

It is thought that the APTT assesses the overall effect of UFH on coagulation, as opposed to the anti-Xa assay, which concentrates on a specific part of coagulation. In addition, for some laboratories, the anti-Xa assay represents an option that is not affordable.

1.4 Interpretation of Results

Interpretation of APTT results is extremely important in ensuring that an accurate diagnosis is made and the best care considered for the patient.

1.4.1 Reference Ranges

Reference ranges for APTT are dependent on reagent/analyzer combination, as well as the population tested (24). Age-related differences in the APTT have been demonstrated with healthy neonates and children having increased reference intervals compared to healthy adults (24–27). The prolongation of the APTT in neonates and children is thought to be caused by a combination of several clotting factors that are decreased in children, rather than one factor in particular (28). In addition, when the same samples are tested using the same analyzer but with different APTT reagents, the reference intervals are different, with the age-specific trend remaining the same (24).

1.4.2 Shortening of the APTT

Shortening of the APTT has until recently been thought to be of no or limited clinical significance. However, a number of recent publications have presented an association between shorter APTTs and venous VTE, rendering the APTT useful in prediction of recurrent VTEs (7, 8). In addition, shortened APTTs have been shown to be associated with increased risk of recurrence of VTE following withdrawal of anticoagulation therapy (29).

Table 1
Factors that lead to the prolongation of the APTT

Hereditary factors (deficiencies of)	Acquired factors (presence of)
Factor VIII, IX, XI, or XII	Lupus anticoagulants
Prekallikrein	Vitamin K deficiency
HMWK	Liver dysfunction
Factor II, V, or X	Coagulation factor inhibitors
Fibrinogen	Disseminated intravascular coagulation (DIC) Heparin Hirudin Argatroban Coumadin Aprotinin Massive transfusion

However, it is important to consider that shortening of the APTT can also be caused in a setting of an acute phase reaction (acute tissue inflammation or trauma). This is a consequence of a temporary increase in the level of factor VIII, with the APTT returning to the expected level after the condition causing the acute phase reaction is resolved.

1.4.3 Prolongation of the APTT

Prolongation of the APTT can be a result of hereditary or acquired factors. These are summarized in Table 1.

The first step in determining the cause of an unexplained APTT prolongation is to perform the APTT in the presence of heparinase, which neutralizes UFH. If the APTT corrects to a value within the reference range for that laboratory, then the presence of UFH is the cause for the prolongation. If the APTT does not correct, then mixing studies are performed, to determine whether the prolongation is due to a factor deficiency (APTT corrected) or due to an inhibitor (APTT remains prolonged).

It is also extremely important to note that "prolongation" of the APTT can be observed if adult reference ranges for APTT are used when pediatric samples are tested.

Prolongation of the APTT can also be caused by the presence of aprotinin (30). This is particularly important in cases where the APTT is used to assess the effect of UFH therapy or the level of coagulation factors in the setting of cardiopulmonary bypass. In this situation, interpretation of results must be performed with caution, and this can be confirmed by the fact that the PT remains unchanged.

2 Materials

2.1 Specimen

Whole blood.

2.1.1 Collection

NCCLS guidelines recommend collection into plastic or siliconized glass tubes containing 3.2% trisodium citrate (e.g., 9 volumes of blood to 1 volume of 0.109 M trisodium citrate) (31). One of the most important aspects of sample collection for an APTT assay involves filling the collection tubes to the correct point (indicated on the tube), as to achieve the adequate ratio of blood sample to anticoagulant. Underfilled or overfilled blood collection tubes should not be used for determination of APTT, because this leads to falsely shortened and prolonged APTT result (see Note 1) (32).

In cases where the APTT is used to monitor UFH therapy, tubes containing citric acid theophylline adenosine, and dipyridamole (CTAD) anticoagulant mixture can be used. This prevents UFH inactivation by the platelet factor 4 released from activated platelets present in whole blood (33).

Once the sample is collected, the tube must be mixed immediately by gentle inversion, to allow for the anticoagulant (usually at the bottom of the tube) to mix appropriately with the sample.

Routine venipuncture is the optimal collection procedure for the APTT assay, as it minimizes sample activation. However, with the recent advancement of point of care technology, finger prick collections are being used more frequently. Care must be taken with such collections, as they can often lead to activation of the sample, and hence extreme care must be taken to avoid difficult collections, whenever possible.

An initial discard is recommended in those situations where blood is collected from a heparinized line. However, to date, there has been no agreement on standardization of the amount of discard for specific clinical situations. The risk of UFH contamination of the sample cannot be completely removed and it is preferable that this situation is avoided whenever possible, by using the peripheral vein. Despite this, the latest data regarding samples drawn from peripherally inserted catheters (PICC) shows that samples collected from this site do not result in clinically significant differences in APTT as compared to the peripheral venous samples (34). The protocol for blood sampling via the PICC line included cleaning the PICC injection port with alcohol wipes, flushing with 20 ml of standard saline, and discarding 5 ml of blood. This finding suggests a protocol that could reduce the need for peripheral venipuncture. However, it is important to note that in the pediatric setting a 5 ml discard volume represents a significant quantity and may not be an optimal method in this setting. Venous access in children can often be extremely difficult and this is often underestimated.

2.1.2 Stability

Once collected, the whole blood sample is prone to activation and this can in turn lead to results that are not representative of the true status of the sample. This is particularly because of the presence of platelets which are easily activated and can then lead to activation of soluble coagulation factors.

The NCCLS guidelines for stability of whole blood samples prior to testing recommend storage at room temperature for 2 h and at 4°C for 4 h.

Non-heparinized plasma samples remain stable for up to 4 h at room temperature, while heparinized samples are stable at the same conditions for up to 2 h. This is due to the fact that UFH can be neutralized by plasma proteins, such as platelet factor 4 (33).

2.1.3 Processing

Recommended centrifugation protocol for obtaining a platelet free plasma sample adequate for coagulation testing includes minimum centrifugation at 2,500 × *g* for 15 min (31).

2.1.4 Storage

Once prepared, the plasma samples can be stored for up to 2 weeks at −20°C and for up to 6 months at −70°C (31). It is important that the plasma sample is separated into smaller aliquots prior to storage. This will allow the sample to freeze quickly and allows for adequate thawing prior to use.

Frozen plasma must be adequately thawed prior to testing (10–15 min in a 37°C water bath) and it is recommended that the testing is performed immediately after thawing. However, in situations where this is not possible, the plasma sample can be stored for 2 h at 4°C prior to use (31).

2.2 Reagents and Reagent Preparation

For commercially available assays, instructions provided by the manufacturer for preparation of reagents and/or instrument should be followed, in order to ensure the validity of the results.

Most reagents used to carry out the APTT assay are not toxic; however working with plasma samples of unknown origin carries a certain level of risk that should be minimized by the use of gloves and eye protection.

2.2.1 APTT Reagent (Platelet Substitute + Particulate Activator)

As mentioned previously, there are many different commercially available APTT reagents. APTT reagents usually come lyophilized and/or are pre-diluted (ready to use), with both stored at 4°C. Lyophilized reagents require reconstitution with distilled water.

It is important that all APTT reagents are mixed well and allowed to stand at room temperature (18–25°C) for approximately 30 min prior to use.

The stability of APTT reagents is manufacturer specific; however 7-day stability at 2–8°C is common.

2.2.2 Calcium Chloride

Calcium chloride ($CaCl_2$) concentration is dependent on each APTT reagent. However, a common concentration of 0.025 M is usually used. This reagent is usually pre-diluted and is stored at 4°C and acclimatized at 18–25°C for approximately 30 min prior to use. This reagent is usually stable for 12 months at 2–8°C.

2.2.3 Control Plasma

The use of control plasma, with a known clotting time (for a particular APTT reagent/analyzer), should be used to ensure that the method has been set up adequately.

2.3 Clot Detection

Automated coagulation analyzers can detect the formation of a stable clot via two mechanisms. Optical measurement involves the change in opacity of the reagent mixture. The mechanical measurement, on the other hand, detects a change in the consistency of the reaction mixture as the clot formation takes place. This particular method of detection is particularly useful for samples obtained from newborns, as it is not affected by the variables that affect light transmission, such as hyperbilirubinemia or lipemia.

3 Methods

3.1 Assay Procedure

The plasma sample is incubated with an APTT reagent containing a platelet substitute (phospholipid) and a particulate activator (silica, celite, kaolin, ellagic acid, polyphenolic polymer). Following an incubation period (approximately 180–240 s), $CaCl_2$ is added and allows the initiation of clot formation. The time required for formation of a stable clot is then recorded.

3.1.1 Automated Assay

1. Plasma sample is loaded onto the analyzer.
2. 50 μl of plasma is mixed with 50 μl of APTT reagent and incubated for 4 min.
3. 50 μl $CaCl_2$ is added to the sample/reagent mixture.
4. The time required for formation of a stable clot is recorded (s).

3.1.2 Manual Assay

Ensure that a water bath is pre-warmed and the temperature stabilized at 37°C and that you have access to a stopwatch (timer) prior to starting the test (see Note 2).

1. Pre-incubate the 0.025 M $CaCl_2$ solution at 37°C.
2. Pipette 0.1 ml test or control plasma into a test tube.
3. Incubate at 37°C for 2 min.
4. Gently mix the APTT reagent by inversion.
5. Pipette 0.1 ml of reconstituted APTT reagent into the test tube with the plasma.
6. Incubate at 37°C for 5 min.
7. Add 0.1 ml of the 0.025 M $CaCl_2$ solution and simultaneously start the timer.

Table 2
Sources of error for the APTT assay

Error	Subheadings	Identification	Cause	Correction
Faulty blood collection	2.1.1	Unexplained prolonged APTT	Difficult venipuncture	If possible, sample needs to be re-collected
Partial clotting of the sample	2.1.1	Presence of a blood clot in whole blood	Late mixing with citrate during collection	Sample must be re-collected
Under- and overfilled collection tube	2.1.1	Observation of the sample volume as compared to the "fill line" indicated on the collection tube		Sample must be re-collected
Evidence of haemolysis	2.1.1	Plasma sample appears red	Difficult collection and/or inappropriate processing	If possible, sample needs to be re-collected
UFH contamination	2.1.1	Unexplained prolonged APTT	Blood collected from heparinized lines	The APTT corrects upon addition of a UFH inhibitor (heparinase, polybrene)
Use of nonspecific (reagent, analyzer, and age) reference ranges	3.2	Unexplained shortened or prolonged APTT	Inappropriate interpretation of the result	Use of appropriate reference ranges

8. Gently tilt the reaction tube back and forth (under water as much as possible) in the 37°C water bath, and continually observe for clot formation. Immediately upon formation of a clot, stop the timer and record the clotting time.

3.2 Interpretation of Results

As previously specified, it is essential that each laboratory establish its own reference values that are specific for the particular APTT reagent, analyzer, and sample combination used in that particular laboratory. This ensures that APTT results can be interpreted correctly, and the best possible care can then be offered to the patient.

4 Notes

1. The major problems/faults related to the APTT assay are related to the pre-analytical variables, such as sample collection, processing, and storage. See Table 2.
2. For manual testing, it is recommended that a duplicate test is performed. The results of the two tests should correlate within 5%.

References

1. Langdell RD, Wagner RH, Brinkhous KM (1953) Effect of anti-hemophilic factor on one-stage clotting tests: a presumptive test for hemophilia and a simple one-stage anti-hemophilic factor assay procedure. J Lab Clin Med 41:637–647
2. Proctor RR, Rapaport SI (1961) The partial thromboplastin time with kaolin. A simple screening test for first stage plasma clotting factor deficiencies. Am J Clin Pathol 36:212–219
3. Cohen AJ, Kessler CM (2002) Haemophilia A and B. In: Kitchens CS, Alving BM, Kessler CM (eds) Consultative haemostasis and thrombosis. WB Saunders, Philadelphia, pp 43–56
4. Roberts HR, Escobar MA (2002) Less common congenital disorders of haemostasis. In: Kitchen S, Alving BM, Kessler CM (eds) Consultative haemostasis and thrombosis. WB Saunders, Philadelphia, pp 57–71
5. Triplett DA (2002) Coagulation abnormalities. In: McClatchey KD (ed) Clinical laboratory medicine, 2nd edn. Lippincott Williams and Wilkins, Philadelphia, pp 1033–1049
6. Arnout J (2001) Antiphospholipid syndrome: diagnostic aspects of lupus anticoagulants. Thromb Haemost 86:83–91
7. Tripodi A, Chantarangkul V, Martinelli I, Buciarelli P, Manucci PM (2004) A shortened activated partial thromboplastin time is associated with the risk of venous thromboembolism. Blood 104:3631–3634
8. Hron G, Eichinger S, Weltermann A, Quehenberger P, Halbmayer WM, Kyrle PA (2006) Prediction of recurrent venous thromboembolism by the activated partial thromboplastin time. J Thromb Haemost 4:752–756
9. Barrowcliffe TW, Gray E (1981) Studies of phospholipid reagents used in coagulation II: factors influencing their sensitivity to heparin. Thromb Haemost 46:634–637
10. Thomson JM, Poller L (1985) The activated partial thromboplastin time. In: Thomson JM (ed) Blood coagulation and haemostasis: a practical guide. Churchill Livingstone, Edinburgh, pp 301–309
11. Olson JD, Arkin CF, Brandt JT (1998) College of American Pathologists Conference XXXI on Laboratory Monitoring on Anticoagulant Therapy: laboratory monitoring of unfractionated heparin therapy. Arch Pathol Lab Med 122:782–798
12. Okuda M, Yamamoto Y (2004) Usefulness of synthetic phospholipid in measurement of activated partial thromboplastin time: a new preparation procedure to reduce batch difference. Clin Lab Haem 26:215–233

13. Kitchen S, Preston FE (1996) The therapeutic range for heparin therapy: relationship between six activated partial thromboplastin time reagents and two heparin assays. N Engl J Med 75:734–739
14. Manzato F, Mengoni A, Grilenzoni A, Lippi G (1998) Evaluation of the activated partial thromboplastin time (APTT) sensitivity to heparin using 5 commercial reagents: implications for therapeutic monitoring. Clin Chem Lab Med 36:975–980
15. Van Cott EM, Laposata M (2001) Coagulation. In: Jacobs DS, DeMott WR, Oxley DK (eds) Laboratory test handbook with key words index. Lexi-Comp, Hudson, pp 327–358
16. Hirsch J, Raschke R (2004) Heparin and low-molecular-weight heparin: the Seventh ACCP Conference on Antithrombotic and Thrombolytic Therapy. Chest 126:188S–203S
17. Baker BA, Adelman MD, Smith PA (1997) Inability of the activated partial thromboplastin time to predict heparin levels. Ann Intern Med 157:2475–2479
18. Brill-Edwards P, Ginsberg JS, Johnston M (1993) Establishing a therapeutic range for heparin therapy. Ann Intern Med 119:104–109
19. Despotis GJ, Summerfield AL, Joist JH, Goodnough LT, Santoro SA, Spitznagel E, Cox JL, Lappas DG (1994) Comparison of activated coagulation time and whole blood heparin measurements with laboratory plasma anti-Xa heparin concentration in patients having cardiac operations. J Thorac Cardiovasc Surg 108:1076–1082
20. Ignjatovic V, Furmedge J, Newall F, Chan A, Berry L, Fong C, Cheng K, Monagle P (2006) Age-related differences in heparin response. Thromb Res 118:741–745
21. Ignjatovic V, Summerhayes R, Gan A, Than J, Chan A, Cochrane A, Bennett M, Horton S, Shann F, Lane G, Ross-Smith M, Monagle P (2007) Monitoring unfractionated heparin (UFH) therapy: which anti factor Xa is appropriate? Thromb Res 120:347–351
22. Kuhle S, Eulmesekian P, Kavanagh B (2007) Lack of correlation between heparin dose and standard clinical monitoring tests in treatment with unfractionated heparin in critically ill children. Haematologica 92:554–557
23. Chan A, Black L, Ing C, Brandao LR, Williams S (2007) Utility of aPTT in monitoring unfractionated heparin in children, Thrombosis Res. 2008;122(1):135–136
24. Monagle P, Barnes C, Ignjatovic V, Furmedge J, Newall F, Chan A, De Rosa L, Hamilton S, Ragg P, Robinson S, Auldist A, Crock C, Roy N, Rowlands S (2006) Developmental haemostasis: impact for clinical haemostasis laboratories. Thromb Haemost 95:362–372
25. Andrew M, Vegh P, Johnston M, Bowker J, Ofosu F, Mitchell L (1992) Maturation of the hemostatic system during childhood. Blood 80:1998–2005
26. Andrew M, Paes B, Milner R, Jonston M, Mitchell L, Tollefsen D, Powers P (1988) Development of the human coagulation system in the healthy premature infant. Blood 72: 1651–1657
27. Andrew M, Paes B, Milner R, Johnston M, Mitchell L, Tollefsen DM, Powers P (1987) Development of the human coagulation system in the full-term infant. Blood 70:165–172
28. Gallisti S, Muntean W, Leschnik B, Myers W (1997) Longer APTT values in healthy children than adults: no single cause. Thromb Res 88:355–359
29. Legnani C, Mattarozzi S, Cini M, Cosmi B, Favaretto E, Palareti G (2006) Abnormally short activated partial thromboplastin time values are associated with increased risk of recurrence of venous thromboembolism after oral anticoagulation withdrawal. B J Haematol 134: 227–232
30. Despotis GJ, Alsoufiev A, Goodnough LT, Lappas DG (1995) Aprotinin prolongs whole blood activated partial thromboplastin time but not whole blood prothrombin time in patients undergoing cardiac surgery. Anesthesia and Analgesia 81:919–924
31. NCCLS (1998) Collection, transport and processing of blood specimens for coagulation testing and general performance of coagulation assays. In: Standards NCCL (ed) 3rd ed NCCLS, 940 West Valley Road, Wayne, Pennsylvania 19087, USA.
32. Reneke J, Etzell J, Leslie S (1998) Prolonged prothrombin time and activated partial thromboplastin time due to underfilled specimen tubes with 109 mmol/L (3.2%) citrate anticoagulant. Am J Clin Pathol 109:754–757
33. Rose VL, Dermott SC, Murray BF, McIver MM, High KA (1993) Decentralized testing for PT and activated PTT using a dry chemistry portable analyzer. Arch Pathol Lab Med 117: 611–617
34. Rondina MT, Markewitz B, Kling S, Nohavec R, Rodgers GM (2007) The accuracy of activated partial thromboplastin times when drawn through a peripherally inserted central catheter. Am J Haematol 82:738–739

Chapter 9

Prothrombin Time/International Normalized Ratio

Vera Ignjatovic

Abstract

Prothrombin time (PT) and/or International Normalized Ratio (INR) is the most commonly used coagulation assay in health care, to diagnose the risk of bleeding and to monitor oral anticoagulation therapy.

This test is based on the principle that in citrated plasma, the addition of a thromboplastin and $CaCl_2$ allows for formation of a stable clot. The time required for the formation of a stable clot is recorded in seconds and represents the actual PT result. INR is calculated from the PT and allows for worldwide standardization of results.

Key words PT, INR, Clotting test

1 Introduction

Prothrombin time (PT) is a coagulation assay that was established by Quick in 1935 (1) to provide a measure of coagulation defect in newborns and jaundiced patients. The use of the term "prothrombin" came from the fact that the test was observed to be sensitive to prothrombin. Since then the assay has been modified for its current use in evaluating the extrinsic coagulation, as well as in monitoring oral anticoagulant therapy.

Clinically, the PT/INR is often performed in conjunction with the activated partial thromboplastin time (APTT) and the fibrinogen assay, with these tests known as the "coagulation screen." This standard set of assays represents the starting point for clinicians when diagnosing a bleeding and/or a clotting disorder and is also useful for pre-surgical assessment of patients, to rule out coagulation defects (2–4).

The PT test specifically involves re-calcification of plasma once the sample has been incubated with the thromboplastin reagent (source of tissue factor), which allows for activation of factor X in the presence of factor VII. This test can therefore be used to detect

Paul Monagle (ed.), *Haemostasis: Methods and Protocols*, Methods in Molecular Biology, vol. 992,
DOI 10.1007/978-1-62703-339-8_9, © Springer Science+Business Media New York 2013

the deficiency of the following factors: factors II, V, VII, and X, as well as fibrinogen. In addition, this assay is used for monitoring oral anticoagulant therapy (warfarin).

1.1 Principle

Activation of the coagulation system in a plasma sample in the presence of tissue factor (apoprotein and phospholipid) and $CaCl_2$ leads to the formation of a stable clot. The time from activation to formation of a stable clot is recorded in seconds, and represents the PT. The thromboplastin used in this assay is complete, unlike the APTT reagent, which lacks the apoprotein.

1.2 Standardization

Despite the fact that the PT assay itself is easy to perform, there are numerous variables that need to be considered. These include the thromboplastin source and concentration, the length of incubation, the buffers used, as well as the method used to measure clot formation. In addition, when the same reagents are used on different coagulation analyzers, different results are obtained. Despite the fact that most PT assays are performed on automated analyzers, standardization of this method represents an important problem.

The sensitivity of PT to detect defects in coagulation is highly dependent on the source and type of tissue factor present in the thromboplastin reagent. There are numerous commercially available PT reagents, with TF from different origin, including rabbit brain, human brain, ox brain, rabbit lung, and human placenta. Reagents that contain recombinant human tissue factor are also available and are in use in some laboratories.

In order to minimize the effect of the differences in thromboplastin reagents available, as well as differences in methods used to carry out the PT, the World Health Organization (WHO) has recommended the use of the International Normalized Ratio (INR) (5, 6). This measure is only recommended for assessment of the PT when monitoring oral anticoagulant therapy (7).

The INR takes into account differences in the sensitivities of different thromboplastins. This value corresponds to the ratio of the PT value of patient plasma to that of the mean normal PT (mean from 20 healthy adults), raised to the International Sensitivity Index (ISI).

$$\text{INR} = (\text{Patient PT}/\text{Mean Normal PT})^{\text{ISI}}$$

The ISI is determined by testing plasma samples obtained from healthy patients and patients on warfarin with the thromboplastin used in the laboratory and with the international reference thromboplastin preparation. The values obtained with the two reagents are plotted on a log–log graph and the slope of the regression line represents the ISI value (8). The ISI values of 1–1.2 represent sensitive thromboplastins, while the thromboplastins with higher ISI are less sensitive to changes in factor levels (9). The calculation of a laboratory-specific ISI is extremely important in the pediatric setting, where the mean normal PT is longer compared to adults (10) who usually represent the mean normal population that is used by the manufacturers.

Despite this attempt of standardization, the INR is still dependent on the concentration of citrate in the sample (11, 12), variation in the thromboplastin (13), instruments (14), as well as the International Sensitivity Index, in terms of manufacturer-specific differences, as well as calibration by the individual laboratories (15, 16).

An ideal PT reagent should have a low ISI (approximately 1.0), be able to identify mild to moderate factor deficiency, be insensitive to heparin in the therapeutic range, and be responsive to depression of factor VII observed in liver disease.

1.3 Clinical Applications

The clinical application of PT is aimed at diagnosing the risk of bleeding (deficiency of factors II, V, VII, and X and fibrinogen), monitoring oral anticoagulant therapy (warfarin), as well as detecting the presence of liver disease and vitamin K deficiency and in diagnosing disseminated intravascular coagulation (DIC) (4).

PT can be used in diagnosis of severe acute and chronic liver disease, where liver dysfunction leads to decreased synthesis and secretion of coagulation factors. However, as an example, the detection of the depression of factor VII observed in liver disease is dependent on the use of a sensitive thromboplastin, with an ISI close to 1.0.

PT is useful in monitoring of warfarin therapy because of the sensitivity of the assay to variations of vitamin K-dependent factors II, VII, and X, whose steady state levels are reduced by warfarin.

In patients that are receiving concomitant treatment with warfarin and heparin, treatment with heparinase ensures that the effect of heparin is abolished (17). This allows for the effect of oral anticoagulant therapy to be investigated independent of heparin.

1.4 Interpretation of Results

Interpretation the PT result is extremely important in ensuring that an accurate diagnosis is made and the best care considered for the patient.

1.4.1 Reference Ranges

Reference ranges for PT are dependent on reagent/analyzer combination, as well as the population tested (10). Age-related differences in the PT have been demonstrated with healthy neonates and children having increased reference intervals compared to healthy adults (10, 18–20).

1.4.2 Shortening of the PT

Shortening of the PT is not usually considered as clinically significant. However, this can occur and/or be observed in presence of a blood clot and cancer (21), as well as in the presence of oral contraceptives (22).

Table 1
Factors that lead to the prolongation of the PT

Hereditary factors (deficiencies of)	Acquired factors (presence of)
Factors II, V, VII, and X	Vitamin K deficiency
Fibrinogen	Liver dysfunction (cirrhosis, hepatitis)
Rare inherited bleeding disorders	Disseminated intravascular coagulation (DIC) Heparin Hirudin Argatroban Vitamin K antagonist (warfarin) Lupus anticoagulants Other drugs (i.e., antibiotics) Post-surgery

1.4.3 Prolongation of the PT

Prolongation of the PT can be a result of hereditary or acquired factors. These are summarized in Table 1. Despite the usefulness of this assay, the PT may often not be sensitive to slight single-factor deficiencies (23).

Unexplained prolonged PT results are potentially significant, because of the low sensitivity of the assay. The first step in determining the cause of an unexplained PT prolongation is to perform the assay in the presence of heparinase, which neutralizes heparin. If the PT corrects to a value within the reference range for that laboratory, then the presence of heparin is the cause for the prolongation. If the PT does not correct, then mixing studies are performed, to determine whether the prolongation is due to a factor deficiency (PT corrected) or an inhibitor (PT does not correct) (4).

It is also extremely important to note that "prolongation" of the PT can be observed if adult reference ranges for APTT are used when pediatric samples are tested.

2 Materials

Pre-analytical error (difficulty of sample collection, type of collection tube, length of storage) is the most common type of mistake associated with the PT assay (see Note 1) (24). As an example, shortening of the PT has previously been observed following collection in borosilicate tubes, combined with prolonged storage at 4°C (25). It is therefore extremely important to consider the information presented in the Subheadings 2.1.1–2.1.4 below.

2.1 Specimen

Whole blood.

2.1.1 Collection

NCCLS guidelines recommend collection into plastic or siliconized glass tubes containing 3.2% trisodium citrate (e.g., 9 volumes of blood to 1 volume of 0.109 M trisodium citrate) (26). One of the most important aspects of sample collection for the PT assay involves filling the collection tubes to the correct point (indicated on the tube), as to achieve the adequate ratio of blood sample to anticoagulant. Underfilled or overfilled blood collection tubes should not be used for determination of PT, because this leads to falsely shortened and prolonged PT result (27).

Once the sample is collected, the tube must be mixed immediately by gentle inversion, to allow for the anticoagulant (usually at the bottom of the tube) to mix appropriately with the sample.

An initial discard is recommended in those situations where blood is collected from a heparinized line. However, to date, there has been no agreement on standardization of the amount of discard for specific clinical situations. The risk of heparin contamination of the sample cannot be completely removed and it is preferable that this situation is avoided whenever possible, by using the peripheral vein.

Routine venipuncture is the optimal collection procedure for the PT assay, as it minimizes sample activation. However, with the recent advancement of point of care technology, finger prick collections are being used more frequently in the adult and pediatric setting (28, 29). Care must be taken with such collections, as they can often lead to activation of the sample and hence extreme care must be taken to avoid difficult collections, whenever possible. In addition, the evacuated collection system for collection has been shown to result in a better sample (decrease in clot formation and hemolysis), compared to the syringe collection (30).

2.1.2 Stability

Once collected, the whole blood sample is prone to activation and this can in turn lead to results that are not representative of the true status of the sample. This is particularly because of the presence of platelets which are easily activated and can then lead to activation of soluble coagulation factors.

The NCCLS guidelines for stability of whole blood samples prior to testing recommend storage at room temperature for 2 h and at 4°C for 4 h. However, it is preferable that the testing is performed within 1 h of venipuncture.

2.1.3 Processing

Recommended centrifugation protocol for obtaining a platelet-free plasma sample adequate for coagulation testing includes minimum centrifugation at 2,500 × *g* for 15 min (26).

2.1.4 Storage

Once prepared, the plasma samples can be stored for up to 2 weeks at −20°C and for up to 6 months at −70°C (26). It is important that the plasma sample is separated into smaller aliquots prior to storage. This will allow the sample to freeze quickly and allow for adequate thawing prior to use.

Frozen plasma must be adequately thawed prior to testing (10–15 min in a 37°C water bath) and it is recommended that the testing is performed immediately after thawing. However, in situations where this is not possible, the plasma sample can be stored for 2 h at 4°C prior to use (26).

2.2 Reagents and Reagent Preparation

For commercially available assays, instructions provided by the manufacturer for preparation of reagents and/or instrument should be followed, in order to ensure the validity of the results.

Most reagents used to carry out the PT assay are not toxic; however working with plasma samples of unknown origin carries a certain level of risk that should be minimized by the use of gloves and eye protection.

2.2.1 Thromboplastin (Tissue Factor + Phospholipid)

As mentioned previously, there are a number of different commercially available PT reagents. These reagents usually contain $CaCl_2$ and come lyophilized and/or are pre-diluted (ready to use), with both stored at 4°C. Lyophilized reagents require reconstitution with distilled water. It is important that all PT reagents are mixed well and allowed to stand at room temperature (18–25°C) for approximately 30 min prior to use.

The stability of PT reagents is manufacturer specific; however, 7–12 day stability at 2–8°C is common.

Some PT reagents (Neoplastine, Diagnostica Stago, France) contain a specific inhibitor of heparin (e.g., polybrene), making the test insensitive to both UFH and LMWH levels up to 1 IU/ml and 1 anti-Xa IU/ml, respectively. This is particularly important in the setting of concomitant heparin and warfarin therapy.

2.2.2 Control Plasma

The use of control plasma, with a known clotting time (for a particular PT reagent/analyzer) should be used to ensure accuracy and the reproducibility of the results obtained.

2.3 Clot Detection

Automated coagulation analyzers can detect the formation of a stable clot via two mechanisms. Optical measurement involves the change in opacity of the reagent mixture. The mechanical measurement, on the other hand, detects a change in the consistency of the reaction mixture as the clot formation takes place. This particular method of detection is particularly useful for samples obtained from newborns, as it is not affected by the variables that affect light transmission, such as hyperbilirubinemia or lipemia.

3 Methods

3.1 Assay Procedure

The plasma sample is incubated with a PT reagent containing thromboplastin and $CaCl_2$. This causes initiation of clot formation and the time required for formation of a stable clot is recorded.

3.1.1 Automated Assay

1. Plasma sample is loaded onto the analyzer.
2. 50 μl of the plasma is incubated for 4 min on the analyzer.
3. 50 μl of PT reagent is added to the plasma.
4. The time required for formation of a stable clot is recorded (s).

3.1.2 Manual Assay

Ensure that a water bath is pre-warmed and the temperature stabilized at 37°C and that you have access to a stopwatch (timer) prior to starting the test. Pre-warm the tubes used for testing at 37°C in the water bath (see Note 2).

1. Pre-incubate the 0.025 M $CaCl_2$ solution at 37°C.
2. Gently mix the thromboplastin reagent by inversion.
3. Pipette 0.1 ml of the thromboplastin in the test tube and incubate at 37°C for 2 min.
4. Pipette 0.1 ml test or control plasma into the test tube with the thromboplastin.
5. Incubate at 37°C for approximately 1 min.
6. Add 0.1 ml of the 0.025 M $CaCl_2$ solution and simultaneously start the timer.
7. Gently tilt the reaction tube back and forth (under water as much as possible) in the 37°C water bath, and continually observe for clot formation. Immediately upon formation of a clot, stop the timer and record the clotting time.

3.2 Interpretation of Results

As previously specified, it is essential that each laboratory establishes its own reference values that are specific for the particular PT reagent, analyzer, and sample combination that are used in that particular laboratory. This ensures that PT results can be interpreted correctly, and the best possible care can then be offered to the patient.

4 Notes

1. Major problems/faults related to the PT assay are related to the pre-analytical variables such as sample collection, processing, and storage (see Table 2).
2. For manual testing, it is recommended that a duplicate test is performed. The results of the two results obtained should correlate within 5%.

Table 2
Sources of error for the PT assay

Error	Subheadings	Identification	Cause	Correction
Faulty blood collection	2.1.1	Unexplained prolonged PT	Difficult venipuncture	If possible, sample needs to be re-collected
Partial clotting of the sample	2.1.1	Presence of a blood clot in whole blood	Late mixing with citrate during collection	Sample must be re-collected
Under- and overfilled collection tube	2.1.1	Observation of the sample volume as compared to the "fill line" indicated on the collection tube		Sample must be re-collected
Evidence of hemolysis	2.1.1	Plasma sample appears red	Difficult collection and/or inappropriate processing	If possible, sample needs to be re-collected
Heparin contamination	2.1.1	Unexplained prolonged PT	Blood collected from heparinized lines	The PT corrects upon addition of a heparin inhibitor (heparinase, polybrene)
Use of nonspecific (reagent, analyzer, and age) reference ranges	3.2	Unexplained shortened or prolonged PT	Inappropriate interpretation of the result	Use of appropriate reference ranges

References

1. Quick J (1935) The prothrombin time in haemophilia and in obstructive jaundice. J Biol Chem 109:74–74
2. Cohen AJ, Kessler CM (2002) Haemophilia A and B. In: Kitchens CS, Alving BM, Kessler CM (eds) Consultative hemostasis and thrombosis. WB Saunders, Philadelphia, pp 43–56
3. Roberts HR, Escobar MA (2002) Less common congenital disorders of hemostasis. In: Kitchen S, Alving BM, Kessler CM (eds) Consultative haemostasis and thrombosis. WB Saunders, Philadelphia, pp 57–71
4. Triplett DA (2002) Coagulation abnormalities. In: McClatchey KD (ed) Clinical laboratory medicine, 2nd edn. Lippincott Williams and Wilkins, Philadelphia, pp 1033–1049
5. Haemostasis (1985) ICSH/ISTH recommendations for reporting prothrombin time in oral anticoagulant control. J Clin Pathol 38: 133–134
6. Standardisation (1983) World Health Organization Expert Committee on Biological Standardization. Thirty third report. Technical report series 687. WHO, Geneva, pp 81–105
7. BCSH (1998) Guidelines on oral anticoagulation: third edition. Br J Haematol 101:374–387
8. Beeser H (1988) Critical evaluation of the so far experience using the WHO model of prothrombin time calibration and outlook for further development. Haemostasis 18:181–182
9. Dalen JE, Hirsh J (1995) ACCP 4th Consensus conference introduction. Chest 108:225–265
10. Monagle P, Barnes C, Ignjatovic V, Furmedge J, Newall F, Chan A, De Rosa L, Hamilton S, Ragg P, Robinson S, Auldist A, Crock C, Roy N, Rowlands S (2006) Developmental haemostasis: impact for clinical haemostasis laboratories. Thromb Haemost 95:362–372
11. Adcock DM, Kressin DC, Marlar RA (1997) Effect of 3.2% vs. 3.8% sodium citrate

concentration on routine coagulation testing. Am J Clin Pathol 107:105–110
12. Duncan EM, Casey CR, Duncan BM, Lloyd JV (1994) Effect of concentration of trisodium citrate anticoagulant on the calculation of the International Normalised Ratio and the International Sensitivity Index of thromboplastin. Thromb Haemost 72:84–88
13. van den Besselaar AM (1993) International standardization of laboratory control of oral anticoagulant therapy: a survey of thromboplastin reagents used for prothrombin time testing. J Heart Valve Dis 2:42–52
14. Cunningham MT, Jonhnson GF, Pennell BJ, Olson JD (1994) The reliability of manufacturer-determined, instrument specific international sensitivity index values for calculating the international normalized ratio. Am J Clin Pathol 102:128–133
15. Craig S, Stevenson KJ, Dufty JM, Taberner DA (1997) Local INR correction: justification for a simplified approach. J Clin Pathol 50:783–789
16. Talstad I (2000) Why is the standardization of prothrombin time a problem? Haemostasis 30:258–267
17. Harenberg J, Reichel T, Malsch R, Hirsh J, Rustagi P (1996) Multicentric evaluation of heparinase on aPTT, thrombin clotting time and a new PT reagent based on recombinant human tissue factor. Blood Coagul Fibrinolysis 7:453–458
18. Andrew M, Paes B, Milner R, Johnston M, Mitchell L, Tollefsen DM, Powers P (1987) Development of the human coagulation system in the full-term infant. Blood 70:165–172
19. Andrew M, Paes B, Milner R, Jonston M, Mitchell L, Tollefsen D, Powers P (1988) Development of the human coagulation system in the healthy premature infant. Blood 72:1651–1657
20. Andrew M, Vegh P, Johnston M, Bowker J, Ofosu F, Mitchell L (1992) Maturation of the hemostatic system during childhood. Blood 80:1998–2005
21. Miller SP, Sanchez-Avalmods J, Stefanski T, Zuckerman L (1967) Coagulation disorders in cancer. I. Clinical and laboratory studies. Cancer 20:1452–1465
22. Gordon EM, Ratnoff OD, Jones PK (1982) The role of augmented Hageman factor (factor XII) titers in the cold-promoted activation of factor VII and spontaneous shortening of the prothrombin time in women using oral contraceptives. J Lab Clin Med 99:363–369
23. Van Cott EM, Laposata M (2001) Coagulation. In: Jacobs DS, De Mott WR, Oxley DK (eds) Laboratory test handbook, 5th edn. Lexi-Comp, Hudson, OH, pp 327–358
24. Plebani M, Carraro P (1997) Mistakes in a stat laboratory: types and frequency. Clin Chem 43:1348–1351
25. Palmer RN, Gralnick HR (1985) Inhibition of cold-promoted activation of the prothrombin time. Studies of new siliconized borosilicate collection tubes in normals and patients receiving warfarin. Am J Clin Pathol 83:492–494
26. NCCLS (1998) Collection, transport and processing of blood specimens for coagulation testing and general performance of coagulation assays. In: Standards NCCL (ed) 3rd edn, NCCLS, 940 West Valley Road, Wayne, Pennsylvania 19087, USA.
27. Reneke J, Etzell J, Leslie S (1998) Prolonged prothrombin time and activated partial thromboplastin time due to underfilled specimen tubes with 109 mmol/L (3.2%) citrate anticoagulant. Am J Clin Pathol 109:754–757
28. Ansell J, Becker R, Becker D, Triplett DA, Cimini C, La Duca F (1995) Accurate and precise prothrombin time measurement in a multicenter anticoagulation trial employing patient self-testing. Blood 86:864a
29. Ignjatovic V, Barnes C, Newall F, Hamilton S, Burgess J, Monagle P (2004) Point of care monitoring of oral anticoagulant therapy in children: comparison of CoaguChek and thrombotest methods with venous international normalised ratio. Thromb Haemost 92:734–737
30. Wiwanitkit V (2002) Rejection of specimens for prothrombin time and relating pre-analytical factors in blood collection. Blood Coagul Fibrinolysis 13:371–372

Chapter 10

Thrombin Clotting Time

Vera Ignjatovic

Abstract

Thrombin clotting time (TCT) is a coagulation assay used to diagnose congenital and acquired fibrinogen deficiency, as well as to identify contamination by heparin, prior to performing additional coagulation assays.

This test is based on the principle that in citrated plasma, the addition of Thrombin allows for formation of a stable clot. The time required for the formation of a stable clot is recorded in seconds and represents the actual TCT result.

Key words TCT, TT, Coagulation test

1 Introduction

Thrombin clotting time (TCT) assay is based on work by Clauss in 1957 (1).

TCT represents a core test in coagulation laboratories (2). Clinically, the TCT is often performed prior to activated partial thromboplastin time (APTT) and prothrombin time (PT), to screen for the presence of heparin. This test is the starting point in diagnosing a bleeding and/or clotting disorder. A prolonged TCT usually leads to additional tests, such as the fibrinogen assay, as well as factor assays, for a specific diagnosis.

TCT measures the time required for formation of a stable clot, following addition of thrombin to citrated plasma. This assay provides the measure of conversion of fibrinogen to fibrin and therefore an estimation of the quantity of fibrinogen. The TCT can therefore detect hypo- and hyperfibrinogenemia, dysfibrinogenemia, as well as drugs that prevent conversion of fibrinogen to fibrin (i.e., heparin, hirudin) (3).

1.1 Principle

Thrombin added to citrated plasma results in the conversion of fibrinogen to fibrin, leading to the formation of a stable clot.

Paul Monagle (ed.), *Haemostasis: Methods and Protocols*, Methods in Molecular Biology, vol. 992,
DOI 10.1007/978-1-62703-339-8_10, © Springer Science+Business Media New York 2013

The time from addition of thrombin to formation of a stable clot is recorded in seconds, and represents the TCT.

1.2 Standardization

The thrombin used in the TCT assay is usually of human or bovine origin. Apart from the origin, the major differences in reagents are related to the sensitivity to heparin, as well as the sensitivity to slight deficiencies in fibrinogen (2). The origin of thrombin reflects on the sensitivity of TCT to heparin, as differences have previously been observed between the TCT performed with thrombin of human and bovine origin (4). The concentration of thrombin used in the assay varies between different laboratories and it is therefore very important to specify the actual concentration of thrombin used in a particular TCT assay. Small variations in the amount of thrombin used lead to marked differences in TCT of heparinized plasma (4).

Despite this variation, the TCT, unlike the APTT and PT assays, does not represent a significant challenge in terms of standardization and it is mostly performed on automated coagulation analyzers.

An ideal TCT reagent should have a high sensitivity to heparin and should be able to detect decrease in the quantity of fibrinogen.

1.3 Clinical Applications

TCT is a useful screening test for quantitative (hypo- and hyperfibrinogenemia), as well as qualitative (modifications of the molecule) abnormalities of fibrinogen. Because the TCT is a function of the available fibrinogen, the test can be used to estimate fibrinogen levels. In addition, it allows for detection of inhibitors against thrombin or fibrin.

TCT performed with high concentration of thrombin has been demonstrated to be more accurate compared to the APTT in monitoring unfractionated heparin UFH therapy (5). The high concentration of thrombin allows for TCT results that are unrecordable with the standard concentration of thrombin to become within the recordable range.

In the pediatric population, TCT was found to correlate better to the anti-Xa activity of UFH, compared to the APTT, confirming the possibility that TCT could in fact be useful in monitoring UFH therapy in this population (6).

TCT can assist in the diagnosis of disseminated intravascular coagulation (DIC) and liver disease when performed in combination with the fibrinogen/fibrin degradation product assay.

Monitoring of hirudin therapy using the APTT is influenced by the presence of heparin, lupus anticoagulants, low concentrations of fibrinogen, as well as increased levels of fibrinogen-fibrin degradation products. A modification of the TCT (quantitative thrombin time) has proved particularly useful in this situation, as it does not respond to factors other than the hirudin itself, and therefore provides an accurate measure of the hirudin concentration in plasma or whole blood (7).

The TCT performed with high concentration of thrombin (high-dose thrombin time) is useful in monitoring UFH therapy during cardiopulmonary bypass (8, 9). In this clinical situation, the high concentration of thrombin can overcome the anticoagulant effect of the high dose of UFH that renders the standard TCT un-recordable.

Diluted TCT where the patient's plasma is diluted with plasma from healthy individuals has shown to be useful in estimating the concentration of drugs such as argatroban, lepirudin, and bivalirudin (10). This version of the assay has been proposed as an alternative to the APTT, for monitoring the levels of direct thrombin inhibitors, particularly because of the insensitivity of the test to lupus anticoagulants and low levels of vitamin K-dependent factors (10).

1.4 Interpretation of Results

Interpretation of TCT results is extremely important in ensuring that an accurate diagnosis is made and the best care considered for the patient.

1.4.1 Reference Ranges

Reference ranges for TCT are dependent on reagent/analyzer combination, as well as the population tested (11). Age-related differences in the TCT have been demonstrated with children having increased reference intervals compared to healthy adults (11–14).

The prolongation of the TCT in neonates and children could be the result of a combination of several clotting factors that are decreased in children, rather than one factor in particular.

1.4.2 Shortening of the TCT

Shortening of the TCT is not usually considered as clinically significant and is usually related to improper sample collection, processing, or storage, as well as improper testing.

The antibiotic ristocetin has been shown to prolonged TCT results, in vitro (15). However, to date there have not been any ex vivo studies confirming whether this observation is valid for patients who are receiving ristocetin.

1.4.3 Prolongation of the TCT

The first step in determining the cause of an unexplained TCT prolongation is to perform the assay in the presence of heparinase, which neutralizes heparin. If the TCT corrects to a value within the reference range for that laboratory, then the presence of heparin is the cause for the prolongation. If the TCT does not correct, then further studies are performed to determine the cause of the prolongation (e.g., fibrinogen assay). See Table 1.

Table 1
Factors that lead to the prolongation of TCT

Hereditary factors (deficiencies of)	Acquired factors (presence of)
Afibrinogenemia	Heparin
Hypofibrinogenemia	Renal dysfunction
Dysfibrinogenemia	Liver dysfunction (cirrhosis, hepatitis) Disseminated intravascular coagulation (DIC) Malignancy Thrombolytic therapy (tPA) Argatroban Hirudin Other drugs (i.e., streptokinase)

2 Materials

Pre-analytical error (difficulty of sample collection, type of collection tube, length of storage) is the most common type of mistake associated with the TCT assay (see Note 1). It is therefore extremely important to consider the information presented in the Subheadings 2.1.1–2.1.4 below.

2.1 Specimen

Whole blood.

2.1.1 Collection

NCCLS guidelines recommend collection into plastic or siliconized glass tubes containing 3.2% trisodium citrate (e.g., 9 volumes of blood to 1 volume of 0.109 M trisodium citrate) (16). One of the most important aspects of sample collection for the TCT assay involves filling the collection tubes to the correct point (indicated on the tube), as to achieve the adequate ratio of blood sample to anticoagulant.

Once the sample is collected, the tube must be mixed immediately by gentle inversion, to allow for the anticoagulant (usually at the bottom of the tube) to mix appropriately with the sample.

Routine venipuncture is the optimal collection procedure for the TCT assay, as it minimizes sample activation.

An initial discard is recommended in those situations where blood is collected from a heparinized line (17). However, to date, there has been no agreement on standardization of the amount of discard for specific clinical situations. The risk of heparin contamination of the sample cannot be completely removed and it is preferable that this situation is avoided whenever possible, by using the peripheral vein.

2.1.2 Stability

Once collected, the whole blood sample is prone to activation and this can in turn lead to results that are not representative of the true status of the sample. This is particularly because of the presence of platelets which are easily activated and can then lead to activation of soluble coagulation factors.

The NCCLS guidelines for stability of whole blood samples prior to testing recommend storage at room temperature for 2 h and at 4°C for 4 h.

2.1.3 Processing

Recommended centrifugation protocol for obtaining a platelet-free plasma sample adequate for coagulation testing includes minimum centrifugation at 2,500 ×*g* for 15 min (16).

2.1.4 Storage

Once prepared, the plasma samples can be stored for up to 2 weeks at −20°C and for up to 6 months at −70°C (16). It is important that the plasma sample is separated into smaller aliquots prior to storage. This will allow the sample to freeze quickly and allow for adequate thawing prior to use.

Frozen plasma must be adequately thawed prior to testing (10–15 min in a 37°C water bath) and it is recommended that the testing is performed immediately after thawing. However, in situations where this is not possible, the plasma sample can be stored for 2 h at 4°C prior to use (16).

2.2 Reagents and Reagent Preparation

For commercially available assays, instructions provided by the manufacturer for preparation of reagents and/or instrument should be followed, in order to ensure the validity of the results.

Most reagents used to carry out the TCT assay are not toxic; however working with plasma samples of unknown origin carries a certain level of risk that should be minimized by the use of gloves and eye protection.

2.2.1 Thrombin

As mentioned previously, the thrombin used in this assay is mostly of human or bovine origin. TCT reagent (thrombin) usually comes lyophilized and is stored at 4°C. The reconstitution is usually performed with addition of distilled water.

It is important that thrombin is mixed well and allowed to stand at room temperature (18–25°C) for approximately 30 min prior to use. The stability of thrombin for the TCT assay is manufacturer specific; however 7-day stability at 2–8°C is common.

2.2.2 Control Plasma

The use of control plasma with a known clotting time (for a particular TCT reagent/analyzer) should be used to ensure that the method has been set up adequately.

2.3 Clot Detection

Automated coagulation analyzers can detect the formation of a stable clot via two mechanisms. Optical measurement involves the change in opacity of the reagent mixture. The mechanical measurement, on the other hand, detects a change in the consistency of the reaction mixture as the clot formation takes place.

This particular method of detection is particularly useful for samples obtained from newborns, as it is not affected by the variables that affect light transmission, such as hyperbilirubinemia or lipemia.

3 Methods

3.1 Assay Procedure

The plasma sample is incubated with thrombin. This causes initiation of clot formation and the time required for formation of a stable clot is recorded.

3.1.1 Automated Assay

1. Plasma sample is loaded onto the analyzer.
2. 100 μl of the plasma is incubated for 4 min on the analyzer.
3. 100 μl of thrombin is added to the plasma.
4. The time required for formation of a stable clot is recorded(s).

3.1.2 Manual Assay

Ensure that a water bath is pre-warmed and the temperature stabilized at 37°C and that you have access to a stopwatch (timer) prior to starting the test. Pre-warm the tubes used for testing at 37°C in the water bath (see Note 2).

1. Pipette 0.1 ml test or control plasma into the test tube.
2. Incubate the sample at 37°C 4 min.
3. Add 0.1 ml thrombin and simultaneously start the timer.
4. Gently tilt the reaction tube back and forth (under water as much as possible) in the 37°C water bath, and continually observe for clot formation. Immediately upon formation of a clot, stop the timer and record the clotting time.

3.2 Interpretation of Results

As previously specified, it is essential that each laboratory establishes its own reference values that are specific for the particular TCT reagent, analyzer, and sample combination that are used in that particular laboratory. This ensures that TCT results can be interpreted correctly, and the best possible care can then be offered to the patient.

4 Notes

1. The major problems/faults related to the TCT assay are related to the pre-analytical variables, such as sample collection, processing, and storage (see Table 2).
2. For manual testing, it is recommended that a duplicate test is performed. The results of the two results obtained should correlate within 5%.

Table 2
Sources of error for the TCT assay

Error	Subheading	Identification	Cause	Correction
Faulty blood collection	2.1.1	Unexplained prolonged TCT	Difficult venipuncture	If possible, sample needs to be re-collected
Partial clotting of the sample	2.1.1	Presence of a blood clot in whole blood	Late mixing with citrate during collection	Sample must be re-collected
Under- and overfilled collection tube	2.1.1	Observation of the sample volume as compared to the "fill line" indicated on the collection tube		Sample must be re-collected
Evidence of hemolysis	2.1.1	Plasma sample appears red	Difficult collection and/or inappropriate processing	If possible, sample needs to be re-collected
Heparin contamination	2.1.1	Unexplained prolonged TCT	Blood collected from heparinized lines	The TCT corrects upon addition of a heparin inhibitor (heparinase, polybrene)
Use of nonspecific (reagent, analyzer, and age) reference ranges	3.2	Unexplained shortened or prolonged TCT	Inappropriate interpretation of the result	Use of appropriate reference ranges

References

1. Clauss VA (1957) Gerinnungsphysiologische schnell methode zur bestimmun des fibrinogens. Acta Haematol 17:237–246
2. Flanders MM, Crist R, Rodgers GM (2003) Comparison of five thrombin time reagents. Clin Chem 49:169–172
3. Bockenstedt PL (1998) Laboratory methods in hemostasis. In: Loscalzo J, Schafer AI (eds) Thrombosis and hemorrhage, 2nd edn. Williams and Wilkins, Baltimore, pp 517–580
4. Ts'ao CH, Raymond J, Kolb T, Lo R (1976) Effects of source and concentration of thrombin, and divalent cations, on thrombin time of heparinized plasma. Am J Clin Pathol 65: 206–212
5. Ray MJ, Perrin EJ, Smith IR, Hawson GA (1996) A proposed model to monitor heparin therapy using the concentrated thrombin time which allows standardisation of reagents and improved estimation of heparin concentrations. Blood Coag Fibrinol 7:515–521
6. Chan A, Black L, Ing C, Williams S, Brandao L, Walter K, Abdelhaleem M (2005) Utility of aPTT in monitoring unfractionated heparin in children. J Thromb Haemost 3, abstract OR360.
7. Reid TJR, Alving BM (1993) A quantitative thrombin time for determining levels of hirudin and hirulog. Thromb Haemost 70: 608–616
8. Shore-Lesserson L, Manspeizer HE, Bolastig M, Harrington D, Vela-Cantos F, DePerio M (2000) Anticoagulation for cardiac surgery in patients receiving preoperative heparin: use of

high-dose thrombin time. Anaesth Analg 90:813–818
9. Wang JS, Lin C, Karp RB (1994) Comparison of high-dose thrombin time with activated clotting time for monitoring of anticoagulant effects of heparin in cardiac surgical patients. Anaesth Analg 79:9–13
10. Love JE, Ferrell C, Chandler WL (2007) Monitoring direct thrombin inhibitors with a plasma diluted thrombin time. Thromb Haemost 98:234–242
11. Monagle P, Barnes C, Ignjatovic V, Furmedge J, Newall F, Chan A, De Rosa L, Hamilton S, Ragg P, Robinson S, Auldist A, Crock C, Roy N, Rowlands S (2006) Developmental haemostasis: impact for clinical haemostasis laboratories. Thromb Haemost 95:362–372
12. Andrew M, Paes B, Milner R, Johnston M, Mitchell L, Tollefsen DM, Powers P (1987) Development of the human coagulation system in the full-term infant. Blood 70:165–172
13. Andrew M, Paes B, Milner R, Jonston M, Mitchell L, Tollefsen D, Powers P (1988) Development of the human coagulation system in the healthy premature infant. Blood 72:1651–1657
14. Andrew M, Vegh P, Johnston M, Bowker J, Ofosu F, Mitchell L (1992) Maturation of the hemostatic system during childhood. Blood 80:1998–2005
15. Aronstam A, Dennis B, Friesen MN, Clark WF, Linton AL, Lindsay RM (1978) Ristocetin and the thrombin clotting time. J Clin Pathol 31:1106–1110
16. NCCLS (1998) Collection, transport and processing of blood specimens for coagulation testing and general performance of coagulation assays. In: Standards NCCL (ed) 3rd edn, NCCLS, 940 West Valley Road, Wayne, PA, USA.
17. Adcock DM, Jensen R, Johns CS, Macy PA (2002) Coagulation handbook. Esoterix Coagulation, Austin, TX

Chapter 11

Thrombin Generation

Leslie R. Berry and Anthony K.C. Chan

Abstract

Generation of thrombin has been established as the critical process leading to coagulation in vivo. Indeed, ex vivo markers of thrombin generation in patients have been useful in detecting thrombosis, while many standard global clot-time tests of haemostasis in blood or plasma samples are simple endpoint measures of the potential to generate thrombin. Thus, there has been a recent surge towards direct measurement of thrombin generation potential in plasma/blood samples as a refined methodology for more precisely assessing procoagulant/anticoagulant/hemorrhagic parameters of the haemostatic status. Presently, however, there is no consensus method for thrombin generation determination. The present treatise gives detailed procedures for available thrombin generation tests, with emphasis on the preferred technology.

Key words Thrombin generation, ETP, Plasma, Blood, Thrombin substrate, Fibrin, Anticoagulant

1 Introduction

Plasma coagulation stems from a cascade of proenzyme activations leading to conversion of prothrombin to thrombin, which in turn reacts with fibrinogen to give the fibrin polymer clot (see Fig. 1) (1). In vivo, control of thrombin generation has long been considered critical given that thrombin is a pivotal factor within the coagulation cascade (2). Apart from its direct role in fibrin production, thrombin can facilitate its own formation by feedback activation of upstream factors V, VIII, and XI (3–5). Furthermore, when bound to thrombomodulin, thrombin can limit factor X and prothrombin activations by generation of activated protein C, which inactivates cofactors Va and VIIIa (6). Thrombin also displays a diverse range of other activities outside of the direct coagulation cascade pathway such as activation of cell receptors (7) and inhibition of fibrinolysis by thrombomodulin-mediated cleavage of thrombin-activatable fibrinolysis inhibitor (8). Over time, inhibition of active free thrombin occurs mainly through the two native plasma protease inhibitors antithrombin (AT) and alpha-2-macroglobulin (A2M). Although

Paul Monagle (ed.), *Haemostasis: Methods and Protocols*, Methods in Molecular Biology, vol. 992,
DOI 10.1007/978-1-62703-339-8_11,

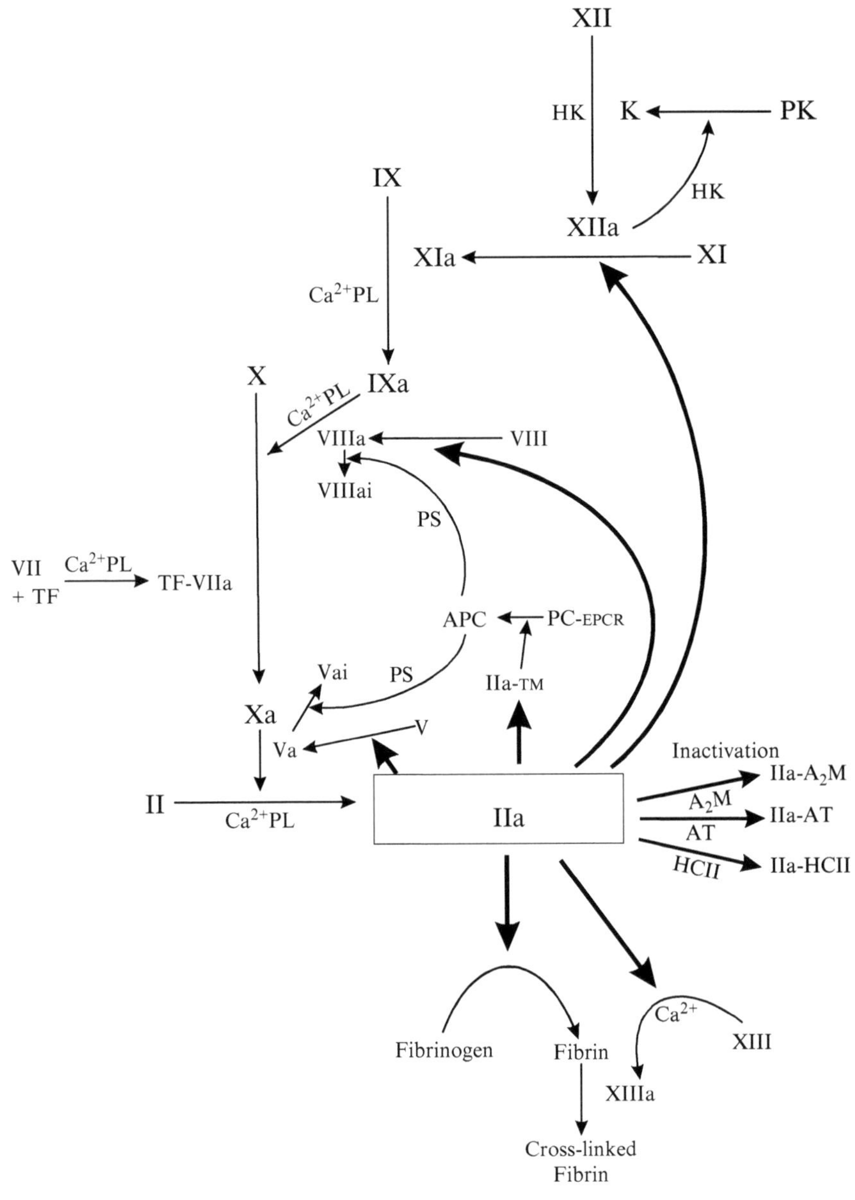

Fig. 1 Coagulation cascade. Thrombin generation proceeds according to the paradigm above with initiation by tissue factor or the factor XII contact phase, inactivation of cofactors by activated protein C + protein S, and neutralization of thrombin by plasma protease inhibitors. Coagulation factors are given as roman numerals. Subscript "*a*" indicates activated factor and subscript "*i*" indicates inactivated factor. *HK* high molecular weight kininogen, *PK* prekallikrein, *K* kallikrein, *PL* phospholipid, *TF* tissue factor, *PC* protein C, *APC* activated protein C, *PS* protein S, *TM* thrombomodulin, *EPCR* endothelial protein C receptor, *AT* antithrombin, *A2M* alpha-2-macroglobulin, *HCII* heparin cofactor II

it has been shown that AT is the main inhibitor of thrombin generated in adult plasma, A2M plays a role comparable to AT for thrombin neutralization in newborns and children (9, 10).

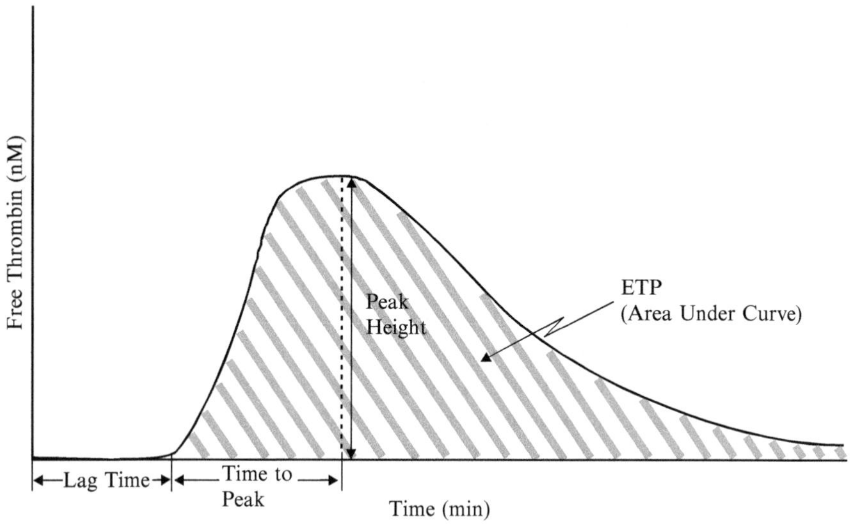

Fig. 2 Thrombin generation time course. Free physiological thrombin activity is generated from recalcified, activated plasma over time in vitro according to a skewed bell-shaped profile. Four major parameters are identified

With more sophisticated understanding of in vivo coagulation pathway mechanisms, there has been a growing groundswell of efforts to directly follow the capacity of plasma samples to generate thrombin upon activation. Early methods used a fibrinogen clot time to measure thrombin expressed in clotting dilute fresh blood samples (11). Although crude in terms of precision, these early studies suggested the general profile for plasma thrombin generation. Plots of thrombin activity versus time show skewed bell curves that can be defined by at least four parameters (Fig. 2). Initially, a phase called the lag time exists which spans the period from addition of calcium + activators to first measurable appearance of functional thrombin. Once detectable thrombin is observed, activity increases sigmoidally to a maximum (Fig. 2). This phase can be characterized by the time to peak (period from initial thrombin activity up to maximum thrombin) and peak height (highest thrombin activity value attained). During the entire thrombin generation phenomenon, native AT and A2M proteins (and to some degree heparin cofactor II) act to neutralize the thrombin produced. By mass action, inhibition accelerates as the amount of available thrombin increases. Thus, at a point approaching maximal conversion of prothrombin (12), inhibition of thrombin predominates relative to formation and the concentration of active molecules falls logarithmically from peak levels down to a final basal equilibrium state (Fig. 2). One measure of the overall potential of the activated sample to generate thrombin is often given as the area under the entire time-course curve (AUC). Although interpretation of the AUC or endogenous thrombin potential (ETP) value may be harder to associate with actual physical molecular mechanisms occurring within the biochemical system, comparison of ETP between samples has a somewhat global feature since it encompasses all of the phases from activation to final endpoint.

Free thrombin generation in plasma samples has been developed in the last 2–3 decades using chromogenic or fluorogenic peptide substrates that are selective for thrombin over other coagulation enzymes. Surveys of the methods used fall into two general categories. Thus, determination of thrombin generation has been done either through discontinuous subsampling of the plasma sample reaction mixture into stop solutions containing substrate or by continuous registration of thrombin activity via substrate in situ. Tripeptide substrates detect thrombin in both the free state and in complex with A2M (which acts as a molecular cage around the enzyme that only restricts macromolecular substrates from contacting the still functional active site) (13). Thus, actual direct measurements that give the physiologically active thrombin at various time points are only achieved by subsampling of reaction mixture into substrate. This is achieved by placing a subsample at time = t into a chelator (to stop further prothrombin conversion) containing either buffer or buffer with added excess AT + heparin, followed by measurement of residual thrombin with substrate. Subtraction of thrombin activity for subsamples with exogenous AT + heparin (thrombin–A2M) from thrombin activity for corresponding subsamples placed in buffer only (free thrombin + thrombin–A2M) yields direct calculation of free thrombin at each time point (14). This methodology is cumbersome and allows for a limited number of time points to construct the thrombin generation profile, but there is assurance that the true uninhibited thrombin is measured in the system being assayed. Unfortunately, subsampling methods do not permit determination of free thrombin in clotting plasma or blood. In an attempt to develop a method that can be automated and may give information in clotting samples, protocols evolved that had substrate included within the activated plasma mixture (15). Laborious subsampling is eliminated and introduction of fluorescent substrates has allowed estimation of thrombin activity in the presence of fibrin. Some debate exists regarding the degree to which optimal measurement of physiologically active thrombin has been established by the in situ substrate, continuous assay of thrombin. Clearly, the subsampling assay hampers large clinical sample assessment and requires strong practical training. However, determination of free thrombin in the continuous thrombin test does not directly detect thrombin–A2M on the time-curve for subtraction from the actual measured total thrombin (continuous tests take the endpoint activity as measured final thrombin–A2M and extrapolate to subtract thrombin–A2M along the curve using estimates involving kinetics of the thrombin + A2M reaction). Unfortunately, in pediatric plasmas with widely varying A2M concentration, accurate determination of free thrombin by indirect means is impeded by uncertainty of true thrombin–A2M generation over time (16).

Procedures to determine thrombin generation are described for direct subsampling detection in macro- or micro-samples, followed by a recent test for continuous registration of thrombin in clotting plasma. Each test is tailored to the sample format being considered. Only continuous assays can be used for the clotting system. However, we do recommend use of subsampling in defibrinated plasma since data provide real measured free thrombin for head-to-head comparison of widely variable samples. Although native fibrin(ogen) needs to be absent for the subsampling, because all samples have the same condition of zero fibrinogen level, comparisons will be matched for this factor.

2 Materials

2.1 Sample Preparation

1. Venous blood samples (9 volumes) are taken using 18–20 gauge needles into 0.109 M (3.2% mass/volume) trisodium citrate dihydrate (1 volume), followed by centrifugation in plastic tubes at 3,000 × *g* for 15 min (preferably at 4 °C) and careful removal of supernatant platelet-poor plasma into plastic (microfuge) tubes (see Note 1).
2. Plasma in plastic tubes can be stored at −80 °C prior to assay (see Note 2).

2.2 Subsampling Protocol

1. 0.02 M HEPES 0.140 M NaCl 0.1 mg/mL bovine albumin (≥99% pure, catalogue # A-7638, Sigma, Mississauga, ON, Canada) pH 7.35 (HBS-BA) is prepared by dissolving NaCl, bovine albumin, and the acid form of HEPES in H_2O, followed by pH adjustment using 4 M NaOH. Storage of HBS-BA is at 4 °C for at least 2 weeks.
2. 0.020 M $CaCl_2$ in HBS-BA is prepared by dissolving $CaCl_2$ to the desired concentration in HBS-BA and kept at 4 °C before use.
3. Reptilase (Batroxobin maranhao®) (Centerchem Inc., Norwalk, CT, USA). Working solutions of reptilase for plasma defibrination are prepared by dissolving 100 units of dry commercial product in 2 mL of H_2O (see Note 3), followed by storage at −20 °C in 100 μL aliquots.
4. Commercial tissue factor reagent Thromborel® S (Dade Behring, Marburg, Germany) is resuspended with H_2O according to the manufacturer. Resuspended reagent can be kept at 4 °C for up to 4 days and is composed of lipidated tissue factor from human placenta that has an estimated activity equivalent to 42.8 nM relipidated recombinant human tissue factor (see Note 4).

5. Dilute tissue factor reagent: mix 1 volume of commercial Thromborel® S with 15 volumes of 0.020 M $CaCl_2$ in HBS-BA.
6. Chelating agent for stopping thrombin generation in plasma reaction mixture time samples is prepared as 5 mM disodium ethylenediaminetetraacetic acid (Na_2EDTA) in H_2O.
7. Stock commercial antithrombin (AT) (Enzyme Research Laboratories, South Bend, IN, USA) has an MW of 59,000 Da and is typically sold in 1–2 mg/mL lots.
8. Stock commercial unfractionated heparin (weight average MW = 15,000) (Leo Laboratories, Ajax, ON, Canada) at 10,000 IU/mL.
9. AT–heparin solution for inhibition of free thrombin: combine stock commercial AT + stock commercial heparin + HBS-BA to give 0.575 mg AT + 20 IU heparin per mL total volume.
10. Human thrombin (MW = 37,000 Da) for use as a standard (Enzyme Research Laboratories).
11. Stock 5 mM S-2238 chromogenic substrate: dissolve dry commercial reagent (25 mg S-2238) (DiaPharma Group Inc, West Chester, OH, USA) in 8 mL of H_2O. Stock S-2238 can be stored at 4°C for at least 1 month.
12. Working substrate solution (constructed on day of assay): mix 1 volume of stock 5 mM S-2238 with 30 volumes of HBS-BA (working substrate is maintained at room temperature when not in use).
13. Stop solution: 50% (volume/volume) acetic acid in H_2O.

2.3 Continuous Protocol

1. Thrombinoscope (Maastricht, Netherlands) provides reagents as part of a kit that can be used to carry out the continuous thrombin generation assay (calibrated automated thrombography). However, some reagents are still required by the investigator. Alternatively, we list materials below for the independent construction of the continuous assay.
2. 0.02 M HEPES 0.140 M NaCl 5 mg/mL bovine albumin pH 7.35 (HBS-BA2) is prepared in a similar manner to that for HBS-BA in the subsampling protocol, and stored frozen at −20 °C until needed.
3. 0.02 M HEPES 60 mg/mL bovine albumin pH 7.35 is prepared similarly to HBS-BA and can be stored for a few days at 4 °C.
4. 1 M $CaCl_2$ is prepared and stored at 4 °C for up to 2 weeks.
5. Z-Gly-Gly-Arg-AMC fluorogenic substrate can be purchased from Bachem (Torrance, CA, USA). Dry fluorogenic product is dissolved in dimethyl sulfoxide to make a 100 mM stock solution that can be stored at 4 °C.

6. Working fluorogenic substrate solution in buffered calcium (Ca–Fl) is prepared fresh at 37 °C on day of assay in a polystyrene tube (Sarstedt, VWR, Mississauga, ON, Canada) by combining in order: 875 μL 0.02 M HEPES 60 mg/mL bovine albumin pH 7.35 + 100 μL 1 M $CaCl_2$ + 25 μL 100 mM substrate in dimethyl sulfoxide, with vigorous vortex mixing between each addition. Final working Ca–Fl is 0.1 M in Ca^{2+} and 2.5 mM in fluorogen.
7. Recombinant tissue factor (rTF) Innovin® (see Note 5) is obtained from Dade Behring (Marburg, Germany).
8. Phospholipid cocktail: phosphatidylserine, phosphatidylethanolamine, and phosphatidylcholine (Avanti Polar Lipids, Alabaster, AL, USA) are combined in a 20%:20%:60% mole ratio, respectively, solvent is removed under N_2 at 45 °C, followed by resuspension in 0.020 M Tris–HCl, 0.150 M NaCl pH 7.4 to a final total phospholipid concentration of 1 mM and extrusion 29 times through a 0.1 μm pore-size polycarbonate filter (Glen Creston Ltd, Stanmore, UK).
9. Working rTF–phospholipid mixture is prepared on day of assay by vortex mixing commercial rTF + phospholipid cocktail + HBS-BA2 to give 30 pM rTF and 24 μM phospholipids.
10. Thrombin–A2M (600 nM in terms of thrombin activity) calibrator from Thrombinoscope BV is obtained for use as a reference of thrombin activity and to correct for variable quenching effects from individual samples of clotting plasma (see Note 6).

2.4 Instrumentation

1. Thrombin generation reactions involving test tube time samples yield 1 mL volumes for determination of thrombin activity following termination of chromogenic substrate reaction with sub-aliquots of time samples. Absorbance at 405 nm of *para*-nitroaniline product can be measured using a cuvette in a wide number of visible range spectrophotometer machines.
2. Measurement of thrombin chromogenic substrate activity in the microtiter plate thrombin generation protocol requires a microtiter plate absorbance spectrophotometer. In the assay described here, the instrumental requirements include ability to maintain plate temperature at 37 °C and make kinetic readings over time to obtain thrombin activity in terms of a rate of substrate cleavage (absorbance/unit time). Several devices are available for this purpose, such as the SpectraMax series from Molecular Devices (Sunnyvale, CA, USA) and the Multiskan from Thermo Fisher Scientific (Ottawa, ON, Canada). Alternatively, if thrombin substrate reaction is carried out at room temperature with endpoint absorbance readings taken after stoppage by acetic acid, several downscale plate readers are sufficient for absorbance measurements (such as Model 680 plate reader from Bio-Rad (Hercules, CA, USA)).

3. Fluorescence measurements in the continuous thrombin registration methods need to be taken at a minimum frequency of 15 s, while heating control at 37 °C is optimal for physiological fibrin clot conditions. A smaller subset of instruments are able to read fluorescence over an entire 96-well plate within the 15 s limit. Potential instruments include the SpectraMax M5 from Molecular Devices. Optionally, the Fluoroskan Ascent from Thermo Fisher Scientific is a versatile and economical machine capable of satisfying the mandatory requirements of this assay.

3 Methods

Choice of reagents and protocols is dependent on whether defibrin(ogen)ated plasma, platelet-poor plasma, or platelet-rich plasma is being used. This holds true regardless of whether subsampling or continuous protocols are being applied. Although some preliminary methods have been proposed for analysis of thrombin generation in whole blood (17), significant issues remain for clotting blood analysis, especially involving the large quenching interferences from hemoglobin and thrombus materials.

3.1 Subsampling Protocol with Test Tube Time Samples (Macrotechnique)

1. If frozen, an aliquot of platelet-poor plasma is thawed at 37 °C and then kept on ice between manipulations (see Note 7).
2. Plasma (500 μL) is defibrinated by heating at 37 °C with working reptilase solution (5 μL) for 10 min in a plastic tube. Fibrin clot is wound out using a 10 μL (3.5 mm I.D.) plastic loop and the resultant plasma placed on ice for another 10 min prior to winding out any further clot formation. Defibrinated plasma is kept on ice prior to use (see Note 8).
3. Tubes (Sarstedt 12 mm × 75 mm polystyrene test tubes) for reaction mixture time points (one per time point) are placed in crushed ice and each filled with 475 μL of 5 mM Na_2EDTA. A control blank for the reaction is prepared by mixing 475 μL of 5 mM Na_2EDTA with 12.5 μL of dilute tissue factor reagent and vigorous vortexing for 1 s, followed by 12.5 μL of defibrinated plasma with vortexing (blank maintained on ice until substrate reaction).
4. For thrombin–A2M time sample measurements, 25 μL of AT–heparin solution is pipetted in tubes embedded in crushed ice.
5. Tubes (12 mm × 75 mm) containing 775 μL of working substrate solution are placed in a 37 °C H_2O bath awaiting assay of thrombin activity in aliquots of Na_2EDTA-neutralized reaction-mixture time samples.
6. Prewarm 200 μL of dilute tissue factor reagent in a polystyrene tube maintained in a 37 °C H_2O bath.

7. Place 150 μL of defibrinated plasma in a 12 mm×75 mm polystyrene tube, and equilibrate for 3 min in a 37 °C H_2O bath.
8. Simultaneously start a clock as 150 μL of prewarmed dilute tissue factor reagent is rapidly added by pipettor (plastic tips) to the 150 μL of defibrinated plasma. Immediately, vigorously vortex the tube+contents for 1 s and replace in the 37 °C bath.
9. At 15, 30, 45, 60, 75, 90, 120, 180, 240, and 300 s after addition of tissue factor to defibrinated plasma, pipet 25 μL of reaction mixture into the 475 μL of cold 5 mM Na_2EDTA, followed immediately by a 1 s vigorous vortex mixing (see Note 9). Keep each tube containing Na_2EDTA-neutralized reaction time sample mixture on ice until reaction time-point subsampling is complete.
10. Once all time samples have been taken, add 25 μL from the reaction blank (step 3) and each Na_2EDTA-neutralized mixture to separate tubes of working substrate, followed by 1 s vigorous vortexing and incubation at 37 °C for 10 min.
11. Following substrate incubation, pipet 200 μL of 50% acetic acid into each tube and vortex rapidly for 1 s.
12. Acetic acid terminated substrate mixtures are allowed to come to room temperature, followed by measurement of the para-nitroaniline absorbance at 405 nm in a cuvette. This resultant chromogenic response gives activity from free thrombin and thrombin–A2M (total thrombin) (18).
13. Determination of thrombin–A2M generated at each time point is achieved by repeating the assay for total thrombin (using the same defibrinated plasma sample), except that each 25 μL plasma-tissue factor time sample is added to 25 μL of AT–heparin solution on ice, followed by immediate 1 s vortex mixing and (after all time sampling is complete) addition of 450 μL of 5 mM Na_2EDTA with vortexing. A control blank is constructed by combining 450 μL of 5 mM Na_2EDTA (on ice) with 12.5 μL of dilute tissue factor reagent, followed by 25 μL of AT–heparin solution and 12.5 μL of defibrinated plasma (with vortex mixing between each addition). Thrombin–A2M substrate activity in the AT–heparin–Na_2EDTA (free thrombin neutralized) samples is then measured in the same manner as for total thrombin.
14. Activity from thrombin standards is determined by reacting 25 μL of commercial human thrombin diluted in HBS-BA (0, 2.5, 5, 10, 20, 30, or 40 nM) with 775 μL working substrate solution in polystyrene tubes at 37 °C for 10 min, followed by neutralization with 200 μL of 50% acetic acid and measurement of the absorbance at 405 nm.

3.2 Subsampling Protocol in Microtiter Plates

1. If frozen, an aliquot of platelet-poor plasma is thawed at 37 °C and then kept on ice between manipulations (see Note 7).
2. Plasma (200 μL) is defibrinated by heating at 37 °C with working reptilase solution (2 μL) for 10 min in a 12 mm × 75 mm polystyrene tube. Fibrin clot is wound out using a 10 μL (3.5 mm I.D.) plastic loop (Thermo Fisher Scientific, Ottawa, ON, Canada) and the resultant plasma placed on ice for another 10 min prior to winding out any further clot formation. Defibrinated plasma is kept on ice prior to use (see Note 8).
3. Microtiter tubes (1 mL, 4.5 mm I.D. × 8.8 mm long, polypropylene tubes, Bio-Rad, Mississauga, ON, Canada) for reaction mixture time points (one per time point) are placed in an open-bottomed microtiter rack (see Note 10) packed in crushed ice and each filled with 190 μL of 5 mM Na_2EDTA. A control blank for the reaction is prepared by mixing 190 μL of 5 mM Na_2EDTA with 5 μL of dilute tissue factor reagent and vigorous vortexing for 1 s, followed by 5 μL of defibrinated plasma with vortexing (blank maintained on ice until substrate reaction).
4. For thrombin–A2M time sample measurements, 10 μL of AT–heparin solution is pipetted into a similar set of titer tubes embedded in crushed ice.
5. In preparation for assay of thrombin activity in Na_2EDTA-neutralized reaction-mixture time samples, place 175 μL of working substrate solution into wells of a 96-well microtiter plate (BD Falcon, polystyrene, 0.3 mL flat-bottom wells) held in a microtiter plate reader maintained at 37 °C (see Note 11).
6. Prewarm 100 μL of dilute tissue factor reagent in a polystyrene tube maintained in a 37 °C H_2O bath.
7. Place 60 μL of defibrinated plasma in a 12 mm × 75 mm polystyrene tube, and equilibrate for 3 min in a 37 °C H_2O bath.
8. Simultaneously start a clock as 60 μL of prewarmed dilute tissue factor reagent is rapidly added by pipettor (plastic tips) to the 60 μL of defibrinated plasma. Immediately, vigorously vortex the tube + contents for 1 s and replace in the 37 °C bath.
9. At 15, 30, 45, 60, 75, 90, 120, 180, 240, and 300 s after addition of tissue factor to defibrinated plasma, pipet 10 μL of reaction mixture into the 190 μL of cold 5 mM Na_2EDTA, followed immediately by a 1 s vigorous vortex mixing (see Note 9). Keep each tube containing Na_2EDTA-neutralized reaction time sample mixture on ice until reaction time-point subsampling is complete.
10. Once all time samples have been taken, using a multichannel pipet add 25 μL from the reaction blank (step 3) and each Na_2EDTA-neutralized mixture to microtiter plate wells containing the 175 μL of working substrate, followed by 1 s mixing

by withdrawal/repipetting of the substrate reaction mixture. Thrombin substrate activity is measured by kinetic absorbance measurements (absorbance/min obtained by readings taken every 15 s) at 405 nm in the microtiter plate reader over 10 min at 37 °C (see Note 12). This resultant chromogenic response gives activity from free thrombin and thrombin–A2M (total thrombin) (18).

11. Determination of thrombin–A2M generated at each time point is achieved by repeating the assay for total thrombin (using the same defibrinated plasma sample), except that each 10 μL plasma-tissue factor time sample is added to 10 μL of AT–heparin solution on ice, followed by immediate 1 s vortex mixing and (after all time sampling is complete) addition of 180 μL of 5 mM Na_2EDTA with vortexing. A control blank is constructed by combining 180 μL of 5 mM Na_2EDTA (on ice) with 5 μL of dilute tissue factor reagent, followed by 10 μL of AT–heparin solution and 5 μL of defibrinated plasma (with vortex mixing between each addition). Thrombin–A2M substrate activity in the AT–heparin–Na_2EDTA (free thrombin neutralized) samples is then measured in the same manner as for total thrombin.
12. Activity from thrombin standards is determined by reacting 25 μL of commercial human thrombin diluted in HBS-BA (0, 2.5, 5, 10, 20, 30, or 40 nM) with 175 μL working substrate solution in microtiter plate wells in the kinetic plate reader at 37 °C over 10 min (see Notes 11 and 12).

3.3 Continuous Protocol

1. Assays are done in Dynex Immulon 2HB polycarbonate round-bottom 96-well plates (VWR).
2. Place 80 μL of plasma into each of two wells.
3. Add 20 μL of working rTF–phospholipid mixture to one well of plasma and 20 μL of 600 nM thrombin–A2M calibrator to plasma in the other well, followed by two cycles of withdrawal/repipetting to mix (minimize bubble formation due to agitation). Incubate in fluorimeter at 37 °C for 5 min.
4. Start reactions by simultaneous addition, with mixing, of 20 μL of Ca–Fl to each well.
5. Start kinetic fluorescence assay in fluorimeter (excitation = 390 nm, emission = 460 nm) with measurements taken every 15 s for a total of 30 min. Under direction of Thrombinoscope® software (Thrombinoscope BV), rate of fluorescence increase between readings in the rTF–phospholipid well is compared to that with thrombin–A2M calibrator to give nM thrombin, which is corrected for thrombin–A2M by an algorithm that takes equilibrium endpoint activity as equivalent to total final thrombin–A2M complexes generated.

	A	*B*	*C*	*D*	*E*
	Time (min)	**Absorbance Total Thrombin**	**Absorbance Thrombin-A_2M**	**Free Thrombin**	**Area**
1	t_0	$Abs_{(T)0}$	$Abs_{(TA)0}$	= (*B1* – *C1*) X[a]	0
2	t_1	$Abs_{(T)1}$	$Abs_{(TA)1}$	= (*B2* – *C2*) X	= ((*D2* + *D1*)/2)(*A2* – *A1*)
3	t_2	$Abs_{(T)2}$	$Abs_{(TA)2}$	= (*B3* – *C3*) X	= ((*D3* + *D2*)/2)(*A3* – *A2*)
:	:	:	:	:	:
N	t_m	$Abs_{(T)m}$	$Abs_{(TA)m}$	= (*BN* – *CN*) X	= ((*DN* + *DN-1*)/2)(*AN* – *AN-1*)

[a]X = (nM Thrombin per Absorbance Unit) x plasma dilution factor in assay

ETP = Σ *E1* + *E2* + … + *EN*

Fig. 3 Calculation of endogenous thrombin potential (ETP) from substrate reaction data. Analysis of thrombin generation data from the subsampling protocol is shown in a spreadsheet format with formulae in cells for calculations. Free thrombin activity (total thrombin chromogenic activity—thrombin–A2M chromogenic activity) is converted to equivalent nM concentration in original plasma by using the thrombin substrate activity derived from the standard curve and the factor for dilution of plasma in the assay. ETP (nM min) is given as the area under the point-to-point curve of free thrombin (in nM) versus time (in min)

3.4 Data Analysis

1. Calculations from raw absorbance data in the subsampling protocol are assisted by use of spreadsheets (such as Microsoft Excel). Mathematical setup for typical analyses of data in cells is given in Fig. 3.
2. In subsampling experiments, free thrombin concentrations in original undiluted plasma at each time point are determined by subtraction of absorbance due to thrombin–A2M from that for total thrombin activity, followed by calculation of the equivalent nM thrombin from a linear regression standard curve corrected for dilution of plasma in the assay (Fig. 3). For the subsampling macro protocol, total dilution factor up to the endpoint absorbance measurement = 1,600 = 2 (for plasma-tissue factor reaction) × 20 (for Na_2EDTA neutralization) × 40 (for acetic acid neutralized substrate reaction). In the case of the microtiter plate subsampling test with kinetic thrombin assay, dilution factor = 320 = 2 (for plasma-tissue factor reaction) × 20 (for Na_2EDTA neutralization) × 8 (for substrate reaction).
3. Thrombinoscope BV provides a dedicated software (Thrombinoscope®) for calculation of the thrombin generation curve; however, spreadsheets can be set up to perform this task as described by Hemker and Beguin (19). In the continuous method, constant activity at endpoint equilibrium is taken as only due to thrombin–A2M. Thus, the total thrombin concentration time course in the rTF–phospholipid sample (calculated by reference to rate of fluorescence increase by the calibrator) is corrected by subtraction of thrombin–A2M (derived by normalizing to zero endpoint activity) to give the free (physiologically active) thrombin versus time curve.

4. Individual parameters are obtained from assessment of the free thrombin generation data files or time course curves prepared from the data.
5. Lag time is taken as the time to first detectable free thrombin measurement.
6. Peak height is the maximum concentration (nM) of free thrombin activity measured over the time course. Correspondingly, the time period from first detectable free thrombin to peak thrombin activity is the time to peak.
7. ETP is area under the free thrombin versus time curve. Total area (nM·min) is computed using the free thrombin concentration at each time point and the trapezoidal rule for summation of area segments under the point-to-point graph. Thus, $\mathrm{ETP} = \sum_{i=1}^{m} \left(\left([\mathrm{IIa}]_i + [\mathrm{IIa}]_{i-1} \right) / 2 \right) \times \left(t_i - t_{i-1} \right)$ where $[\mathrm{IIa}]_i$ is free thrombin concentration in nM at time point i; t_i, time in min at time point i; m, total number of time-point samples taken from the reaction mixture; $[\mathrm{IIa}]_{i-1}$ and t_{i-1} are thrombin concentration and time at the point immediately prior to time point i; and $[\mathrm{IIa}]_{i-1}$ is the control blank value for the t_{i-1} zero time when $i = 1$.

3.5 Data Interpretation

1. In order to assess the impact of thrombin generation parameter values on haemostatic condition of patients, normal ranges need to be established. Some sense of the boundary levels for peak height and area under the curve in adult plasma using the microtiter plate method given here have been recently published by our group (20). A very similar technique has given excellent data to assess ETP throughout childhood (21). Systematic international studies of continuous thrombin generation are underway to establish a technology with uniform parameter values (22).
2. At this time, general comments can be made about implications of parameter variation from normal populations.
3. Increase in lag time and time to peak, along with modest decrease in peak height and/or ETP, can be observed in factor deficiencies (such as FVIII) (23) or at certain levels of direct thrombin inhibitors (20).
4. Heparin anticoagulants increase lag time, decrease peak height, and decrease ETP (20).
5. Prothrombotic activity can lead to decreased lag time and increased ETP (14, 22).
6. From neonatal stages, through childhood up to adulthood, there is a continuous increase in ETP (21).

4 Notes

1. Plasma samples are prepared by methodology appropriate for the assay protocol. For example, various additives may be included at time of blood collection to prevent activation of or neutralize activated factors in the blood in order to limit consumption of nonactivated coagulation proenzymes. However, the general procedure will use simple citrate chelation to halt coagulation prior to analysis.
2. Storage of samples is important in determination of absolute thrombin generation activity values due to the effect of conditions on stability of plasma components (22). Thus, for assay consistency in any set of samples, all plasmas should be maintained under the same storage conditions (by convention, rapid freezing at −80 °C of freshly prepared plasma).
3. Previously, Arvin (Ancrod, Knoll Pharma, Markam, ON, Canada) was used as defibrinating agent following the same protocol as with reptilase. Stock solutions (35 units/mL) were composed of the commercial reagent mixed 1:1 volume with glycerol, and 5 μL of Arvin in glycerol was reacted with 500 μL of plasma. Arvin can still be obtained on request from Neurobiological Technologies Inc. (Edgewater, NJ, USA).
4. We have compared Thromborel S reagent preparations with purified recombinant human tissue factor in phosphatidyl choline/phosphatidyl serine using a simple recalcified plasma clot time assay. From a range of dilutions, it was calculated that undiluted Thromborel S stock reagent prepared according to the manufacturer contains an equivalence of 42.8 nM recombinant tissue factor.
5. Recombinant tissue factor (rTF) concentrations in the commercial reagent are determined using the Actichrome® tissue factor activity assay from American Diagnostica (Montreal, QE, Canada).
6. Alternatively, thrombin–A2M reference calibrator can be prepared by reacting 900 nM human thrombin (Enzyme Research Laboratories) + 1,500 nM human A2M (Sigma) in HBS-BA2 for 1 h at 37 °C, followed by supplementation with human AT (300 nM final) + unfractionated heparin (2 U/mL final) to neutralize any thrombin not captured by A2M. The resultant product is assayed for activity with S-2238 substrate versus thrombin standard (see Subheading 3.2, step 12) and diluted with HBS-BA2 to 600 nM (in terms of thrombin).
7. Freshly thawed plasma is stable on ice during the day of assay and is preferably not refrozen for future use.
8. Defibrinated plasma is stable on ice for up to 2 h without significant change in thrombin generating potential.

9. For neutralizing plasma-tissue factor reaction mixture subsamples with Na_2EDTA, the aliquot should be removed from the 37 °C reaction mixture about 2 s prior to the required time for thrombin generation stoppage, followed by addition to 5 mM Na_2EDTA precisely at the preset termination time. Thus, time apart from the 37 °C condition prior to EDTA treatment is minimized and calcium chelation occurs at the desired time point for assay of generated thrombin activity.
10. Leave a space between each row of 10 titer tubes containing Na_2EDTA for easy manipulation during time sample addition from the plasma-tissue factor reaction mixture.
11. Substrate reactions may also be carried out at room temperature; however thrombin activity will be decreased which lowers sensitivity.
12. Alternatively, if the microtiter plate reader does not possess kinetics software, the substrate reaction can be terminated after 10 min by addition of 50 μL of 50% (volume/volume) acetic acid (with mixing), followed by endpoint absorbance measurement at 405 nm.

Acknowledgments

The authors would like to thank Helen Atkinson for assistance in preparation of figures. Anthony Chan is supported by McMaster Children's Hospital/Hamilton Health Sciences Foundation Chair in Pediatric Thrombosis and Hemostasis.

References

1. Daubie V, Pochet R, Houard S, Philippart P (2007) Tissue factor: a mini-review. J Tissue Eng Regen Med 1:161–169
2. Menear K (1999) Direct thrombin inhibitors: current status and future prospects. Expert Opin Investig Drugs 8:1373–1384
3. Ofosu FA, Sie P, Modi GJ, Fernandez F, Buchanan MR, Blajchman MA, Boneu B, Hirsh J (1987) The inhibition of thrombin-dependent positive-feedback reactions is critical to the expression of the anticoagulant effect of heparin. Biochem J 243:579–588
4. Ofosu FA, Liu L, Feedman J (1996) Control mechanisms in thrombin generation. Semin Thromb Haemost 22:303–308
5. Naito K, Fujikawa K (1991) Activation of human blood coagulation factor XI independent of factor XII: factor XI is activated by thrombin and factor XIa in the presence of negatively charged surfaces. J Biol Chem 266:7353–7358
6. Dahlback B (1995) The protein C anticoagulant system: Inherited defects as basis for venous thrombosis. Thromb Res 77:1–43
7. Leger AJ, Covic L, Kuliopulos A (2006) Protease-activated receptors in cardiovascular diseases. Circulation 114:1070–1077
8. Boffa MB, Koschinsky ML (2007) Curiouser and curiouser: recent advances in measurement of thrombin-activatable fibrinolysis inhibitor (TAFI) and in understanding its molecular genetics, gene regulation, and biological roles. Clin Biochem 40:431–442
9. Schmidt B, Mitchell L, Ofosu FA, Andrew M (1989) Alpha-2-macroglobulin is an important progressive inhibitor of thrombin in neonatal and infant plasma. Thromb Haemost 62:1074–1077
10. Andrew M, Mitchell L, Vegh P, Ofosu F (1994) Thrombin regulation in children differs from adults in the absence and presence of heparin. Thromb Haemost 72:836–842
11. Macfarlane RG, Biggs R (1953) A thrombin generation test: the application in haemophilia and thrombocytopenia. J Clin Pathol 6:3–8
12. Berry LR, Klement P, Andrew M, Chan AKC (2003) Effect of covalent serpin-heparinoid

complexes on plasma thrombin generation on fetal distal lung epithelium. Am J Respir Cell Mol Biol 28:150–158

13. Sottrup-Jensen L (1989) Alpha-macroglobulins: structure, shape and mechanism of protease complex formation. J Biol Chem 264:11539–11542
14. Streif W, Paes B, Berry L, Andrew M, Andreasen RB, Chan AKC (2000) Influence of exogenous factor VIIa on thrombin generation in cord plasma of full-term and pre-term newborns. Blood Coag Fibrinol 11:349–357
15. Hemker HC, Al Dieri R, de Smedt E, Beguin S (2006) Thrombin generation, a function test of the haemostatic-thrombotic system. Thromb Haemost 96:553–561
16. Ignjatovic V, Greenway A, Summerhayes R, Monagle P (2007) Thrombin generation: the functional role of alpha-2-macroglobulin and influence of developmental haemostasis. Br J Haematol 138:366–368
17. Tappenden KA, Gallimore MJ, Evans G, Mackie IJ, Jones DW (2007) Thrombin generation: a comparison of assays using platelet-poor and -rich plasma and whole blood samples from healthy controls and patients with a history of venous thromboembolism. Br J Haematol 139:106–112
18. Berry L, Andrew M, Post M, Ofosu F, O'Brodovich H (1991) A549 lung epithelial cell line synthesize anticoagulant molecules on the cell surface and matrix and in conditioned media. Am J Resp Cell Mol Biol 4:338–346
19. Hemker HC, Beguin S (1995) Thrombin generation in plasma: its assessment via the endogenous thrombin potential. Thromb Haemost 74:134–138
20. Lau A, Berry LR, Mitchell LG, Chan AK (2007) Effect of substrate and fibrin polymerization inhibitor on determination of plasma thrombin generation in vitro. Thromb Res 119:667–677
21. Monagle P, Barnes C, Ignjatovic V, Furmedge J, Newall F, Chan A, De Rosa L, Hamilton S, Ragg P, Robinson S, Auldist A, Crock C, Roy N, Rowlands S (2006) Developmental haemostasis. Impact for clinical haemostasis laboratories. Thromb Haemost 95:362–372
22. Dargaud Y, Luddington R, Gray E, Negrier C, Lecompte T, Petros S, Hogwood J, Bordet J-C, Regnault V, Siegemund A, Baglin T (2007) Effect of standardization and normalization on imprecision of calibrated automated thrombography: an international multicentre study. Br J Haematol 139:303–309
23. Parmar N, Berry LR, Paredes N, Chan AKC (2005) Effect of heparins on thrombin generation in hemophilic plasma supplemented with FVIII, FVIIa, or FEIBA. Clin Lab 51: 157–166

Chapter 12

Activated Clotting Time (ACT)

Stephen Horton and Simon Augustin

Abstract

The standard assay for monitoring anticoagulation during extracorporeal life support (ECLS) is the activated clotting time (ACT) test, with celite, kaolin, and glass beads being the most commonly used activators to initiate contact activation. The point-of-care ACT test has been the preferred test in catheterization labs and cardiac theatres because it has a number of advantages over laboratory tests (Spinler et al., Ann Pharmacother 39(7–8):1275–1285, 2005):

–Shorter time between sampling and results.
–Smaller blood sample size.
–Availability to have test performed by non-lab personnel.
–Reduced errors associated with sample mislabeling/mishandling.
–Decreased risk of sample degradation with time.

There are other coagulation monitoring tests available; however these are usually specific and do not take into account the global picture of the entire clotting system. The standard coagulation tests (prothrombin time (PT), activated partial thromboplastin time, thrombin time (TT), and fibrinogen level) are plasma tests measuring plasma haemostasis and not patient haemostasis. The ACT measurement uses whole blood, thereby incorporating the importance of platelets and phospholipids in the role of coagulation. Many of the problems with the haemostatic system during ECLS are caused by the activation of platelets, which are not detected by standard tests.

Because an ACT test is nonspecific there are many variables such as hypothermia, platelets, aprotinin, GP IIb/IIIa antagonists, haemodilution, etc. that can alter its results. For this reason it is important to gain an understanding as to how these variables interact for meaningful interpretation of the ACT test result.

Key words Activated clotting time, Coagulation monitoring, Whole blood coagulation time, Hemotec, Hemochron, MAX-ACT

1 Introduction

The activated clotting time (ACT) is a commonly used point-of-care coagulation test used in almost all cardiac theatres across the world to monitor the coagulation of blood, usually from the effect of heparin. During various medical procedures there is a need to control blood coagulation. Blood which remains fluid throughout the normal circulatory system solidifies when it interacts with a foreign

Paul Monagle (ed.), *Haemostasis: Methods and Protocols*, Methods in Molecular Biology, vol. 992,
DOI 10.1007/978-1-62703-339-8_12,

material or a damaged blood vessel. This is natural to prevent haemorrhage. During most vascular procedures that involve surgical manipulation of the vascular tissue this blood clotting can be detrimental and cause frequent complications to the procedure. To inhibit the haemostatic response for cardiac surgery with cardiopulmonary bypass and prevent consumption of platelets and clotting factors a prophylactic dose of anticoagulant, most commonly unfractionated heparin, is used. Unfractionated heparin is the anticoagulant of choice in most cardiac centers because it has a short half-life and is easily reversed. During longer procedures the short half-life, blood component replacement/dilution, and the patient's individual interaction can alter the effective time course of heparin. As well as unfractionated heparin intensive efforts have been made to reduce the haemostatic activation and inflammation that extracorporeal support can produce. These include the use of antifibrinolytic agents, the protease inhibitor aprotinin, platelet inhibitors, and foreign surface manipulation (1).

Monitoring and stabilizing the coagulation profile of cardiac patients, particularly those on extracorporeal life support (ECLS), is one of the major challenges in successfully supporting these patients over a period of days to weeks. Haemorrhage is among the most frequent complications encountered in ECLS, particularly in neonates where they may have coagulation factor levels substantially lower than adults as well as greater haemodilution. Excessive anticoagulation can potentiate bleeding with the risk of inadequate anticoagulation leading to thrombosis and vessel occlusion. In these circumstances, such as in the catheterization lab, cardiac theatres, or during ECLS, a point-of-care method for assessing anticoagulation is required, to monitor and maintain an optimum level of anticoagulation. The most utilized test is the ACT. Despotis determined that some cardiac centers are still using fixed dosing schemes, which are limited because of lack of confirmation of adequate anticoagulation (2). The ACT is a test of whole blood coagulation that gives a single parameter for interpretation. Because it is nonspecific there are many variables (hypothermia, platelets, aprotinin, GP IIb/IIIa antagonists, haemodilution) (3) and various coagulopathies that can alter the result. ACTs are indicative of inhibition of contact and common pathway (X–Xa) activation rather than inhibition of the extrinsic coagulation pathway (see Chapter 1) (4).

ACT test was the preferred test in catheterization labs and cardiac theatres because it has a number of advantages over lab tests including (5):

–Shorter time between sampling and results.
–Smaller blood sample size.
–Availability to have test performed by non-lab personnel.
–Reduced errors associated with sample mislabeling/mishandling.
–Decreased risk of sample degradation with time.

It has been shown that point-of-care testing was as effective as standard laboratory testing with reduced occurrence of blood product usage when compared to clinician discretion (6).

Hattersley first proposed the use of the ACT test in 1966 for a number of coagulation disturbances, including those receiving therapeutic heparin (7). It was also reported in a survey of 81 US ECMO centers that all use heparin for anticoagulation and 80% use ACT to monitor the anticoagulation. In addition, cardiac patients for whom the drug is most commonly used often have a propensity for underlying consumptive coagulopathies due to liver impairment, or low cardiac outputs (8). This may not be due to ECLS anticoagulation or its management, as 68% of extracorporeal membrane oxygenation (ECMO) patients were found to have a clotting factor deficiency prior to ECMO support (9).

ACT is an important test of the clotting system that is quick, easy, and a point-of-care test, which gives a single result from which all the intricacies of the coagulation system are incorporated. The ACT tube has an activator substance that will activate factor XII through contact activation. The main activator substances used are celite (diatomaceous earth), kaolin, or glass beads, which all have large surface areas for contact. The essence of the test is to completely activate the intrinsic coagulation cascade and measure the time it takes for generation of a fibrin clot. The machine heats the sample to 37°C. Depending on the type of machine being used, movement is created whether through rotation of the sample tube (Max-ACT, Hemochron), a plunger (Hemotec), or through pressure (Hemochron Jr.). As a clot forms it imparts resistance onto a plunger (Hemotec), onto a free rolling bar in the sample tube (Max-ACT, Hemochron), or impedes flow of the blood (Hemochron Jr.). The end result is the time taken for the sample to form a clot which is detected photo-optically (Hemotec, Hemochron Jr) or electromagnetically (Max-ACT, Hemochron).

It is important to recognize that the standard coagulation tests (prothrombin time (PT), activated partial thromboplastin time (aPTT), thrombin time (TT), and fibrinogen level) are plasma tests measuring plasma haemostasis and not patient haemostasis. The ACT measurement uses whole blood, thereby incorporating the importance of platelets and phospholipids in the role of coagulation.

The MAX-ACT (Helena laboratories, Beaumont, TX, USA) uses a "cocktail" formulation of activators (celite, glass beads, and kaolin) for maximal stimulation of factor XII. It also incorporates a dual endpoint detection mechanism with magnetic sensors at 0 and 90° to give greater consistency in results. There may be variable patient reactivity to different types of activator, so by using three activators this is minimized, providing more reproducible results.

The Hemochron Jr. Signature Whole Blood Microcoagulation System also uses a combination of activators in its cuvette: silica, kaolin, and phospholipids for a more sensitive ACT measurement. This device has been developed slightly differently than the standard ACT machines because of its capillary action cuvette, which only requires a drop of blood for its test. Up to 234 patients and 85 quality control tests can be stored on the device for later printing or downloading. This device also measures PT, aPTT, and INR. It is a unique instrument that self-calibrates through its internal software, so no user calibration of the device is necessary.

While running an ACT test it must be appreciated that it is a whole blood coagulation test, with many variables that can alter the test's result. Two variables in cardiac theatres are patient hypothermia and use of aprotinin. Its use can lead to an underestimation of the anticoagulation status as aprotinin causes a prolongation of both the celite and, to a lesser extent, the kaolin ACT.

Aprotinin is a bovine lung-derived serine protease inhibitor. It acts as an inhibitor of human trypsin, plasmin, human kallikrein and tissue kallikrein, and contact phase activation, reducing fibrinolysis and attenuating the inflammatory response. It also indirectly preserves platelets while on CPB by minimizing fibrinolysis activation (10, 11). Khan also found that aprotinin prevented protease-dependant platelet aggregation (12).

Aprotinin has been known to alter the ACT times of cardiac patients depending on the type of activator used by the ACT machine (13–15). There has been much speculation as to the reason for this; Wang suggested that the increase in ACT in the presence of aprotinin for celite-ACT over kaolin-ACT was the ability of aprotinin to bind to the celite activator. This artificially alters the ACT by decreasing the activator concentration present with a prolongation from approximately 500 to 700 s (13). Dietrich examined the effect of adding aprotinin to heparinized whole blood in the presence of either kaolin or celite activator. These samples were then tested for aprotinin concentrations. He found that the highly positively charged aprotinin molecule was attracted to the highly negatively charged kaolin and to a lesser extent the minor negatively charged celite. In this environment there is significantly less aprotinin to inhibit contact activation in the kaolin test tube, which would demonstrate a lower ACT measurement (14).

Hypothermia can also affect an ACT result. There was a prolongation of ACT using celite, kaolin, and a mixture (celite, kaolin, glass bead) activators when patients on CPB were cooled to 28°C (15).

The reasons hypothermia may cause this ACT prolongation are reversible platelet membrane dysfunction and partially inhibited platelet adhesion. The coagulation system is inhibited because it relies on enzymatic activity, which is reduced proportionately with decreasing temperature (16). There is also a significant prolongation of ACT conducted at room temperature compared to in a heat block at 37°C (17). Haemodilution can result in a prolonged ACT measurement despite lack of adequate heparin concentration in the patient. Conversely the ACT measurement could be shortened during haemodilution due to reduced antithrombin (AT) (4). This outcome was supported by Hashimoto with AT supplementation reducing thrombin activity during CPB (18).

Other anticoagulants have been measured via ACT; the use of low-molecular-weight heparin (LMWH) has increased in the catheterization laboratory because of fewer side effects, particularly heparin-induced thrombocytopenia (19). Marmur found that the use of an ACT assay is beneficial in monitoring coagulation using intravenous dalteparin (20).

2 Materials

The ACT may be performed on a number of bedside analyzers that each has its own specific cuvettes for loading samples. Importantly the results from each separate analyzer are not interchangeable.

The following analyzers are commonly used:

1. MAX-ACT, Helena Laboratories, Texas, USA.
2. Medtronic ACT Plus, Medtronic, Minneapolis, USA.
3. Hemochron Jr., International Technidyne Corporation (ITC), New Jersey, USA.
4. Hemochron Response, ITC, New Jersey, USA.

3 Methods (See Note 1)

3.1 MAX-ACT (21)

1. Allow the heating block time to stabilize to 37°C ± 0.5.
2. Open the MAX-ACT test tube containing the kaolin, celite, and glass particles and fill with 0.5 ml of blood (see Note 2). Close the tube lid. Do not agitate the tube but place directly into the test well opening of the machine.
3. Once the presence of the tube is detected the timer will automatically start. Rotate the tube 4–5 times to assist mixing. Once the clot is detected a buzzer will sound and the result is displayed (see Note 3).

3.2 Medtronic ACT Plus (22) (See Note 4)

1. Warm the cartridge to 37°C ± 0.5 in the heat block for at least 3–5 min before using.
2. Tap the cartridge to suspend the reagent. Always fill HR channel first and the HR-HTC channel second.

   For HRACT—add 0.4 ml sample to each cartridge channel; between the fill lines of the cartridge.

For LRACT—add 0.2 ml sample to each cartridge channel; between the fill lines of the cartridge.

For HTC—add 0.4 ml sample to each cartridge channel; between the fill lines of the cartridge.

3. Insert cartridge into the analyzer and move into the closed position to start the test. The test will finish when an audible alarm is heard once the clot is detected.

3.3 International Technidyne Corp. Hemochron Jr. Signature Whole Blood Microcoagulation System (23)

1. The operator inserts a cuvette for the test into the instrument and then enters information about the sample (if desired). After the cuvette has warmed to 37°C ± 1.0, the instrument beeps, signaling the operator that a blood sample can be added to the cuvette and the test started.
2. Place a drop of blood into the sample well of the cuvette (see Note 5).
3. When a clot is detected, the instrument beeps once. Final results of the test are calculated and displayed.

It is standard for ACT instruments to allow a printout of the results with the time and date, some also allowing the patient ID or details of the test to be printed. There is also usually a communication port for downloading results to a computer for storage or analysis.

3.4 International Technidyne Corp. Hemochron Response (24)

1. Dispense the sample into the test tube and simultaneously press the *START* key. A beep will signal the start of the test and timing of the test begins.
2. Mix the contents of the test tube.
3. Insert the test tube in the well. Quickly rotate the tube clockwise one revolution. The screen will briefly display DETECTING MAGNET PLEASE WAIT.
4. Wait for message to disappear, while the instrument verifies that the magnet is moving freely in the tube. When verified, the green detector light will illuminate.

When clot formation is detected, the instrument beeps and the test name and results are displayed (see Note 6).

4 ACT Interpretation

ACTs are more indicative of inhibition of contact activation rather than providing information about the degree of inhibition of the extrinsic coagulation pathway and heparin levels during CPB (4). Prolonged ACTs can be found with coagulation activation even though there is a decrease in heparin levels. This condition can lead to a progressive consumptive coagulopathy. Because of this there have been investigations into improving the correlation between ACTs to heparin concentration (as measured by chromogenic assay of the plasma anti-Xa activity). This has been found by using a plasma-supplemented (equal mixture of patient blood and fresh frozen plasma (FFP)) modified kaolin ACT (mACT) (25). The correlation to the non-haematocrit corrected values of the chromogenic assay was $r = 0.43$ for the kaolin ACT and $r = 0.69$ for the mACT. Recently efforts have been made to improve the correlation of ACT with heparin concentrations. It is of interest to compare a recent in-house study of kaolin ACT results with those of the MAX-ACT in a number of different clinical situations. When a paired *t*-test of ACT results between the two methods was undertaken for all samples (CPB and VAD, $n = 88$) and subsets of this group treated with either aprotinin ($n = 13$) or VAD ($n = 15$) alone, in all circumstances the MAX-ACT was lower ($p < 0.05$). The corresponding correlations for these groups were $r = 0.75$, $r = 0.48$, and $r = 0.22$. This demonstrates that there is a difference in the way that ACT results for the same sample can be affected by differing conditions and techniques. Supplementation of FFP to the kaolin ACT (mACT) resulted in an improved correlation of the ACT to heparin anti-XA activity ($r = 0.43$ to $r = 0.69$) (see Note 7).

Interestingly all mACT measurements were within measurement device range (<1,000 s), whereas approximately 20% of ACTs (no FFP) exceeded 999 s (outside device range) and therefore are not valid, suggesting that when FFP is not added some ACT measurements are prolonged due to haemodilution. The depletion of the plasma coagulation system by haemodilution and consumption has a major influence on ECLS ACTs. Apart from the variation in individual response to heparin (caused by different levels of AT, cell binding, or binding to platelet factor IV), haematocrit influences plasma chromogenic assays, as it determines the volume unfractionated heparin can be utilized in.

It is important to appreciate the codependence of inflammation and coagulation and hence the effect that anti-inflammatories have on ACTs. CPB results in an inflammatory response, with one of the sites of biologic activity being the endothelial cell. In response to cytokines, ischemia, abnormal shear stresses, activated platelets, and other stimuli, tissue factor is expressed on the endothelial cell surface. Blood flow is maintained by the balance of haemostasis and fibrinolysis, an interdependent network of cascading enzymatic reactions. The critical aspect of the coagulation pathway is thrombin generation with fibrin polymerization as its end point. Thrombin catalyzes conversion of fibrinogen to fibrin, activates fXIII and platelets, and positively feeds back into upstream factors. Tissue factor (TF) exposure, either from vessel wall damage or activated platelets and leucocytes, generates thrombin; thus inflammation can initiate coagulation. TF and fVIIIa form a complex to activate fX, which with fVa cleaves a small amount of prothrombin to thrombin. This causes platelet, fV, fVIII, and fXI activation increasing thrombin formation. Foreign surface contact results in activation of high-molecular-weight kininogen, plasma kallikrein, and fXII, with additional fXII activation via a positive feedback loop from kallikrein.

fIXa (previously activated by TF-VIIa, fXIa on platelet surface, or artificial surface fXII activation) and fVIIIa complex on the platelet surface (in the presence of calcium) further activates fX and with fVa generates a thrombin burst. This burst rather than initial thrombin production becomes the crucial process in haemostasis. Inhibition of the whole body inflammatory response will lead to a decrease in thrombin generation, which will result in further decrease of inflammation. The rises that occur in ACT results when anti-inflammatories are used can be understood to occur as a result of the reduced expression of procoagulants on the vascular cell surfaces and tissue factor pathway inhibition, with corresponding reduction of thrombin generation (26).

Our concepts of anticoagulation during CPB and the information derived from the ACT must recognize the variations caused by the degree of inflammatory and surface contact activation. The heparin–AT complex has the ability to inhibit the intrinsic pathway factors IXa, Xa, and XIIa, and the common pathway factor Xa, as well as thrombin. When the patient is exposed to an inflammatory stimulant such as ECLS (as demonstrated by elevated interleukin-6 (IL-6) and interleukin-8 (IL-8) levels) thrombin generation is ongoing and may be insufficiently inhibited by heparin-induced AT activation (27). The inflammatory stimulus may continue during support with a subsequent ongoing increase in thrombin production. As thrombin concentration rises there is a decrease in the effect of circulating heparin. This initiates a shifting of the slope to the right of the heparin dose–response curve (HDRC). As the severity of the inflammatory response is unpredictable, the heparin concentration cannot be determined by the use of the HDRC (26). Even though the ACT cannot be relied on as an indicator of heparin concentration, we may be able to use the ACT to gain insight into the effects of thrombin formation and the state of the haemostatic mechanism during and after ECLS, as the ACT is related to the variables that influence thrombin formation (i.e., rising thrombin concentration and AT).

The ACT is proportional to the concentrations of heparin and AT ([HEP–AT]) and inversely proportional to the thrombin concentration [T]. As these variables change so will the ACT; however the slope does not, thus falling ACT result from a decreasing [HEP–AT] or a rising [T]. Thus thrombin generation due to the inflammatory response can contribute to heparin resistance. Also as the ACT post protamine normalizes if [T] is increased, but offset by increased HEP–AT, the HEP–AT may inhibit the intrinsic pathway at the time it is most needed. The intrinsic pathway is necessary for clot growth and maintenance, with continuing inhibition creating the typical clinical picture of generalized microvasculature bleeding that is seen after ECLS heparinization with or without reversal by protamine. Additional protamine will lower the [HEP–AT]; however released thrombin furthers the inflammatory response. As [T] decreases the [HEP–AT] ratio will shift resulting in increased ACTs and contribute to the phenomenon known as the heparin rebound effect. This term was used to describe increased ACTs after what was considered an appropriate protamine dose (protamine 1.1 mg/mg heparin given) and an initial lowered response of the ACT with a subsequent elongation of the ACT.

To attenuate thrombin generation during ECLS it is possible to use anti-inflammatories such as aprotinin. It reduces CPB-induced monocyte and leucocyte expression of integrin Mac-1 and also inhibits tissue factor VIIa complex. Thus the ACT changes associated with this decrease in thrombin generation take on the characteristics of the APTT-HDRC. As the ACT is representing a cellular APTT, because the inflammatory induced thrombin generation occurs at the surface of vascular cells, the decrease in Mac-1 expression and tissue factor pathway inhibition due to aprotinin can be described as a decrease in the vascular cell contribution to thrombin generation. The exponential rise in ACT is not aberrant but rises when cell-derived thrombin generation is decreased, as procoagulant and proinflammatory agents diminish and heparin-induced antithrombin activity increases.

5 Conclusion

Values from different ACT machines although intrinsically repeatable are not always in agreeance between the machines (28). It is therefore advised for an individual hospital to develop its own therapeutic ranges and protocol, and use the same ACT machine through all departments to derive consistent results.

ACTs are the most widely used assays, as point-of-care tests of coagulation, because they are inexpensive, convenient, and give a single result for a global whole blood coagulation measurement. While being the mainstay of cardiac theatres around the world it is unrealistic to believe that all coagulation derangements can be summed up with a single assay, which only describes the primary fibrin strand formation. However ACTs are a good first option when a patient is bleeding because of the rapid response time. As the laboratory-based, point-of-care assays become more reliable and are able to be performed at the bedside, their specificity may diminish ACT use.

The anti-Xa laboratory test indirectly assesses heparin concentration rather than the anticoagulant effect; a test that measures the whole blood coagulation time therefore may be more beneficial in patients undergoing cardiac surgery as well as percutaneous coronary interventions. The advantage of an ACT over an anti-Xa assay is that it is a point-of-care test, which takes minutes rather than hours, and anti-IIa effects that occur to varying degrees with LMWH, and maximally with unfractionated heparin, are not determined with an anti-Xa test. There are several point-of-care analyzers on the market, or in clinical trials, that are designed to investigate the full pathway of the clot formation. From fibrin strand formation to the fibrinolytic breakdown of the clot, a comprehensive analysis of the coagulability of the patient is undertaken (29).

It has been shown how the use of the Sonoclot Coagulation and Platelet Function Analyzer can be used to predict postoperative haemorrhage from a point-of-care system. The Sonoclot system also obtains an ACT value, which was found not to be significant in predicting blood loss. The main aspect in the patients with excessive bleeding was not the primary clot formation, but the variables later in the clotting process which the ACT does not incorporate, the platelet–fibrin interaction and clot retraction (30). The Thromboelastograph 5000 (TEG®) (Haemoscope, Niles, IL, USA) is another point-of-care test similar to the Sonoclot analyzer in that it measures several variables throughout the dynamics of the clot formation to give a global picture. This device helps to determine the causes of a coagulopathy and target the treatment needed for improved patient haemostasis. Use of the TEG® system can provide the benefits of reduced transfusion volume and reduced number of patients receiving transfusions over conventional coagulation assays (31).

Devices such as the TEG or Sonoclot, that are able to give a significant amount of information (including ACTs) efficiently by the bedside, are of great benefit in scenarios where there is considerable blood loss in a short period of time.

By identifying factor deficiency, allowing appropriate factor replacement, patient morbidity should improve and blood product use reduce, allowing the resources to be better utilized.

6 Notes

1. Manufacturer's guidelines for maintenance and quality control often involve monthly or yearly temperature calibrations as well as timing and sensor calibrations with no sample. These cuvettes can be obtained from the manufacturer.
2. Do not use a needle on the syringe when filling ACT tubes as this can prematurely activate the coagulation cascade.

3. If the result is thought to be unusually prolonged, another sample should be taken, especially if there is heparin in the sample line (heparin/saline flush).

   A two-syringe technique to obtain the sample should be used:

   a. Initially remove three times the dead space, usually 5–7 ml of the line in the first syringe, to be confident that heparin or dilution effect from the flush in the line has been eliminated.
   b. Take a second syringe to obtain the sample from the line. Just before filling the ACT tube discard the first quarter of 1 ml from the syringe in case it is contaminated.
4. The Medtronic ACT Plus has a choice of cuvettes depending on the machine's clinical application. They have a high range (HR), low range (LR), and a heparinase test cartridge (HTC). The HR cuvettes are usually used during cardiopulmonary bypass while the LR cuvettes are used during ECMO or dialysis monitoring. The HDT cuvette has the ability to eliminate the heparin effect of a sample to determine if there is an underlying coagulopathy independent of residual heparin in the patient. This HDT cuvette is run concurrently alongside a routine ACT cuvette. Heparinase negates the effect of heparin, enabling the difference between the two ACT measurements to ascertain whether there is residual heparin in the patient or a coagulation factor deficiency, thus enabling the appropriate treatment to be determined, either extra protamine or clotting factor transfusion (FFP, cryoprecipitate, platelets).
5. Fill the sample well from the bottom up. Add enough blood so that the lower wall of the center sample well is completely filled. If the meniscus of the blood sample extends above the lower wall, push the excess blood into the overflow area. A transfer needle can be used to transfer blood.
6. If the expiration date on a barcode label on the test tube is exceeded, the test will be aborted. After *START* is pressed, the operator can enter the patient ID or add notes.
7. Use of FFP.

   A prolonged ACT could be attributable to an abnormally high haematocrit (i.e., low plasma volume) as the reduced plasma volume results in less plasma clotting factors, hence a greater anticoagulant effect (17). The ACT can be improved in this case by giving a unit of FFP, which increases clotting factors.

   FFP is also used to treat a low ACT due to the lack of AT available for heparin to bind to, reducing the effect of heparin. This is overcome via the administration of FFP, thereby increasing the concentration of AT in the patient, increasing heparin's effectiveness.

References

1. Royston D (1996) Preventing the inflammatory response to open-heart surgery: the role of Aprotinin and other protease inhibitors. Int J Cardiol 53(suppl):S11–S37
2. Despotis GJ, Gravlee G, Filos K, Levy J (1999) Anticoagulation monitoring during cardiac surgery. Anesthesiology 91:1122–1151
3. Ammar T, Scudder LE, Coller BS (1997) In vitro effects of platelet Glycoprotein IIb/IIIa receptor antagonist c7E3 Fab on the activated clotting time. Circulation 95:614–617
4. Despotis GJ, Summerfield AL, Joist JH et al (1994) Comparison of activated coagulation time and whole blood heparin measurements with laboratory plasma anti-Xa heparin concentrations in patients having cardiac operations. Thorac Cardiovasc Surg 108: 1076–1082
5. Spinler SA, Wittkowsky AK, Nutescu EA, Smythe MA (2005) Anticoagulation monitoring part 2: unfractionated heparin and low-molecular-weight heparin. Ann Pharmacother 39(7–8):1275–1285
6. Avidan MS, Alcock EL, Da Fonseca J, Ponte J, Desai JB, Despotis GJ, Hunt BL (2004) Comparison of structured use of routine laboratory tests or near-patient assessment with clinical judgement in the management of bleeding after cardiac surgery. Br J Anaesth 92:178–186
7. Hattersley PG (1966) Activated clotting time of whole blood. JAMA 196:436–440
8. Graves DF, Chernin JM, Kurusz M, Zwischenberger JB (1996) Anticoagulation practices during neonatal extracorporeal membrane oxygenation: survey results. Perfusion 11:461–466
9. McManus ML, Kevy SV, Bower LK, Hickey PR (1995) Coagulation factor deficiencies during initiation of extracorporeal membrane oxygenation. J Pediatr 126:900–904
10. MIMS on-line (2003) Copyright MIMS Australia Pt. Ltd. http://www.mims.com.au
11. van Oeveren W, Harder MP, Roozendaal KJ, Eijsman L, Wildevuur CRH (1990) Aprotinin protects platelets against the initial effect of cardiopulmonary bypass. J Thorac Cardiovasc Surg 99:788–797
12. Khan TA, Bianchi C, Voisine P, Sandmeyer J, Feng J, Sellke FW (2005) Aprotinin inhibits platelet aggregation and thrombosis. Ann Thorac Surg 79:1545–1550
13. Wang JS, Lin CY, Hung WT, Karp RB (1992) Monitoring of heparin-induced anticoagulation with kaolin-activated clotting time in cardiac surgical patients treated with Aprotinin. Anesthesiology 77(6):1080–1084
14. Dietrich W, Jochum M (1995) Effect of celite and kaolin on activated clotting time in the presence of Aprotinin: activated clotting time is reduced by binding of Aprotinin to kaolin. J Thorac Cardiovasc Surg 109:177–186
15. Machin D, Devine P (2005) The effect of temperature and Aprotinin during cardiopulmonary bypass on three different methods of activated clotting time measurement. J Extra Corpor Technol 37(3):265–271
16. Wolberg AS, Meng ZH, Monroe DM 3rd, Hoffman M (2004) A systematic evaluation of the effect of temperature on coagulation enzyme activity and platelet function. J Trauma 56(6):1221–1228
17. Kase PB, Dearing JP (1985) Factors affecting activated clotting time. J Extra Corpor Technol 17(1):27–30
18. Hashimoto K, Yamagishi M, Sasaki T, Nakano M, Kurosawa H (1995) Heparin and Antithrombin III levels during cardiopulmonary bypass: correlation with subclinical plasma coagulation. Ann Thorac Surg 58:799–805
19. Kadakia RA, Baimeedi SR, Ferguson JJ (2004) Low-molecular-weight heparins in the cardiac catheterization laboratory. Tex Heart Inst J 31(1):72–83
20. Marmur JD, Anand SX, Bagga RS, Fareed J, Pan CM, Sharma SK, Richard MF (2003) The activated clotting time can be used to monitor the low molecular weight heparin dalteparin after intravenous administration. J Am Coll Cardiol 41:394–403
21. Operation manual. MAX-ACT activated clotting time test. Helena Laboratories point of care. Beaumont, Texas, USA
22. Operation manual. Hemotec ACT II activated clotting time test. Medtronic. Minneapolis, MN, USA
23. Instrument operator manual. Hemochron Jr.signature whole blood microcoagulation system – International Technidyne Corporation. Edison, NJ, USA
24. Instrument operator manual, HEMOCHRON® response activated clotting time test – International Technidyne Corporation. Edison, NJ, USA
25. Koster A, Despotis G, Gruendel M, Fischer T, Praus M, Kuppe H, Levy J (2002) The plasma supplemented modified activated clotting time for monitoring of heparinization during cardiopulmonary bypass: a pilot investigation. Anesth Analg 95:26–30

26. Gil W (2001) Inflammo-coagulatory response, extrinsic pathway thrombin generation and a new theory of activated clotting time interpretation. Perfusion 16:27–35
27. Horton SB, Butt WW, Mullaly RJ, Thuys CA, O'Connor EB, Byron K, Cochrane AD, Brizard CP, Karl TR (1999) IL-6 and IL-8 levels following cardiopulmonary bypass are not affected by surface coating. Ann Thorac Surg 68:1751–1755
28. Bosch YPJ, Ganushchak YM, de Jong DS (2006) Comparison of ACT point-of-care measurements: repeatability and agreement. Perfusion 21:27–31
29. El Rouby S, Cohen M, Gonzales A, Hoppensteadt D, Lee T, Zucker ML, Khalid K, LaDuca FM, Fareed J (2006) The use of Hemochron® Jr. Hemonox™ point of care test in monitoring the anticoagulant effects of enoxaparin during interventional coronary procedures. J Thromb Thrombolysis 21:137–145
30. Yamada T, Katori N, Tanaka K, Takeda J (2007) Impact of Sonoclot hemostasis analysis after cardiopulmonary bypass on postoperative hemorrhage in cardiac surgery. J Anesth 21:148–152
31. Shore-Lesserson L, Manspeizer HE, DePerio M, Francis S, Vela-Cantos F, Ergin MA (1999) Thromboelastography-guided transfusion algorithm reduces transfusions in complex cardiac surgery. Anesth Analg 88:312–319

Part IV

Examples of Tests for Bleeding Disorders

Chapter 13

Factor XIII Assays

Stephen Opat, Jenny Butler, Erica Malan, Elizabeth Duncan, and Huyen A.M. Tran

Abstract

Factor XIII (FXIII) deficiency is a rare cause of bleeding and pregnancy loss that is easily treated with plasma products. Reliable assays for FXIII are necessary not only for the diagnosis of deficiency state but also to guide prophylaxis and replacement therapy in patients during times of increased risk. Diagnostic tests for FXIII activity whilst not technically demanding have a number of pitfalls including limited sensitivity and overestimation of activity at the lower end. Despite these shortcomings the performance of these assays is adequate for the diagnosis and management of the majority of patients with clinically significant deficiency.

Key words Factor XIII assay, Coagulation factor

1 Introduction

Factor XIII (FXIII), a member of the transglutaminase family of enzymes, is responsible for stabilizing the fibrin clot by forming intermolecular covalent bonds between fibrin monomers (1). It circulates as heterotetramer composed of two catalytic A subunits synthesized in the liver, bone marrow, and placenta, and two non-catalytic B subunits synthesized in the liver (2). Following activation by thrombin, FXIII forms a thioester bond with a protein-bound glutamine residue, releasing ammonia. This thioester intermediate reacts with an amine group from a protein-bound lysine, or other primary amine resulting in an isopeptide bond. This reaction results in cross-linking (see Fig. 1) of several targets in addition to fibrinogen, including α_2 antiplasmin, fibronectin, and collagen leading to increased mechanical clot strength and resistance to proteolytic degradation. Other targets for FXIII include osteopontin, factor V, thrombospondin, vinculin, and endothelial cell receptors $\alpha V\beta_3$ integrin and VEGFR-2 suggesting a role in angiogenesis, atherosclerosis, and inflammation. FXIII is particularly important

Paul Monagle (ed.), *Haemostasis: Methods and Protocols*, Methods in Molecular Biology, vol. 992,
DOI 10.1007/978-1-62703-339-8_13, © Springer Science+Business Media New York 2013

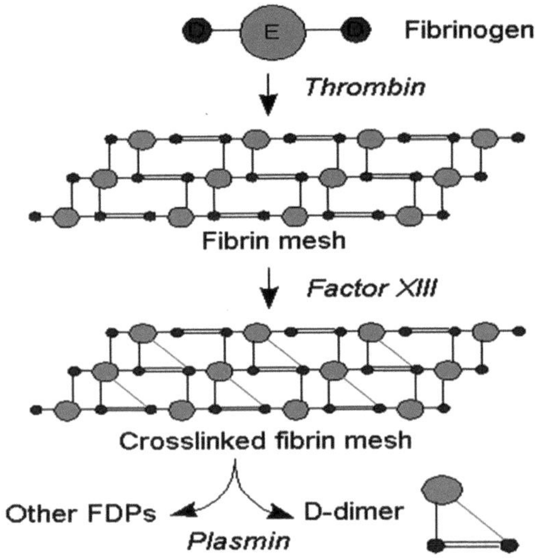

Fig. 1 Factor XIII leads to the formation of cross-linked fibrin mesh

for the maintenance of pregnancy where fibrin–fibronectin cross-linking is necessary to support the formation of the cytotrophoblastic shell at the site of placental implantation (3).

1.1 Deficiency of Factor XIII

FXIII deficiency is a rare autosomal recessive disorder affecting approximately one in one million (4). Patients with FXIII deficiency have been found to have a variety of mutations (missense and nonsense), deletions, and insertions resulting in premature chain termination and splicing abnormalities, which predominantly affect the A subunit (95% of cases) (5). Acquired FXIII deficiency has also been described in several disease states including acute leukemia, severe liver disease, disseminated intravascular coagulation, and inflammatory bowel disease, but bleeding is rare. Increased levels have been noted in some studies involving patients with arteriovascular disease (6, 7).

Severe deficiency is characterized by a haemorrhagic diathesis, recurrent pregnancy loss, and defective wound healing. Intracranial haemorrhage occurs in up to 40% of effected individuals (8).

The long plasma half-life of FXIII (7–12 days) makes prophylaxis a practical option. Reliable assays for FXIII are necessary not only for the diagnosis of deficiency state but also to guide prophylaxis and replacement therapy in patients during times of increased risk for bleeding, such as surgery and pregnancy.

1.2 Assays

Several assays for FXIII activity have been established with several commercial kits available using various methodologies. Clot solubility is most commonly performed using in-house methods with common laboratory reagents (see Table 1).

Table 1
Factor XIII assays

Type of assay	Principle	Methodology	Application
Qualitative assays	Clot solubility in urea, acetic acid, or chloroacetic acid.	In-house method‡ Stago.	Routine laboratory.
Functional assays	Transglutaminase-mediated ammonium ion release. Synthetic amine incorporation into a fibrin clot. Clot strength and resistance to fibrinolysis by thromboelastography.	Berichrom FXIII assay‡. Pefakit factor XIII incorporation assay.	Routine laboratory. Routine laboratory. Research laboratory.
Immunologic assays	Sensitive factor XIII assay by ELISA. Factor XIII antigen latex immunoassay. Factor XIII assay by immunodiffusion.	AssayMax FXIII ELISA kit. HemosIL factor XIII antigen. Binding site RID.	Research laboratory. Routine laboratory. Routine laboratory.
Genotyping	PCR for DNA mutations.		Reference laboratory.

The level of FXIII required for normal haemostasis is uncertain. Some studies have reported that levels as low as 2–5% are adequate for effective haemostasis while others have demonstrated a mild increase in surgical bleeding with levels between 5 and 40% (9). The reliability of FXIII assays using different methodologies, particularly at the lower end, may partially explain these differences in bleeding phenotype (10).

1.2.1 Factor XIII Screening Test/Clot Solubility Assay

The clot solubility assay (Table 1) is the most widely used FXIII screening test in routine laboratories (11). It has been performed using a number of different methodologies: Clotting may be activated using calcium, thrombin, thromboplastin, or combinations, and clot lysis demonstrated using urea, acetic acid, or monochloacetic acid. There are also substantial variations in the concentrations, volumes, and sources of reagents and normal ranges (12).

The major shortcoming of these assays is their limited sensitivity which may result in failure to identify patients with clinically significant deficiency (2–40% activity) (9). There is some evidence supporting the use of the thrombin/acetic acid method, since this combination has been reported to identify patients with levels less than 10% compared with the calcium/urea method which may only be abnormal with levels less than 1–5% (12). However calcium-based screening methods are currently the most commonly performed.

1.2.2 Berichrom Factor XIII Activity

The Berichrom FXIII activity assay (Table 13.1) is rapid and easy to adapt to clinical chemistry analyzers; however it also has a number of shortcomings including low sensitivity and overestimation of FXIII levels at the lower end (<10%). One study identified an average 8% increase in levels using this methodology compared with a sensitive immunoassay. Metabolism of NADH through alternative pathways and plasma turbidity due to hyperfibrinogenemia are thought to be some of the mechanisms for these observations in patients with severe deficiency. Despite these limitations this assay is still useful to identify the vast majority of patients with clinically important deficiency and acts as a guide for replacement therapy.

2 Factor XIII Screening Assay

2.1 Principle

Plasma is clotted by the addition of calcium chloride, and then incubated with urea or acetic acid solution. Acetic acid and urea will dissolve the clot in the absence of adequate levels of FXIII. Approximately 2% of the normal level of FXIII is sufficient to protect the clot against the action of acetic acid and approximately 1% is sufficient for protection against urea.

2.2 Reference Intervals

"Normal" or "Reduced," given in interpretative comments. >2% FXIII is sufficient to stabilize clots. This level is quoted from the literature.

2.3 Equipment and Reagents

2.3.1 Equipment

37°C incubator or water bath.

Glass tubes.

Parafilm.

2.3.2 Reagents

BDH calcium chloride solution 25 mM (diluted 1/40 in sterile water from 1 M stock).

30% urea solution: 30 g urea dissolved in distilled water to a final volume of 100 ml.

2% acetic acid solution: Concentrated glacial acetic acid (analytical grade) diluted 1:50 (1 ml acetic acid added to 49 ml distilled water).

Owren's buffer pH 7.35 (Dade-Behring B4234-25) or equivalent.

2.4 Specimen Requirements

2.4.1 Sample Required

3.5 ml sample; 9 parts whole blood:1 part 0.11 M (3.2%) trisodium citrate dihydrate.

The sample must not contain heparin as this will interfere with the clot formation.

2.4.2 Sample Preparation

Prepare platelet-free plasma by centrifugation at 2,300×*g* for 15 min at 10–20 °C.

Remove plasma, taking care not to contaminate with platelet pellet, and aliquot into approximately 0.5–1.0 ml volumes in two (if possible) or more storage tubes. Label tubes with patient's name, laboratory number, and date of sample. Store plasma at −70 °C.

Fresh or frozen plasma may be assayed. If frozen, thaw samples at 37 °C for approximately 5–10 min prior to assay.

2.5 Quality Control Plasma

Negative control—pooled normal plasma currently in use. Tested in parallel with patient.

Buffer control: Buffer added during clot solubility test—to check for clot stability in the absence of urea and acetic acid. Proceed to report patient samples if normal plasma result has "normal" FXIII; proceed to troubleshooting if result is abnormal, i.e., <2%.

If a source of FXIII-deficient plasma is available, either purchased commercially or from archived samples, it is useful to run this at regular intervals, and especially when training new staff. Cost and limited availability probably prohibit this QC being run with every test.

2.6 Procedure

2.6.1 Preparation

Prepare reagents as described in Subheading 2.3.2.

2.6.2 Quality Control

QC plasma is tested in parallel with patient sample (as the test requires an overnight incubation the QC is not performed before the patient test).

2.6.3 Patient Information and Sample Preparation

Select patient samples to be tested.

Label tubes adequately with patient's name and the chemical added (buffer, urea, or acetic acid).

2.6.4 Sample Testing

1. Place 200 μl of test plasma into three glass tubes. Glass tubes must be used as the clot will adhere to the bottom of plastic ones.
2. In parallel, add 200 μl of control plasma to each of the three tubes.
3. Add 200 μl of calcium chloride solution to each tube. Record the time calcium is added.
4. Mix and leave to clot for 30 min at 37 °C. *Note: The incubation time of 30 min must be exact. Do not exceed by >5 min*. Prolonged incubation (e.g., >35 min) will decrease the sensitivity of the test to FXIII deficiency.
5. To the first tube of each set add 2.5 ml of Owren's buffer. To the second tube of each set add 2.5 ml of urea solution and to the third tube of each set add 2.5 ml of acetic acid solution.

Cap tubes. Record the time each solution is added.

6. Invert each tube (preferably only once) to ensure that the clots are floating freely in the solution. After the addition of buffer, urea, or acetic acid the clots must be free floating. If gentle inversion fails to detach the clot use a plastic pipette to dislodge it.
7. Incubate at 37 °C. Observe after the first hour and again after overnight incubation.
8. A deficiency of FXIII is indicated by the complete dissolution of the clots in tubes with urea and acetic acid.
9. An adequate level of FXIII is shown by the presence of the clots after the overnight incubation.
10. If FXIII is reduced and the urea and/or acetic acid tubes show dissolution of clots, the buffer tube should still contain a clot.
11. Record details of clot stability (+ve, clot present) or lysis (−ve, clot absent) in routine workbook.

If clot is PRESENT, there WAS resistance to dissolution by ACETIC ACID and/or UREA.

If clot is ABSENT, there WAS NOT resistance to dissolution by ACETIC ACID and/or UREA.

2.6.5 Calculation of Results

The test is normal if the clots do not dissolve.

If acetic acid dissolves the clot it is considered that there is <2% of FXIII. If the clot is also dissolved by urea, <1% of FXIII is present.

If acetic acid dissolves the clot but not urea, the FXIII level is 1–2%.

If urea dissolves the clot but not acetic acid, an error in the test setup is likely to have occurred as this combination is not theoretically possible. Repeat the test.

2.6.6 Interpretation

Low levels of FXIII are diagnostic of a bleeding disorder caused by the failure of clots to stabilize.

If acetic acid dissolves the clot it is considered that there is <2% of FXIII. If the clot is also dissolved by urea, <1% of FXIII is present. If acetic acid dissolves the clot but not urea, the FXIII level is 1–2%.

If buffer dissolves the clot it is possible that the plasma sample contains a physiological/therapeutic agent or cause resulting in clot instability that is unrelated to a FXIII deficiency.

In rare cases the screening test may show clot lysis in the acetic acid tube and a stable clot in urea, but the plasma has a normal FXIII level by activity assay. This is due to increased levels of an acid protease in the plasma, which is activated in the acetic acid solution and able to lyse the fibrin clot (13).

2.6.7 Reporting Results

Results of clot solubility are entered for ACETIC ACID/UREA as "dissolved"/"not dissolved."

If a low level is found a mixing study should be performed to exclude an inhibitor.

3 Factor XIII Activity Assay [14]

3.1 Principle

FXIII contained in the patient's plasma sample is activated by the addition of thrombin in the presence of a peptide to inhibit clot formation. Plasma must be used as fibrin is required to accelerate FXIII activation.

FXIIIa cross-links a specific peptide substrate with glycine ethyl ester, releasing ammonia (see Eq. 2), which subsequently participates in the oxidation of NADH to NAD (see Eq. 3). The fall in NADH is measured by monitoring its absorbance at 340 nM. The rate of the change in absorbance (ΔA/min) after reaching the linear phase is proportional to the FXIII activity.

1. FXIII activation.

   Thrombin, Ca^{2+}

$$\text{Factor XIII} \rightarrow \text{Factor XIIIa.} \quad (1)$$

2. Transglutaminase reaction.

   FXIIIa.

$$\text{Glycine ethyl ester} + \text{peptide substrate} \rightarrow \text{conjugate} + \text{NH3.} \quad (2)$$

3. Indicator reaction.

   Glutamate dehydrogenase (GLDH).

$$\text{NH3} + \text{NADH} + \alpha\text{-ketoglutarate} \rightarrow \text{NAD} + \text{glutamate.} \quad (3)$$

3.2 Reference Interval

0.70–1.40 U/ml.

3.3 Equipment and Reagents

3.3.1 Equipment

Unicel DXC800 (Beckman-Coulter) or other photometer capable of measuring absorbance at 340 nM.

37 °C incubator or water bath.

Plastic tubes.

3.3.2 Reagents

Berichrom FXIII kit (Code No. OWSU): Reagents for the photometric determination of FXIII kit:

NADH Reagent: Dissolve in 5 ml of distilled water.

Activator reagent (bovine thrombin and additives): Reconstitute with 5 ml of NADH. Reconstituted solution stable for 6 months when stored at −20 °C.

Detection reagent (GLDH, glycine ethyl ester, peptide): Dissolve in 5 ml of distilled water. Reconstituted solution stable for 6 months when stored at −20 °C.

3.4 Specimen Requirements

3.5 ml sample; 9 parts whole blood:1 part 0.11 M (3.2%) trisodium citrate dihydrate.

3.4.1 Sample Required

Centrifuge at 2,300 × *g* for 10 min at 8 °C for plasma separation.

Viability: Test within 2 months when stored frozen at −20 °C.

3.4.2 Sample Preparation

Standard plasma: Any standard plasma with an assigned FXIII value is suitable.

3.5 Quality Control Plasma

Normal plasma: Commercial control with normal FXIII level.

Abnormal plasma: Commercial control with reduced FXIII level.

3.6 Procedure

Prepare the reagents as described in Subheading 3.3.2.

3.6.1 Preparation

QC plasma is tested in parallel with patient sample.

3.6.2 Quality Control

Calculate the total volume of reagent mixture required allowing 300 μl per plasma (sample, control, or standards) for single testing.

3.6.3 Sample Testing

Prepare the reagent mixture by combining equal parts of activator reagent and detection reagent and warm to 37 °C in water bath.

Load reagent mixture plasma samples, controls, and standard onto Unicel DXC800 according to manufacturer's instruction and process.

Note: Familiarity with the DXC800 or an equivalent instrument is mandatory. Duplicate testing is recommended.

3.6.4 Suggested Settings for DXC800

Start read: 300 s.
End read: 600 s.
Dispense volume: 300 μl.
Sample volume: 30 μl.
Reaction type: Rate 1.
Units: mAbs/min.
Reaction direction: Negative.
Maths model: Linear.
Primary wavelength: 340 nM.
Secondary wavelength: 700 nM.

3.6.5 Calculation of Results

FXIII activity is calculated using the following equation:

$$\text{Factor XIII activity} = \frac{\text{Assigned value of standard plasma (U / ml)}}{\Delta A_{\text{Standard}} / \text{min(measured by instrument)}} \times \Delta A_{\text{Sample}}.$$

The ratio of the assigned FXIII value of standard plasma (U/ml) over $\Delta A_{Standard}$/min (measured by instrument) is called the F_L factor and may be used to calculate the activity of patient and control samples as follows:

$$F\ XIII_{Sample}\left(U / ml\right) = F_L \times \Delta A_{Sample}.$$

Alternatively the results can be calculated using a standard curve in place of the calculation with the F_L factor. Doubling dilutions of the standard plasma are prepared in isotonic saline to cover an approximate range from 100 to 10%.

As the assay is nonlinear at the lower end, levels below 10% should be reported as "<10%."

Reject run if controls are outside acceptable limits.

4 Significance

Marked deficiency of FXIII activity is seen with congenital deficiency, and in patients with acquired inhibitors which may occur following exposure to certain drugs (phenytoin, penicillin, isoniazid, and valproate) or plasma products. Milder deficiency may be seen in patients with disseminated intravascular coagulation, liver disease, leukemia, Henoch–Schönlein purpura, inflammatory bowel disease, prematurity, plasmacytoma, and following recent surgery (15).

References

1. Ichinose A (2001) Physiopathology and regulation of factor XIII. Thromb Haemost 86:57–65
2. Ariens RA, Lai TS, Weisel JW, Greenberg CS, Grant PJ (2002) Role of factor XIII in fibrin clot formation and effects of genetic polymorphisms. Blood 100:743–754
3. Asahina T, Kobayashi T, Okada Y, Goto J, Terao T (2000) Maternal blood coagulation factor XIII is associated with the development of cytotrophoblastic shell. Placenta 21: 388–393
4. Peyvandi F, Mannucci PM (1999) Rare coagulation disorders. Thromb Haemost 82:1207–1214
5. Ivaskevicius V, Seitz R, Kohler HP, Schroeder V, Muszbek L, Ariens RA, Seifried E, Oldenburg J (2007) International registry on factor XIII deficiency: a basis formed mostly on European data. Thromb Haemost 97:914–921
6. Kloczko J, Wojtukiewicz M, Bielawiec M, Zarzycka B, Kinalska I (1986) Plasma factor XIII and some other haemostasis parameters in patients with diabetic angiopathy. Acta Haematol 76:81–85
7. Kloczko J, Wojtukiewicz M, Bielawiec M, Zuch A (1988) Alterations of haemostasis parameters with special reference to fibrin stabilization, factor XIII and fibronectin in patients with obliterative atherosclerosis. Thromb Res 51:575–581
8. Board PG, Losowsky MS, Miloszewski KJ (1993) Factor XIII: inherited and acquired deficiency. Blood Rev 7:229–242
9. Seitz R, Duckert F, Lopaciuk S, Muszbek L, Rodeghiero F, Seligsohn U (1996) ETRO Working Party on Factor XIII questionnaire on congenital factor XIII deficiency in Europe: status and perspectives. Study Group. Semin Thromb Hemost 22:415–418
10. Bolton-Maggs PH, Perry DJ, Chalmers EA, Parapia LA, Wilde JT, Williams MD, Collins PW, Kitchen S, Dolan G, Mumford AD (2004) The rare coagulation disorders–review with guidelines for management from the United Kingdom Haemophilia Centre

Doctors' Organisation. Haemophilia 10: 593–628
11. Mitchell Lewis S, Bain BJ, Bates I (eds) (2006) Dacie and Lewis practical haematology, Vol. 1, 10th edn. Churchill Livingstone, Philadelphia
12. Jennings I, Kitchen S, Woods TA, Preston FE (2003) Problems relating to the laboratory diagnosis of factor XIII deficiency: a UK NEQAS study. J Thromb Haemost 1:2603–2608
13. Ragaz S, Kemp G, Furlan M, Beck EA (1976) Bleeding disorder with abnormal wound healing, acid-soluble clots and normal factor XIII. Thromb Haemost 36:537–541
14. Dade-Behring (2005) Berichrom FXIII In: Reagents for the photometric determination of Factor XIII p6, Dade Behring, Marburg, Germany
15. Colman RW (ed) (2006) Hemostasis and thrombosis, basic principles and clinical practice, Vol. 1, 5th edn. Lippincott, Williams & Wilkins, Philadelphia

Chapter 14

Fibrinogen

Linda J. Stang and Lesley G. Mitchell

Abstract

Fibrinogen is the final essential building block of the clotting process. Thus, all of the preliminary "cause and effect" events in the clotting cascade rely on the work of this molecule to measure their success. The most commonly used laboratory method for measuring fibrinogen is the Clauss fibrinogen assay. The Clauss fibrinogen assay is a quantitative, clot-based, functional assay. The assay measures the ability of fibrinogen to form fibrin clot after being exposed to a high concentration of purified thrombin. Plasma samples are pre-diluted which minimize assay interference from substances like heparin and fibrinogen degradation products. In brief, the diluted plasma is incubated at 37°C prior to the addition of the pre-warmed (37°C) thrombin reagent. From the exact moment of the addition of thrombin, the time to clot is measured. The clotting time in seconds is interpolated from a standard curve made using various dilutions of assayed standard plasma. The following chapter includes detailed information on the Clauss fibrinogen assay. Other fibrinogen assays used include fibrinogen levels derived from prothrombin time assays and antigenic methods. Fibrinogen measurements using the prothrombin time and antigenic based assays are described in brief.

Key words Fibrinogen, Thrombin reagent, Clauss method, Standard curve, Alert value, Hypofibrinogenemia

1 Introduction

The first report identifying fibrinogen was by Dr. Olaf Hammarsten (1841–1932) who elucidated the fact that the precursor to fibrin is fibrinogen, which will clot when exposed to thrombin. Also, Dr. Hammarsten demonstrated that fibrinogen is insoluble in H_2O and that it will precipitate from plasma when dialyzed against H_2O (1). Another characteristic of fibrinogen was first observed in 1947 and again in 1959 in that when plasma is frozen and then thawed, the fibrinogen is the last protein to return to solution (2, 3). Isolating the remaining precipitate from the cold plasma results in a small volume rich in fibrinogen as well as factor VIII. The technique for making cryoprecipitate continues to be used today in blood processing centers.

Paul Monagle (ed.), *Haemostasis: Methods and Protocols*, Methods in Molecular Biology, vol. 992,
DOI 10.1007/978-1-62703-339-8_14, © Springer Science+Business Media New York 2013

Fibrinogen is produced in the liver and has a half-life of approximately 3–4 days (4). Considered to be an acute-phase reactant, fibrinogen exhibits increased levels in various systemic inflammatory conditions. Circulating fibrinogen exhibits some heterogeneity related to enzyme degradation and genetic influence, whereby not every molecule is fully functional in formation of a clot (5). Thus, assays of clottable fibrinogen may show disparity with antigenic assays even with samples from normal healthy patients.

The fibrinogen molecule consists of three subunits denoted as Aα, Bβ, and γ occurring in pairs for a total of six subunits. When fibrinogen is exposed to thrombin, the conversion of fibrinogen to fibrin results in the α-subunit releasing two fibrinopeptides denoted as fibrinopeptide A (FPA). Following the release of FPA, the β-subunit also releases two subunits denoted accordingly as fibrinopeptide B (FPB). Other than some reports in the literature that fibrinopeptide B has the ability to sensitize and increase DNA synthesis in smooth muscles, very little work has been published on the possible functional attributes of the fibrinopeptides released (6, 7). With thrombin cleaving of FPA and FPB the newly formed fibrin monomers now lack the negatively charged fibrinopeptides which had previously caused the molecules to repel each other. The monomers can now link initially end to end and then side to side (4). The fibers blend into a crisscross mesh-like pattern which essentially produces a "net," capable of entrapment of erythrocytes, platelets, and clot-bound thrombin. The density of the mesh net can be affected by physical conditions present (pH, temperature etc.). The fibrin polymer formed from the fibrin monomer is then further modified by factor XIII which changes the hydrogen bonds to covalent bonds, thus strengthening and stabilizing the clot (4). The stabilization of the clot is critical for haemostasis as indicated by the fact that congenital deficiencies of factor XIII result in bleeding disorders at birth.

Familial afibrinogenemia is a term used to describe patients with complete lack of fibrinogen or only small amounts of measurable fibrinogen. The condition is extremely rare. Patients who are heterozygotes with afibrinogenemia are asymptomatic. Homozygote afibrinogenemia is generally a result of consanguinity (8).

Hypofibrinogenemia as defined by low but detectable levels usually <1.0 g/L results in relatively mild bleeding (see Note 1) (9). Inherited dysfibrinogenemia, with circulating fibrinogen molecules that are present but not functional, has been documented in at least 250 patients. Symptoms range from patients with bleeding diathesis, asymptomatic patients, to the other extreme, thrombophilic patients (10). Improperly functioning molecules may also be as a consequence of excessive glycosylation of the fibrinogen molecule, likely as a result of liver disease (11). Acquired conditions are much more common than congenital disease and are related to impaired production (e.g., liver disease), increased consumption (e.g., post cardiac bypass surgery), or increased destruction (e.g., fibrinolytic system anomalies). There have been a few reports of autoantibodies that inhibit the formation of fibrin from fibrinogen by varying mechanisms depending on the antibody specificity. Inhibition of release of a polypeptide causing abnormal monomer polymerization, inhibition of the connection between fibrin monomers, or inhibition of the formation of the cross-links between α-chains (12–14). In addition, there have been rare reports of alloantibodies following transfusion (15).

As clinically relevant decreases in fibrinogen are rare, measurement of fibrinogen is not frequently requested by physicians (see Note 2). However, recent large studies have indicated that elevated fibrinogen levels are associated with increased risk for cardiovascular disease (16). Therefore, in the near future, measurement of fibrinogen may be increased in hospital laboratories as part of routine clinical care.

2 Materials

2.1 Clauss Assay Reagents

See Table 1 for details of specific reagents.

Owren's buffer recipe (0.02 mol/L, pH 7.4 ± 0.05) (17). To a 2 L volumetric flask with approx 1 L of type 1 dH_2O, add

Table 1
Clauss assay reagents

Reagent	Variations
Thrombin or thrombin calcium—reconstitute according to manufacturer's product insert	Thrombin concentrations will vary between commercial preparations (35–100 U/mL) and can be either human or bovine Reagents are usually lyophilized Commercial thrombin preparations are recommended over in-house preparations, for increased stability (see Note 3)
Owren's barbital (or Veronal) buffer	Available commercially (or see described recipe) Equivalent buffers may be used
Standard assayed plasma (calibrator)	Generally standards are assayed against an international standard The method of assay, used to determine the assayed plasma value, should be similar to the method being performed in the local laboratory (see Note 4)
Control plasma-2 levels; normal and abnormal low—reagent is usually lyophilized; reconstitute according to manufacturer's product insert	QC should be run at minimum, for two different levels on the calibration graph, ensuring the slope of the trend line to be appropriate (see Note 5)

430 mL of 0.1 mol/L HCl and then 11.7 g of sodium diethylbarbiturate and 14.7 g NaCl. Stir until dissolved. Add dH_2O to just under 2 L, and adjust pH to 7.4 with 1 N HCl. Add dH_2O for a final volume of 2 L. Buffer is stable 3–6 months when stored at 4°C, and check for contamination prior to each use (see Note 6).

3 Methods

Fibrinogen can be directly assayed by numerous methods including clot based, immunological, clottable protein, and nephelometric. The most common assay is a clot-based assay which utilizes a dilution of patient's plasma in which the clotting time is inversely proportional to the concentration of fibrinogen. This method, commonly referred to as the Clauss assay, uses a high concentration of thrombin, which minimizes interference from heparin and FDPs (see Notes 7–9) (18). The Clauss method is recommended for use in the clinical lab. Other methods such as ELISA or nephelometry are useful in research settings or certain clinical circumstances such as diagnosing dysfibrinogenemia (11). In addition, some coagulation analyzer reagent combinations have the capability of deriving the fibrinogen concentration from the optical density change that occurs during another coagulation assay. The prothrombin time assay is usually used for this purpose, likely due to the speed of thrombin generation and the ensuing fibrin formation. The assay has the advantage of no additional cost for reagent or consumables and is currently being used in a varying number of clinical labs and appears to be more popular in certain countries than others. However, this assay may give higher estimates than the Clauss and may be inaccurate in anticoagulated patients and with certain disease states (19).

For the purposes of the current review chapter, the majority of information listed pertains to the Clauss clot-based assay. The less commonly used assays are briefly discussed.

3.1 Clauss Assay for Fibrinogen

The Clauss fibrinogen assay is a quantitative, clot-based, functional assay. It measures the ability of fibrinogen to form fibrin after being exposed to a high concentration of purified thrombin. Plasma samples are pre-diluted which minimizes assay interference from substances like heparin and FDPs. In brief, the diluted plasma is incubated at 37°C prior to the addition of the pre-warmed (37°C) thrombin reagent. From the exact moment of the addition of thrombin, the time to clot is measured. This clotting time in seconds is interpolated from a standard curve made using various dilutions of assayed standard plasma (see Notes 10–12).

Table 2
Summary of commercially available reagents for performing a Clauss fibrinogen assay

Product	Origin/calcium content	Concentration	Unfractionated heparin interference	FDP interference
Diagnostica Stago STA Fib 5	Human thrombin + calcium	80 U/mL Final = 26.6 U/mL	>2 U/mL	>130 μg/mL
Diagnostica Stago STA Fib 2	Human thrombin + calcium	40 U/mL Final = 13.3 U/mL	>1 U/mL	>130 μg/mL
HemosIL Fibrinogen-C	Bovine thrombin + calcium	35 U/mL Final = 11.7 U/mL	>1 U/mL	>100 μg/mL
HemosIL QFA Thrombin	Bovine thrombin	100 U/mL Final = 33.3 U/mL	>2 U/mL	Not specified
Dade Behring Multifibren U	Bovine thrombin + calcium	50 U/mL Final = 33.3 U/mL	>2 U/mL	Not specified
Dade Fibrinogen Determination	Bovine thrombin	100 U/mL Final = 33.3 U/mL	>1 U/mL	>100 μg/mL
Amax Fibrinogen	Bovine thrombin	75 U/mL Final = 25 U/mL	Not specified	Not specified
BioMerieux Fibriquik	Bovine thrombin	100 U/mL Final = 33.3 U/mL	>0.6 U/mL	>100 μg/mL
BioMerieux MDA Fibriquik	Bovine thrombin	Not specified	>0.6 U/mL	>100 μg/mL

3.2 Commercially Available Clauss Reagents

There are multiple commercially available reagents for performing fibrinogen assays (see Table 2). However, there are marked differences in both the types of reagents (e.g., bovine or human thrombin) and concentrations depending on the distribution company. The differences in reagents result in differences in the sensitivity to heparin and/or FDPs as well as potential differences in sensitivity to fibrinogen levels. In Table 2, the differences in the reagents in the various methods are listed. Please note that final concentrations take into consideration the individual procedures contained in the respective package inserts or are the current recommendations for the corresponding clinical analyzers (see Note 13).

3.3 Sample Requirements

Sodium citrate plasma, (for specifics see "Specimen Requirements"), 9 parts blood to 1 part trisodium citrate (3.2% or 0.105–0.109 mol/L). Adjust the citrate concentration for patients with hematocrit >0.55 L/L. Platelet-poor plasma can be prepared at room temperature by centrifugation at 1,700 × *g* for 10 min (producing platelet-poor plasma with a resulting plasma platelet count of <10×10^9/L). Sample can be stored at room temperature for 8 h, or frozen at −70°C for long-term storage (up to 6 months) followed by thawing at 37°C for 5–10 min (time needed is dependent on the volume frozen; ensure all flocculation has dissolved and sample is well mixed prior to analysis) (see Notes 14 and 15).

3.4 Standard Curve

(a) Input into analyzer the predetermined standard curve from reagent manufacturer (see Note 16) OR

(b) Standard plasma—assayed against an international standard.

Dilute the standard plasma in Owren's buffer as follows: 1/6, 1/10, 1/20, 1/40.

Calibration curves should include at least three dilutions performed in duplicate; 4 or 5 individual dilutions are preferable and will produce a standard curve with a broader working range. These dilutions can be modified slightly as long as a trend line can be produced with an R2 value of >0.995 on a log/log graph. The 1/20 dilution represents the 100% point of the calibrator value (some manufacturers recommend other dilutions to represent the 100% point—i.e., 1/10). Standard curves should be generated for each new lot number of reagent or change in analyzer.

When performing the Clauss assay on an automated analyzer, results are calculated automatically by the software. However, when performing a Clauss assay manually or on a semiautomated analyzer the graphs must be generated by the user. Although the relationship of the clotting time to fibrinogen concentration is logarithmic, it is important to note that determining patient's results is more accurate if a graph with a linear/linear relationship is used. Examples of standard curves for fibrinogen are shown in Fig. 1. A table of data with a calibrator assay value of 3.00 g/L was used. Both the logarithmic scale and the linear scale with a power trend line are shown; each graph is included to inform the user that a logarithmic scale is sometimes difficult to read corresponding fibrinogen values for a given clotting time. Linear graphs generally have more options for *x* and *y* scale on automated graphing programs.

The steps involved in performing the assay are detailed in Table 3.

3.5 Expected Results

The reference range for the normal adult population is 2.0–4.0 g/L. Each laboratory should establish its own normal range from a minimum of 40 normal subjects, including a wide age range from both sexes. Samples from patients should not be included in the reference range determination as the levels of fibrinogen may be increased in the patient population, as fibrinogen is an acute-phase reactant.

Dilution of Standard	Fibrinogen (g/L)	Clotting time (seconds)
1/40	1.50	36.0
1/20	3.00	17.5
1/10	6.00	8.5
1/6	10.00	5.8

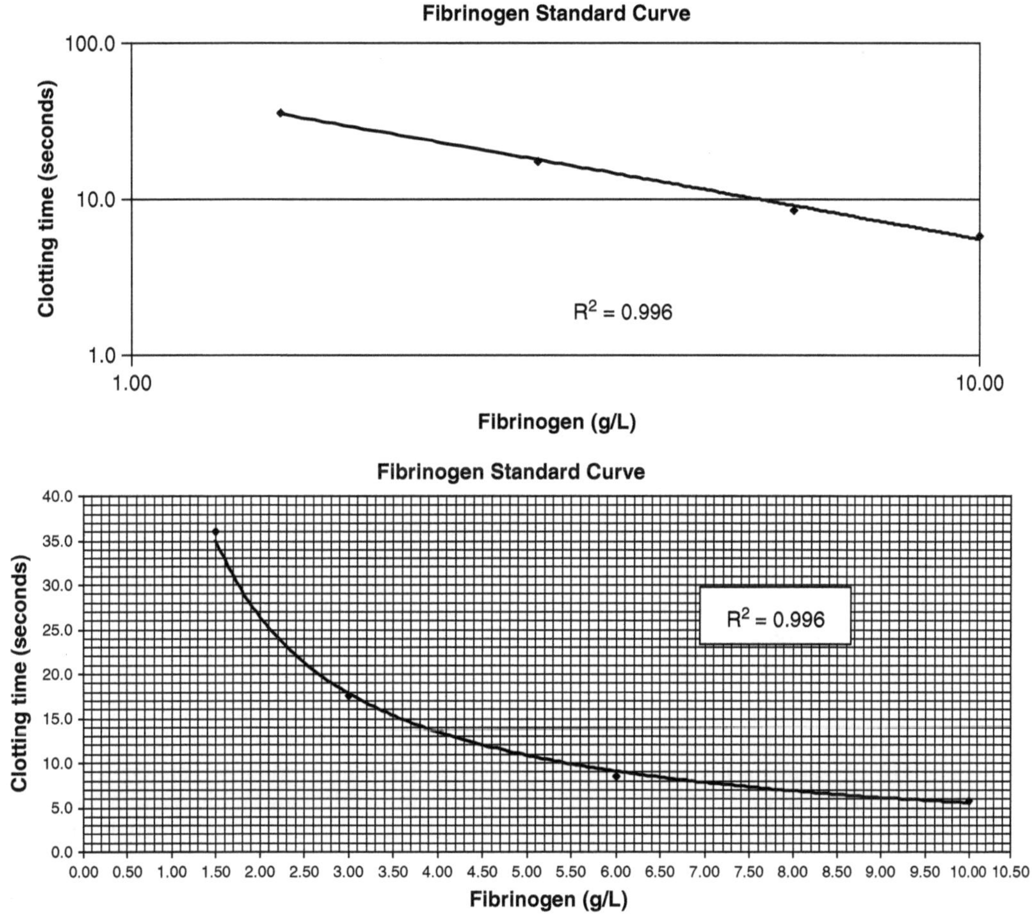

Fig. 1 Example of a standard curve for fibrinogen plotted on both the logarithmic scale and the linear scale

3.6 Fibrinogen Derived from PT Assays

Calibration is performed by using standard plasma (or multiple standard plasmas). A graph is plotted with fibrinogen concentration against optical density. The optical change for each patient sample is then read off the graph, generating a fibrinogen value. When using this assay, ensure that suitable reference ranges are generated for the instrument/reagent combination, as they may differ from the Clauss assay.

3.7 Antigenic Fibrinogen Assays

There are currently numerous commercially available antigenic fibrinogen assays. These assays are usually in the format of a competitive sandwich enzyme immunoassay (ELISA) and can be useful in the diagnosis of dysfibrinogenemia; nonfunctional as well as functional molecules will be quantified.

Table 3
The steps in performing a Clauss fibrinogen assay

Step	Details/variations/comments
1. Add 100 μL to each of two sample cups, for each dilution of the standard plasma (i.e., 1/6, 1/10, 1/20, 1/40)	Volume can be doubled to accommodate analyzer minimum volumes, if necessary. Use double volumes for all steps Manufacturer volume recommendations may vary
2. Incubate for 4 min at 37°C	This incubation time may vary by analyzer
3. Add 50 μL of pre-warmed (37°C) thrombin reagent. Begin timing precisely at the addition of the thrombin	Automated analyzers will generally warm the required amount of reagent just before use
4. Using the 1/20 dilution as the "100%" point, plot fibrinogen concentration (*x*-axis) against time to clot in seconds (*y*-axis) on a log–log graph	If assigned calibrator value is 3.00 g/L, then 1/6 = 10.00 g/L; 1/10 = 6.00 g/L; 1/20 = 3.00 g/L; -1/40 = 1.50 g/L Use both of the individual values from each calibrator dilution
5. Dilute control samples 1/20 in the Owren's buffer. Mix well. Follow steps 1–3 above for each control sample	25 μL of control material in 475 μL of buffer Reconstitute controls according to manufacturer's instructions 2 control levels—low and normal control are recommended
6. Read the fibrinogen concentration off graph for the corresponding seconds of each control value	Average the duplicate readings Duplicates should check within 10% of each other
7. If the low control clotting time in seconds is greater than the highest point on the standard curve, dilute the low control 1/10 in Owren's buffer Repeat steps 1–3 as above	Automated analyzers will usually have the capability of reflex testing to allow re-dilution (at a lower or higher dilution) of samples that are not within the range of the standard curve The mathematical corrector for a 1/10 dilution is to multiply the fibrinogen value by (0.5) If very low values of fibrinogen cause a reflex test and smaller dilutions are made on that reflex test, the low QC level should reflect this range and alternate dilution
8. Verify the controls are within allowable limits before proceeding to patient samples	See Note 5
9. Dilute patient sample(s) 1/20 in the Owren's buffer. Mix well	
10. Repeat steps 1–3 as above for patient samples	Average the duplicate readings Duplicates should check within 10% of each other

(continued)

Table 3 (continued)

Step	Details/variations/comments
11. For patient samples with clotting times: Shorter than the lowest standard dilution, dilute at 1/60 (multiply the value read off the graph by a factor of 3) Higher than the highest standard dilution, dilute using a 1/10 (multiply the value read off the graph by a factor of 0.5)	The patient clotting time in seconds must fall between the lowest and highest standard; values should not be extrapolated beyond the highest or lowest point. Linearity outside these points has not been defined An alternative dilution of the patient sample may also be used, provided that the clotting time is within the range of the standard curve, with the appropriate mathematical corrector used to calculate the results

Wells of a microtiter plate are coated with polyclonal (or monoclonal) antibody to fibrinogen. After a blocking step, dilutions of standard, control(s) and samples are added to the plate. Following incubation and washing, a solution containing a second conjugated antibody (i.e., streptavidin peroxidase or horseradish peroxidase conjugated) against fibrinogen is added. After a second incubation and washing step, the substrate is added followed by a stop solution and the absorbance is read on an ELISA plate reader.

4 Notes

1. Critical or alert values for fibrinogen are generally below the level of 1.00 g/L. As a general rule, the Transfusion Medicine Department will not release cryoprecipitate for infusion unless the fibrinogen has fallen below 1.00 g/L. When plasminogen activators are being administered and the fibrinogen level is being used as an indicator of therapy the assay values desired may be in this critical range (0.50–1.00 g/L) (20).
2. There is a general assumption that the PT and PTT can be used as a screening test to rule out a low fibrinogen. However, this assumption is probably incorrect. Studies in our laboratory determined the sensitivity of the PT and PTT to fibrinogen concentration by using plasma from a congenitally fibrinogen-deficient donor spiked with different concentrations of normal plasma. The data showed that fibrinogen concentrations of 0.45 g/L which are well below critical levels result in a normal PTT value, if all other factors are present in normal amounts. In fact, when fibrinogen levels are as low as 0.15 g/L, the PTT is only elevated by a few seconds (unpublished data).

   In the same experiments using PT INR, a fibrinogen of 0.76 g/L will produce a normal INR. A level of 0.45 g/L fibrinogen will increase the INR by only 0.2 from the top of the normal range. To produce an INR that has a significant increase (2.0), the fibrinogen level would need to drop to 0.15 g/L (unpublished data).

3. Stability is greatly increased by the use of commercial reagents; therefore, in-house preparations of pure thrombin are not recommended. Current commercially available fibrinogen reagents, which are essentially thrombin or a thrombin and calcium chloride mix, are stable for approximately 4–5 days at 15°C. In contrast, purified thrombin is relatively unstable, and solutions at a concentration of 4–5 U/mL last only about 1 h at 2–8°C.
4. When choosing standard plasma for use with photo-optical analyzers, avoid reference plasmas that are markedly turbid, as turbidity may interfere with the linearity of the standard curve. As well, severely lipemic or icteric patient samples may cause interference with photo-optical methods.
5. The QC material and/or reagent used for fibrinogen seems to be more sensitive to changes in the dH_2O source used by the coagulation lab, than other QC/reagent combinations in use for PT, PTT, or other specialized coagulation clot-based assays. In-house distillers as well as hospital wide distilled water systems (type II dH_2O) have on occasion proven problematic. One recommended water source that has provided more stable QC data is an "ultrapure water system" which produces type I water.
6. The sodium diethylbarbiturate needed for the Owren's buffer is a controlled substance in many countries, and thus requires a significant amount of paper work/permissions, etc. to obtain the product. Commercially available buffer is generally much easier to attain.
7. Some commercially available fibrinogen reagents contain both heparin neutralizers and a high concentration of thrombin that helps to eliminate interference from heparinized patients. However, there is usually a maximum heparin level stated in the product insert (i.e., 1.0 or 2.0 U/mL), for which the reagent is capable of producing an accurate result. In certain clinical settings heparin levels will exceed maximum limits. For example, fibrinogen assays during cardiopulmonary bypass are sometimes clinically necessary, but the level of heparinization of these patients will almost certainly exceed the stated maximum heparin level for a given product. These circumstances have the potential to produce a falsely low fibrinogen result and heparin removal from the sample with an absorbent or enzyme may be needed.
8. Interference from direct thrombin inhibitors (DTI) (i.e., lepirudin, Argatroban, etc.) should be investigated for reagents in use in each respective laboratory as the interference is likely dependent on thrombin concentration of the reagent. As a portion of the thrombin will be directly and immediately inhibited

by the DTI, there must be adequate thrombin remaining to initiate the clotting reaction. If there is ample thrombin in the reagent, the fibrinogen values obtained may not be affected. In our laboratory using a commercial reagent containing 80 U/mL of human thrombin, fibrinogen values were not affected for concentrations of lepirudin and Argatroban between 0.3 and 2.0 mg/mL (unpublished data). However other investigators have found interference in some commercially available reagents at similar DTI concentrations (21). Origin of the thrombin (bovine vs. human) may also affect the degree of interference.

9. Increased levels of FDPs may result in false low or falsely increased levels depending on the type of fibrinogen assay being performed. Underestimation may occur in a clot-based assay; overestimation may occur in a total protein or antigenic assay (22). Each manufacturer of clot-based assays will usually have defined limits above which the FDPs may interfere.
10. The initial 1/20 dilution of the patient's plasma produces a so-called "weak" or "wispy" clot. In comparison, for a PT or PTT assay, no dilution of patient sample is made prior to assay; thus the clot is much stronger. For mechanical analyzers (and optical, if possible), the sensitivity of the clot detection system should be altered such that a "weaker" clot can be detected accurately. Therefore, patients with very low fibrinogens produce a clot that is even more delicate and should be tested at a lesser dilution that is within the linear range of the standard curve to ensure accurate results.
11. Duplicate clotting times are generally recommended for automated fibrinogen assays in contrast to other routine coagulation assays.
12. Extrapolation of results outside the standard curve is never recommended for any coagulation assay. Therefore, different dilutions of the patient plasma should be made so that the clotting time falls within the standard curve.
13. When using a random access analyzer, it is necessary to verify that carryover of the fibrinogen reagent does not occur. The high levels of thrombin in the reagent would cause significant change in the subsequent assay if any thrombin were to remain on the reagent pickup probe. Therefore, the fibrinogen assay should be included in any initial carryover verification.
14. Samples collected on patients with DIC or on thrombolytic therapy should be processed in a timely manner, as prolonged storage may result in a falsely low fibrinogen level caused by plasmin proteolysis. Alternatively, the samples can be collected into tubes containing a plasmin inhibitor such as aprotinin.
15. Frozen samples need to be fully thawed to avoid cryoprecipitate formation. As cryoprecipitate contains fibrinogen patients' results have the potential to be inaccurate.

16. Owing to improved stability of current fibrinogen reagents, some manufacturers provide a standard curve that has been predetermined in their laboratory, which is then input into the clinical laboratory's automated coagulation analyzer and used for the entire lot of reagent. Although this method of standard curve preparation is generally not used in the coagulation laboratory, it has proven to be reliable and accurate for fibrinogen assays.

Acknowledgments

Funding support was from the Canadian Institute of Health Research (L Mitchell Grant#114981).

References

1. Owen CA Jr (2001) Fibrinogen. In: Wl N, Bowie EJW (eds) A history of blood coagulation. Rochester, Minnesota, pp 19–26
2. vanCreveld S, Verder HA, Pascha CN, Kroeze WF (1959) The separation of AHF from fibrinogen. Thromb Diath Haemorrh 3:572–577
3. Ware AG, Guest MM, Seegers WH (1947) Fibrinogen, with special reference to its preparation and certain properties of the product. Arch Biochem 13:231–236
4. Brown BA (1980) Coagulation. Hematology. Lea and Febiger, Philadelphia, pp 115–150.
5. Nieuwenhuizen W, Mossesson MW, De Maat MPM (2001) Fibrinogen: XVIth International Fibrinogen Workshop. Ann NY Acad Sci 645.
6. Gladner JA (1968) The action of fibrinogen. In: Laki K (ed) Marcel Dekker, Fibrinogen, pp 87–115
7. Sturge J, Carey N, Davies AH, Powell JT (2001) Fibrin monomer and fibrinopeptide B act additively to increase DNA synthesis in smooth muscle cells cultured from human saphenous vein. J Vasc Siurg 33:847–853
8. Owen CA Jr (2001) Inherited coagulation factor deficiencies. A history of blood coagulation. Rochester, Minnesota, p 127
9. Brown BA (1980) Diseases. Hematology. p 256.
10. Haverkate F, Samama M (1995) Familial dysfibrinogenemia and thrombophilia. Report on a study of the SSC subcommittee on fibrinogen. Thromb Haemost 73:151–161
11. Mackie IJ, Kitchen S, Machin SJ, Lowe GD (2003) Guidelines on fibrinogen assays. Br J Haematol 121:396–404
12. Hoots WK, Carrell NA, Wagner RH, Cooper HA, McDonagh J (1981) A naturally occurring antibody that inhibits fibrin polymerization. N Engl J Med 304:857–861
13. Marciniak E, Greenwood MF (1979) Acquired coagulation inhibitor delaying fibrinopeptide release. Blood 53:81–92
14. Rosenberg RD, Colman RW, Lorand L (1974) A new haemorrhagic disorder with defective fibrin stabilization and cryofibrinogenaemia. Br J Haematol 26:269–284
15. de Vries A, Rosenberg T, Kochwa S, Boss JH (1961) AM J Med 30:486–494
16. Lowe GD, Rumley A (1999) Use of fibrinogen and fibrin D-dimer in prediction of arterial thrombotic events. Thromb Haemost 82:667–672
17. Procedure for the determination of fibrinogen in plasma; approved guideline. 2nd edn. CLSI(NCCLS). 21(18):H30-A2
18. Clauss A (1957) Rapid physiological coagulation method in determination of fibrinogen. Acta Haematol 17:237–246
19. Laffen M, Manning R (2006) Investigation of haemostasis. In: Lewis SM, Bain BJ, Bates I (eds) Practical hematology. Elsevier, Philadelphia, pp 401–422
20. Ludlam CA, Bennett B, Fox KA, Lowe GD, Reid AW (1995) Guidelines for the use of thrombolytic therapy. Haemostasis and thrombosis task force of the British Committee for standards in haematology. Blood Coagul Fibrinolysis 6:273–285
21. Gosselin RC, King JH, Janatpur KA et al (2004) Effects of pentasaccharide (fondaparinux) and direct thrombin inhibitors on coagulation testing. Arch Pathol Lab Med 128:1142–1145
22. Lowe GD, Rumley A, Mackie IJ (2004) Plasma fibrinogen. Ann Clin Biochem 41:430–440

Chapter 15

Platelet Counting

Sylvain Salignac, Véronique Latger-Cannard, Nicole Schlegel, and Thomas Pierre Lecompte

Abstract

Platelet counting is a daily basic hematological analysis of crucial interest in many clinical situations. Historical manual techniques (phase-contrast microscopy) have been replaced by automated techniques (impedance or optical analyzers) more rapid and precise. More recently, flow cytometry techniques using labeled monoclonal antibodies have been proposed as reference techniques. Nevertheless, pre-analytical and analytical variables should be respected to obtain reliable results and avoid validation pitfalls.

Key words Platelet count, Hematology analyzers, Platelet disorders, Thrombocytopenia, Thrombocytosis

1 Introduction

Platelet counting is a crucial, basic, and daily analysis, for clinical and research purpose. A deficiency of number and/or functions of platelets may lead to a life-threatening bleeding. A significant increase of platelet number may reveal either a benign or malignant disease. Normal reference ranges of platelet count are comprised between 150 and 450 G/L, except for very preterm babies who have lower platelet counts. The knowledge of method and hematology analyzers (HA) used allows avoiding analytical pitfalls.

2 Materials

2.1 Blood Sampling

Performing an accurate blood count requires an appropriate sample mixed with the correct volume of a suitable anticoagulant. In most cases, platelet count is performed with peripheral venous blood obtained by venepuncture. It is also possible to use capillary blood obtained by skin punctures in babies, young infants, and more rarely in adults with poor veins. Capillary blood samples are more susceptible of clotting, and platelet counts performed with

Paul Monagle (ed.), *Haemostasis: Methods and Protocols*, Methods in Molecular Biology, vol. 992,
DOI 10.1007/978-1-62703-339-8_15,

capillary blood are often lower than those performed on venous blood (see Note 1).

2.1.1 Anticoagulant

The anticoagulant of choice is K_2EDTA (ethylenediaminetetraacetic acid) or K_3EDTA. K_2 is recommended by the International Council for Standardization in Hematology (ICSH), at a final concentration of 1.5–2.2 mg/mL (ICSH 1993).

It is also possible to count platelets using trisodium citrate, ACD (citric acid, citrate, dextrose), CTAD (citrate, theophylline, adenosine, dipyridamole), or even heparin as anticoagulant in case of pseudothrombocytopenia.

2.2 Unopette® Commercial Device

Unopette® system (Becton Dickinson, Franklin Lakes, NJ, USA) is composed of a capillary tube used for blood drawing and a reservoir containing ammonium oxalate as anticoagulant. This system can be used either for anticoagulated blood obtained by venepuncture or for capillary blood.

3 Methods

3.1 Platelet Counting: Nonautomated Methods

3.1.1 Manual Phase-Contrast Microscopy

Manual phase-contrast microscopy method has been described in 1953 (1). After lysis of red blood cells, platelets are counted in a counting chamber called hemocytometer (Malassez or Thoma) with a phase-contrast microscope. The commercial device Unopette® system makes this technique easier (see Note 2).

Manual phase-contrast microscopy is time consuming and unprecise, particularly if platelet count is low. Typical interobserver coefficient of variations is in the range of 10–25% (2). This method is still recognized as the reference method but the International Society of Laboratory Hematology (ISLH) has proposed a new reference method using flow cytometry analysis using platelet-specific fluorochrome-labeled monoclonal antibodies (a mixture of anti-CD41 and anti-CD61) (3). Using this method, platelet count is not altered by dilution errors.

3.1.2 Platelet Counting from a Blood Film

It is possible to evaluate platelet count from a stained blood film (see Note 3). This technique is indirect and gives only an estimation of the count. Nevertheless, it is possible to have a look at platelet morphology and to detect fibrin strands, platelet clumps, or leukocyte satellitism.

3.2 Platelet Counting: Automated Methods

3.2.1 Impedance Platelet Count

The development of "Coulter principle" by Wallace Coulter in 1953 has permitted the first red and white blood cell counting and has been used later for platelet counting (late 1970s). "Coulter principle" is based on the increase in electrical impedance when a blood cell in a conducting solution passes through a small aperture encompassed by two electrodes (Fig. 1). Blood cells are very poor conductors of electricity. The impedance increase is proportional

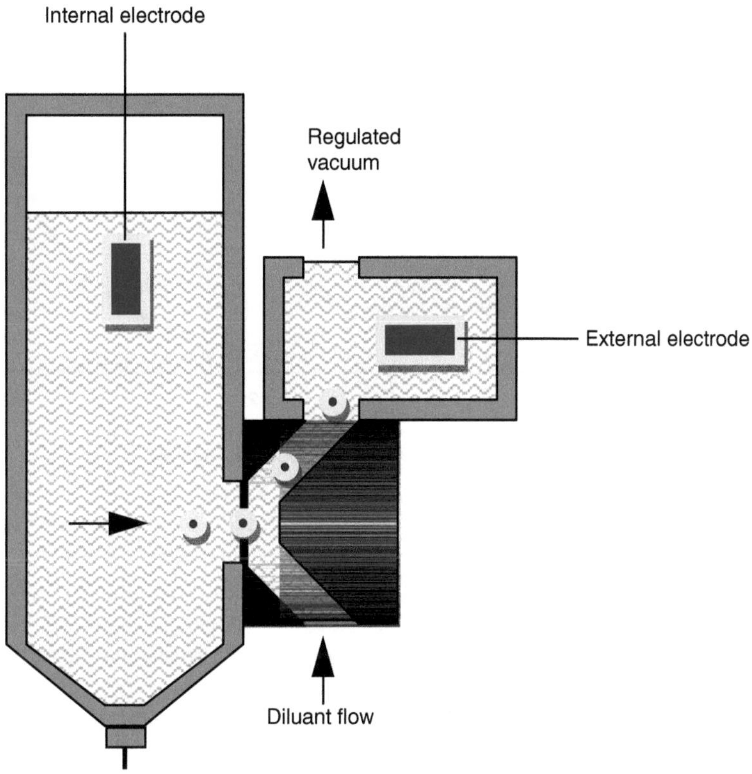

Fig. 1 Measuring chamber (coulter principle)

to the cell volume. This method allows individual cells counting and volume determination. Cells should pass one by one through the aperture to avoid coincidence, which would lead to inaccurate platelet count. To avoid or at least to reduce this phenomenon, coincidence correction and hydrodynamic focusing (directing cells to the center of the aperture) have been developed on some analyzers during the 1970s.

Beckman Coulter analyzers that are currently available count particles with a volume between 2 and 20 femtoliters (fL) in 3 different measurement chambers. Histograms of platelet volume distribution are obtained and a lognormal curve is fitted. Platelet count is derived from this curve and extrapolated between 0 and 70 fL. Fitting of the curve is an indicator of quality of the count and distribution. Presence of giant platelets leads to a typical curve fitting and the count is underestimated. Algorithms have been developed to minimize these problems or at least to warn the user about potentially incorrect results. HA such as Sysmex, Horiba Medical (Pentra®), and Abbott (Cell-Dyn®) use impedance technology too.

A major disadvantage of the impedance method is the impossibility to distinguish large platelets from extremely small red cells or fragments of red cells. Beckman Coulter analyzers use an "interference zone" (24–36 on Coulter analyzer), to flag the possibility of an

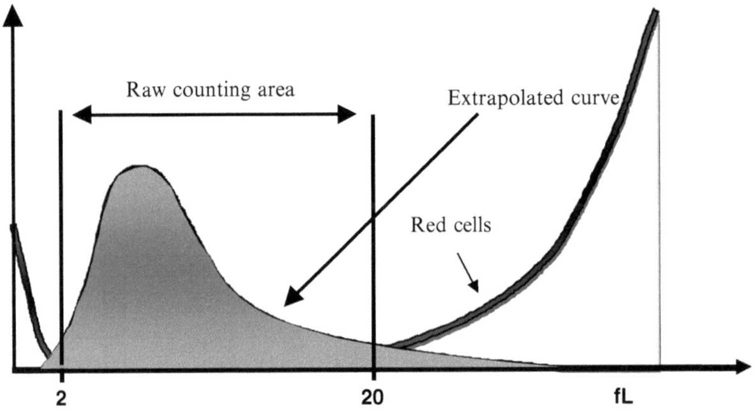

Fig. 2 Counting area and "interference zone" on Coulter analyzer

interference on platelet count due to red cells (Fig. 2). Another disadvantage of the impedance method is the risk of underestimating platelet count when large platelets are present.

3.2.2 Optical Platelet Count

Optical light scatter methods have been developed after the impedance method and are based on light diffraction. Initially, one-dimensional platelet analysis has been developed followed by two-dimensional method. Principle is based on flow cytometry system in which the cells pass through a laser beam and permit a cell by cell analysis of volume and structure (in two-dimensional method). Platelets are sphered without modification of their volume before analysis (sodium dodecyl sulfate and glutaraldehyde). The measure is based on Mie theory of light scattering for homogenous spheres (4).

Two-Dimensional Laser Light Scatter

ADVIA 120 and 2120 (Siemens) measure two angles of laser diffraction, 2–3° converted into volume (platelet size) and 5–15° converted into refractive index (platelet density) (5, 6). This technology allows the differentiation of large platelets and cellular fragments and the measurement of platelets between 1 and 60 fL (Fig. 3).

Cell-Dyn 4000 and Cell-Dyn Sapphire instruments (Abbott) used an optical platelet count but at different angles (7° and 90°) than Siemens system. Simultaneously, an impedance count is performed and compared to optical count. In case of discrepancies, an alert flag suggests an interference phenomenon.

Optical Fluorescence Platelet Counting

Sysmex XE-2100 analyzer can optionally use an optical fluorescence count performed in the reticulocyte channel in addition to the impedance count. It uses a fluorescent dye to stain nucleic acids of reticulocytes and platelets. Since this optical count is not always more accurate than impedance count, a switching algorithm has been designed to report the most accurate platelet count.

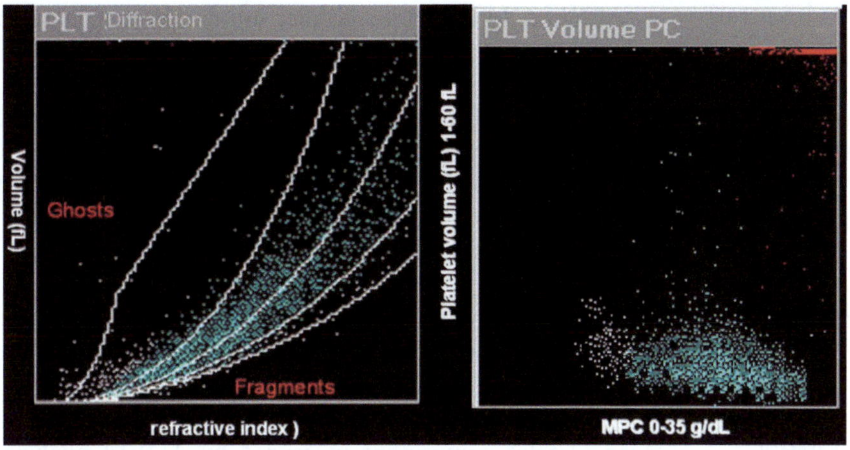

Fig. 3 ADVIA 120 and 2120 (Siemens) platelet scattergram

3.3 Flow Cytometry

Immunological counting of platelets by FCM is proposed now as a new reference method (7). Platelets are labeled with a specific antibody (anti-GPIIbIIIa or anti-GPIb) bound to a fluorochrome and then analyzed. Platelet quantitation is the result of the ratio between labeled events (platelets) and red cells (2) and labeled events and beads (known number) introduced in the counting tube. This method is the most sensitive and reproducible. It is particularly helpful in cases of low platelet count (<50 G/L) in order to increase the precision of the results and adjust the threshold of platelet transfusions to reliable very low platelet counts such as 5–10 G/L (8).

3.4 Comparison and Limits in Case of Low Platelet Count

A number of reports have compared different analyzers between them and versus manual method (9) and more recently immunological platelet counting (10, 11). They highlight the inaccuracies of HA in platelet counting when platelet count is below 20 G/L. These inaccuracies would be responsible for different decision regarding transfusion of platelets. Segal published in 2005 (12) a large multicenter study about platelet count in severe thrombocytopenia comparing HA counting with a FCM method. There was an overestimation by most analyzers. When platelet is normal, in these cases optical method may not be superior to impedance counts.

3.5 Additional Platelet Parameters and Clinical Applications

3.5.1 Mean Platelet Volume

MPV is derived from platelet size distribution curve and is analogous to mean red cell volume (MCV). MPV depends largely on analyzers (technology and calibration) (13). Therefore MPV normal ranges vary with each analyzer (see Note 4).

MPV rises over time because a majority of platelets swell in EDTA within the first 6 h (14). Impedance-based analyzers are not able to count large platelets and underestimate MPV when large platelets are present.

MPV could be helpful to discriminate the mechanism, central or peripheral, of thrombocytopenia (see Note 5).

3.5.2 Large Platelets Percentage

Sysmex XE-2100 calculates the platelet large cell ratio (P-LCR), i.e., the number of platelets with a volume greater than 12 fL divided by the total number of platelets. It is also possible to calculate this ratio on ADVIA analyzer for platelets with a volume greater than 20 fL.

3.5.3 Platelet-Crit

PCT derives from the MPV and the platelet count. It is analogous to red cells hematocrit and is not really useful in clinical and laboratory practice.

3.5.4 Mean Platelet Component

Mean platelet component measured by ADVIA analyzers corresponds to platelet density (refractive index converted into platelet density) and provides information on platelet activation (reduced when activated) (15). The problem is a possible in vitro artifactual activation due to anticoagulant, storage, and blood-drawing conditions. Therefore a specific protocol should be followed for the measurement of MPC (14). Some reports evaluate the possibility to use MPC for patients with coronary artery disease (16) or myelodysplasia (17).

3.5.5 Reticulated Platelets

Reticulated platelets (R.Plt.) are the youngest platelets which contain RNA, and are analog to reticulocytes for red cells. Their number reflects the thrombopoiesis rate and could be useful to distinguish between a central (decreased R.Plt.) and a peripheral (increased) thrombocytopenia. This count is possible on Sysmex XE-2100 (immature platelet fraction, IPF) using a nucleic dye in the optical platelet count channel (18). The automated IPF could be useful in optimizating platelet transfusions in patients undergoing chemotherapy or transplantation (19).

3.6 Validation Tricks of Platelet Counting

Despite the improvement of instrument hardware and software, the systematization of cleaning and background counting procedures, and the generalization of quality and control of data, all HA may be affected by spurious measurements (20). Printed platelet counting may be biologically validated only in the condition that all following criteria are respected: fitted lognormal volume distribution curve, curve starting and returning to baseline, absence of flag.

3.6.1 Pre-analytical Variables

All steps from blood drawing to platelet analysis may generate spurious platelet counts. The venepuncture site should be considered carefully. Analysis of diluted samples (blood drawn in the proximity of a drip or from a line) leads to spuriously low platelet count.

The anticoagulant/blood ratio should follow the manufacturer's recommendations. The recommended time between blood sampling and analysis should be below 6 h at room temperature

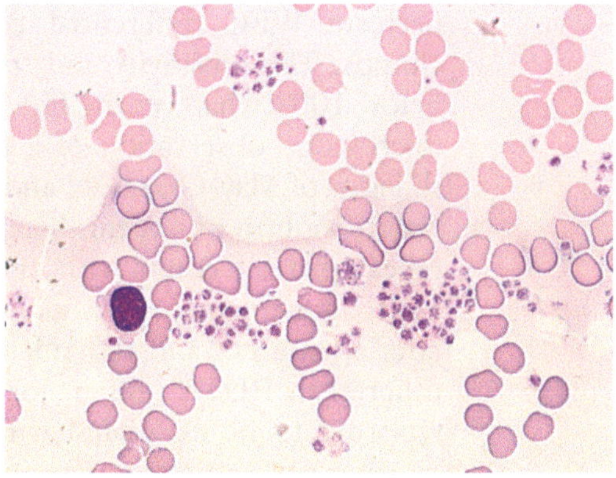

Fig. 4 Platelet clumps visualized by light microscopy on a blood smear

(24 h at 4°C). Increased concentration of anticoagulant (tube not full because of difficult venepuncture) or overtime between sampling and analysis may change platelet volume and consequently may affect platelet count (underestimation).

Inadequate mixing blood sample with anticoagulant or difficult venepuncture may initiate coagulation leading to platelet clumps by stimulation by thrombin and aggregates (see Note 6).

3.6.2 Pseudothrombocytopenia Related to the Anticoagulant

EDTA-dependent pseudothrombocytopenia (EDP) is the most frequent cause of pseudothrombocytopenia related to the anticoagulant and is characterized by a falsely low platelet count caused by an in vitro platelet clumping at room temperature (Fig. 4). EDP is thought to be due to the presence of antiplatelet autoantibodies that recognize platelet antigens (GPIIb/IIIa complex or more precisely GPIIb) modified by or exposed (cryptoantigens) to the combined action of EDTA and room temperature (21).

EDP is not associated with any hemorrhagic tendency. The prevalence rate of EDP was reported to be 0.07–0.20% and was higher in hospitalized patients (1.9%) than in outpatients (0.2%). This phenomenon is transient and may vary with time. It is not related to any peculiar disease and is observed in various clinical situations. Some reports suggested that there was a possible relationship with either autoimmune pathology or cancers. The mechanism of antibody production is yet unknown.

HA do not enumerate platelets in the large clumps and the platelet count corresponds to the count of small clumps. HA generally generate a flag such as "platelet clumps" or "large platelets." In addition, if platelet clumps reach the size of WBC, falsely elevated WBC counts may be observed. Platelet clumps are usually detected by HA that analyze WBC populations in order to perform a WBC differential count (see Note 7). By contrast HA that do not perform WBC differential count frequently overlook platelet clumps. The sensitivity and specificity of "platelet clump" flag is below 100% whatever the HA. When EDP is suspected by a flag, a microscope observation of a freshly drawn blood drop between slides or of May-Grunwäld and Giemsa stained blood smear is crucial to confirm or not this hypothesis. Then, it is recommended to repeat platelet count with another blood sample using another anticoagulant such as trisodium citrate, CTAD (citrate, theophylline, adenosine, and dipyridamole). Nevertheless, anticoagulants other than EDTA (citrate, oxalate, and heparin) have also been reported to be associated with EDP. In these cases, immediate dilution without any anticoagulant or collecting blood using the Unopette® system and observation by phase-contrast microscopy is recommended (see above). If temperature-dependent agglutinins are present, it is recommended to draw and keep the blood sample at 37°C until analysis.

An extremely rare form of platelet agglutination has been reported that is anticoagulant and temperature independent.

3.6.3 Pseudothrombocytopenia Related to Platelet Satellitism Around WBC

Platelet satellitism is characterized by the adherence of platelets around normal or abnormal WBC in EDTA-anticoagulated blood samples, which may lead to false thrombocytopenia. This phenomenon is very rare (1 of 12,000 blood cell counts) and is generally unrelated to any specific disease. Its clinical significance is not known. Polymorphonuclear neutrophil (PMN) is the WBC mostly implied in this phenomenon which may result from an interaction between immunoglobulin G (IgG) or IgM autoantibodies and PMN. The bridge between platelets and PMN has been reported to involve platelet cryptic antigen on GPIIb and Fcγ receptors or CD16 on PMN (22). Platelet satellitism around monocytes, basophils, lymphocytes, or lymphoma cells has been also described (23).

HA are diversely mistaken by this anomaly. Flagging is inconstant. A careful observation of the WBC differential scattergram may reveal abnormal localization of PMN (overlap between PMN and lymphocytes in impedance-type HA or larger PMN in laser-beam HA or WBC with high peroxidase activity on Bayer-Siemens HA).

3.6.4 Large Platelets

Heterogeneity of platelet size with the presence of large platelets is often encountered during pregnancy and in many hematological disorders such as myeloproliferative or myelodysplastic syndromes (see Chapter 16). Large platelets correspond also to young platelets when megakaryocytopoiesis is stimulated. Determination of the accurate platelet size is crucial for the diagnosis of inherited thrombocytopenias since the most commonly used classification is based on both platelet size (see Chapter 16) and the presence or absence of extra-platelet features (24). A number of inherited thrombocytopenias are misdiagnosed as immune thrombocytopenia purpura, leading to inappropriate laboratory exploration and to inadequate and possibly deleterious therapies.

Variation of platelet size may affect both the log curve of platelet volume distribution and the MPV. Indeed, impedance-type counters analyze particles ranging from 2 to 20–30 fL although laser-type instruments (type ADVIA 2120, Siemens) are able to count larger particles (until 60 fL). When large platelets are present, impedance HA are not able to count them by the curve fitting and extrapolation. This lead to false thrombocytopenia and false MPV, which is primordial since management of bleeding is based at least on platelet count. Some HA provide immunological platelet counts (Abbott) or platelet RNA fluorescent staining (Sysmex). Platelet count can be also assessed by using classical hematimetric chamber and phase-contrast microscopy or by FCM associated with platelet-specific immunostaining.

3.6.5 Cryoglobulins

Cryoglobulins are immunoglobulins or immune complexes able to precipitate at a temperature lower than 37°C (see Note 8). The precipitates are solid particles of various size and shape. These particles are dissolved again at 37°C. A trouble can be visible sometimes in plasma after sedimentation. Cryoglobulins can lead to an overestimation of the platelet count or the leukocyte count depending on the size of the particles. The overestimation of the leukocyte count was the first to be described (25) but the overestimation of the platelet count is the most frequent and can be very important (26). Very rare perturbations of hemoglobin measurement have been described. Cryoglobulins can be seen on MGG blood smears or in fresh whole blood examined at microscope between slides. The aspects can be variable (amorphous or stained material between red blood cells or inside leukocytes). When using ADVIA analyzers, these particles are at the origin of "events" in the ghosts' zone on the platelet graph and/or an arrow-like aspect between "LUC zone" on the PEROX graph (Fig. 5).

If the blood sample is warmed during 30 min at 37°C and analyzed again, the interference disappears generally. If not, a new blood sample should be drawn into a pre-warmed tube kept at 37°C till the analysis is performed. Cryofibrinogen may have the same consequences.

3.6.6 Lipids

An abnormal presence of lipids in blood may have various origins: parenteral nutrition, intralipid infusion as therapeutic agents, hyperchylomicronemia either postprandial or relative to endogenous dyslipidemia, or a consequence of l-asparaginase treatment. These lipid abnormalities induce formation of micellae, with heterogeneous constitution and size, and can be misdiagnosed as platelets (27, 28).

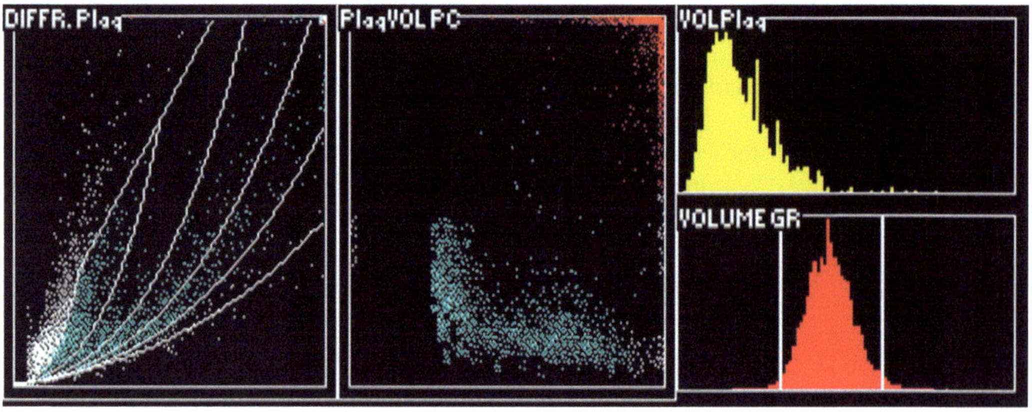

Fig. 5 Interference of cryoglobulin on platelet count

The analysis of lactescent blood by ADVIA analyzers disturbs mainly the leukocyte graphs.

Impedance HA are mistaken by these microparticles. They analyze them as events of very small size that contaminate the distribution curve of the platelet volume at its origin.

In case of exogenous dyslipidemia, it is recommended not to validate platelet count and to control it with another blood sample. In case of endogenous dyslipidemia, it can be proposed to substitute lactescent plasma by an equivalent volume of isotonic solution before new analysis.

3.6.7 Fragmented RBC

Fragmented red blood cells include erythrocytes with very small size generated in anemias with iron deficiency, microspherocytosis or fragments of erythrocytes, and schistocytes occurring in thrombotic microangiopathies or burns. Impedance HA are usually unable to differentiate the erythrocyte fragments from the platelets and count them as large platelets, interfering with the extrapolation zone of platelet analysis. They generate flags "platelet clumps" or "large platelets." Optical HA such as the ADVIA 2120 counter (Siemens), which measures volume and composition simultaneously, is theoretically able to differentiate the platelet from these fragments owing to diffraction analysis. In very rare cases microcytic hypochromic erythrocytes can be confused with platelets.

Some analyzers can avoid this trap owing to their ability of platelet counting after immunolabeling (Abbott) or RNA labeling (Sysmex). In other cases, platelet count can be assessed by classical hematimetric chamber and phase-contrast microscopy counting or by FCM associated with specific immunostaining.

3.6.8 Cytoplasmic Fragments of Nucleated Cells

Cytoplasmic fragments can be generated by any abnormal cell, either myeloid or lymphoid (lymphocytic lymphoma, hairy cell leukemia) due to the fragility of these cells. These are anucleated cellular fragments, with small volume and heterogeneous granularity according to their cell origin. They can have a platelet-like behavior (29). Such interference should be suspected in two situations. A discrepancy between platelet count and clinical situation (bleeding in a patient with normal platelet count or not correlated with the platelet count) should lead to discuss the validity of the platelet count. A careful observation of the blood smear detects these cytoplasm fragments and helps to estimate the platelet count. In these situations, light microscope counting can be unreliable due to the difficulty to distinguish the refringency of the platelets from that of the cell fragments. Platelet counting using flow cytometry with platelet-specific antibodies should be considered as the most adequate and precise method (coefficient of variations <5%) (3).

The detection of this analytic trap is crucial from a clinical point of view to better manage platelet transfusions. The risk to ignore this interference is to delay the treatment of thrombocytopenia and to expose the patient to a life-threatening bleeding risk.

3.6.9 Microorganisms

Bacteria or yeast may be observed on peripheral blood smears and may lead to spuriously elevated platelet counts and disturb the white blood cell (WBC) differential count if they clumped together. A large number of such microorganisms have been shown to be implicated (30).

4 Notes

1. Blood samples from neonates and young children may contain small clots frequently.
2. Draw blood with the capillary, push it in the small container (containing ammonium oxalate as diluent), wait 10–15 min (lysis of red cells), and then fill the hematimetric chamber with diluted blood using the capillary. Platelet count is calculated taking in account the blood dilution in the Unopette (1p100), the volume of the hematimetric chamber, and the number of its squares that have been counted. For instance, for Malassez chamber divided into 100 small squares, the formula is the following: Platelet count = number of platelets counted × 100 × 100/number of small squares counted.
3. The principle is to calculate the ratio platelets number/erythrocytes number and then to determine the platelet count from the erythrocyte count.
4. Personal data show that for a healthy population, MPV varies according to the HA used: mean MPV (fL) is 8.81, 10.76, and 8.86 for ADVIA, XE-2100, and LH750, respectively. The difference between ADVIA/LH750 and XE-2100 is 1.9 approximately, corresponding to 20% approximately.

5. MPV of a majority of peripheral thrombocytopenias is higher than the MPV of central thrombocytopenias (31, 32).
6. Clots should be searched for by transferring the blood sample very carefully into an empty tube.
7. Platelet aggregates can be detected also by analyzing the leukocyte distribution curve ("shouldering" with impedance HA or spindle shape on "perox cytogram" with ADVIA HA). If the leukocyte differential count is not necessary, the presence of platelet aggregates can be ignored.
8. Cryoglobulins are detected at +4°C in the laboratory, but they can precipitate between +11°C and +37°C, and therefore they can disturb blood cells count.

5 Conclusion

The validation of platelet count should take in account a number of pre-analytical factors, such as human errors in sample identification, site of venepuncture, inadequate mixing prior to analysis, and/or analytical factors such as quality control failure or abnormalities in cleaning procedures of HA. The criteria for validating platelet count should consider the respect of fitted lognormal volume distribution curve and the presence of a curve starting and returning to baseline. The absence of flag should be recommended to avoid that spurious platelet count are delivered to the physicians.

References

1. Brecher G, Schneiderman M, Cronkite EP (1953) The reproducibility and constancy of the platelet count. Am J Clin Pathol 23:15–26
2. Harrison P (2000) Progress in the assessment of platelet function. Br J Haematol 111:733–744
3. Harrison P, Ault KA, Chapman S, Charie L, Davis B, Fujimoto K et al (2001) An interlaboratory study of a candidate reference method for platelet counting. International Society of Laboratory Hematology Task Force for the Reference Platelet Count. Am J Clin Pathol 115:448–459
4. Tycko DH, Metz MH, Epstein EA, Grinbaum A (1985) Flow-cytometric light scattering measurement of red blood cell volume and hemoglobin concentration. Appl Opt 24:1355
5. Kunicka JE, Fischer G, Murphy J, Zelmanovic D (2000) Improved platelet counting using two-dimensional laser light scatter. Am J Clin Pathol 114:283–289
6. Harris N, Kunicka J, Kratz A (2005) The ADVIA 2120 hematology system: flow cytometry-based analysis of blood and body fluids in the routine hematology laboratory. Lab Hematol 11:47–61
7. Harrison P, Horton A, Grant D, Briggs C, Machin S (2000) Immunoplatelet counting: a proposed new reference procedure. Br J Haematol 108:228–235
8. Norris S, Pantelidou D, Smith D, Murphy M (2003) Immunoplatelet counting: potential for reducing the use of platelet transfusions through more accurate platelet counting. Br J Haematol 121:605–613
9. Stanworth SJ, Denton K, Monteath J, Patton WN (1999) Automated counting of platelets on the Bayer ADVIA 120 analyser. Clin Lab Haematol 21:113–117
10. Trabuio E, Valverde S, Antico F, Manoni F, Gessoni G (2009) Performance of automated platelet quantification using different analysers in comparison with an immunological reference

method in thrombocytopenic patients. Blood Transfus 7:43–48
11. Hong KH, Kim MJ, Lee KW, Park KU, Kim HS, Song J (2009) Platelet count evaluation using three automated haematology analysers compared with the immunoplatelet reference method, and estimation of possible inadequate platelet transfusion. Int J Lab Hematol 31:298–306
12. Segal HC, Briggs C, Kunka S, Casbard A, Harrison P, Machin SJ et al (2005) Accuracy of platelet counting haematology analysers in severe thrombocytopenia and potential impact on platelet transfusion. Br J Haematol 128:520–525
13. Ntaios G, Papadopoulos A, Chatzinikolaou A, Girtovitis F, Kaiafa G, Savopoulos C, Hatzitolios A (2009) Evaluation of mean platelet volume in the differential diagnosis of thrombocytopenia. Int J Lab Hematol 6:688–689
14. Brummitt DR, Barker HF (2000) The determination of a reference range for new platelet parameters produced by the Bayer ADVIA120 full blood count analyser. Clin Lab Haematol 22:103–107
15. Macey MG, Carty E, Webb L, Chapman ES, Zelmanovic D, Okrongly D et al (1999) Use of mean platelet component to measure platelet activation on the ADVIA 120 haematology system. Cytometry 38:250–255
16. Cooke J, Murphy T, McFadden E, O'Reilly M, Cahill MR (2009) Can mean platelet component be used as an index of platelet activity in stable coronary artery disease. Hematology 14:111–114
17. Brummitt DR, Barker HF, Pujol-Moix N (2003) A new platelet parameter, the mean platelet component, can demonstrate abnormal platelet function and structure in myelodysplasia. Clin Lab Haematol 25:59–62
18. Briggs C, Kunka S, Hart D, Oguni S, Machin SJ (2004) Assessment of an immature platelet fraction (IPF) in peripheral thrombocytopenia. Br J Haematol 126:93–99
19. Briggs C, Hart D, Kunka S, Oguni S, Machin SJ (2006) Immature platelet fraction measurement: a future guide to platelet transfusion requirement after haematopoietic stem cell transplantation. Transfus Med 16:101–109
20. Zandecki M, Genevieve F, Gerard J, Godon A (2007) Spurious counts and spurious results on haematology analysers: a review. Part I: platelets. Int J Lab Hematol 29:4–20
21. Bizzaro N (1995) EDTA-dependent pseudothrombocytopenia: a clinical and epidemiological study of 112 cases, with 10-year follow-up. Am J Hematol 50:103–109
22. Bizzaro N, Goldschmeding R, von dem Borne AE (1995) Platelet satellitism is Fc gamma RIII (CD16) receptor-mediated. Am J Clin Pathol 103:740–744
23. Latger-Cannard V, Debourgogne A, Montagne K, Plénat F, Lecompte T (2009) Platelet satellitism and lympho-agglutination as presenting finding in marginal zone B-cell lymphoma. Eur J Haematol 83:81–82
24. Balduini CL, Cattaneo M, Fabris F, Gresele P, Iolascon A, Pulcinelli FM et al (2003) Inherited thrombocytopenias: a proposed diagnostic algorithm from the Italian Gruppo di Studio delle Piastrine. Platelets 88:582–592
25. Emori HW, Bluestone R, Goldberg LS (1973) Pseudo-leukocytosis associated with cryoglobulinemia. Am J Clin Pathol 2:202–204
26. Fohlen-Walter A, Jacob C, Lecompte T, Lesesve JF (2002) Laboratory identification of cryoglobulinemia from automated blood cell counts, fresh blood samples, and blood films. Am J Clin Pathol 4:606–614
27. Cantero M, Conejo JR, Jimenez A (1996) Interference from lipemia in cell count by hematology analyzers. Clin Chem 42:987–988
28. Kabutomori O, Iwatani Y, Kabutomori M (1999) Effects of hypertriglyceridemia on platelet counts in automated hematologic analysis. Ann Int Med 130:452
29. van der Meer W, MacKenzie MA, Dinnissen JW, de Keijzer MH (2003) Pseudoplatelets: a retrospective study of their incidence and interference with platelet counting. J Clin Pathol 56:772–774
30. Kim HR, Park BR, Lee MK (2008) Effects of bacteria and yeast on WBC counting in three automated hematology counters. Ann Hematol 87:557–562
31. Bowles KM, Cooke LJ, Richards EM, Baglin TP (2005) Platelet size has diagnostic predictive value in patients with thrombocytopenia. Clin Lab Haematol 27:370–373
32. Numbenjapon T, Mahapo N, Pornvipavee R, Sriswasdi C, Mongkonsritragoon W, Leelasiri A et al (2008) A prospective evaluation of normal mean platelet volume in discriminating hyperdestructive thrombocytopenia from hypoproductive thrombocytopenia. Int J Lab Hematol 30:408–414

Chapter 16

Platelet Morphology Analysis

Véronique Latger-Cannard, Odile Fenneteau, Sylvain Salignac, Thomas Pierre Lecompte, and Nicole Schlegel

Abstract

Platelets are very small blood cells (1.5–3 μm), which play a major role in primary haemostasis and in coagulation mechanisms. Platelet characterization requires their counting (see Chapter 15) associated with accurate morphology analysis. We describe the major steps in order to correctly obtain stained blood films, which can be analyzed by optical microscope. Platelet morphology abnormalities are found in acquired malignant hematological diseases such myeloproliferative or myelodysplastic syndromes and acute megakaryoblastic leukemia. A careful analysis of the platelet size and morphology, by detecting either normal platelets with or without excessive anisocytosis, microplatelets, or large/giant platelets, will contribute to inherited thrombocytopenia diagnosis and gather substantial data when looking for an acquired platelet disorders.

Key words Platelets, Morphology, Thrombocytopenia, Platelet disorders, Inherited thrombocytopenia

1 Introduction

Platelets are discoid anucleated cells originating from fragmentation of megakaryocyte cytoplasm. Each megakaryocyte produces several thousand of platelets, leading to a rather stable intra-individual platelet count of 150–400 giga per liter (G/L) during the whole life. Platelet half-life is 7–12 days. Senescent platelets are eliminated by macrophages. Platelets play a major role in primary haemostasis and participate actively in coagulation. Performing an accurate platelet count and a correct morphology analysis requires that an appropriate sample from the patient, mixed with the adequate amount of a suitable anticoagulant, is delivered to the laboratory without undue delay. After blood smear preparation and staining, blood films should be examined by an experienced hema tologist—pathologist—technician who will describe platelet size and morphology and deliver a tentative diagnosis in face of

Paul Monagle (ed.), *Haemostasis: Methods and Protocols*, Methods in Molecular Biology, vol. 992,
DOI 10.1007/978-1-62703-339-8_16, © Springer Science+Business Media New York 2013

thrombo-cytopenia or bleeding. The final diagnosis should take into account the platelet count and morphology and the clinical data.

2 Materials

2.1 Venous Blood Drawing

1. Blood specimens can be obtained with a needle and an evacuated tube or with either a needle or a winged blood collection cannula (a "butterfly"). A 19 or 20 gauge needle is suitable for an adult and a 21 or 23 gauge for a child or an adult with small veins.
2. In children a cutaneous antalgic preparation can be applied at the site selected for venepuncture 1 h before blood drawing.
3. In neonates or very young children or children with poor veins capillary blood can be obtained from a wound of the heel or a finger made by a sterile lancet.

2.2 Anticoagulant

1. The anticoagulant recommended by the International Committee for Standardization in Haematology (ICSH) is K_2EDTA (ethylenediamine tetra-acetic acid) at a final concentration of 1.5–2.2 mg/mL. Both dry EDTA and EDTA in solution may be used.
2. Anticoagulated blood should be fully, carefully, and thoroughly mixed in order to respect manufactory's dilution (see Note 1).
3. EDTA acts by its chelating effect on the calcium molecules, which are essential for coagulation.

2.3 Blood Film Making and Staining, Fixation, and Mounting

1. Ideally, glass slides should be frosted at one end on both sides, in order to avoid the loss of the patient's name or identifying number during staining. Glass slides must be clean and free of grease.
2. A hot-air blower or a fan can be used for rapidly drying blood films.
3. Blood film staining can be performed by a manual technique, a staining machine, or an automated blood counter.
4. The stain most commonly used is a combination of Giemsa's (G) stain with May-Grünwald (MG) stain designated May-Grünwald-Giemsa (MGG). MGG dye is a mix of an acidic dye, eosin, and, a basic one, methylene blue. MG stains platelet cytoplasm and granules mainly. G dye is a mix of an acidic dye, eosin, and, a basic one, methylene azure. G dye stains platelet nuclei and azurophilic granules. Phosphate buffer pH is 6.6.
5. Absolute methanol can be used for fixation.
6. Coverslips and neutral mountant miscible with xylene are used for mounting.

2.4 Optic Microscope

1. A binocular microscope used for examining platelet morphology needs three different objectives: 10×, 40×, and 100× (immersion oil).
2. Immersion oil is necessary for 100× objective.

3 Methods

3.1 Venous Blood Collection (See Note 2)

1. The identity of the patient should be carefully checked before blood collection. Tubes should be labelled after blood collection.
2. Venous blood is usually obtained from peripheral venous blood from a vein in the antecubital fossa. In case of difficult access, other puncture sites such as veins of the dorsum of the hand or foot veins can be tried.

3.2 Blood Film Making (See Note 2)

1. Ideally, blood films should be made immediately after blood drawing and it is usually recommended that the delay between venepuncture and blood film staining being less than 4 h.
2. A drop of anticoagulated blood is placed near one end of the slide and a clean coverslip held at about a 45° tilt is used to spread out the drop and create a uniform film.
3. Once prepared, the blood smear should be dried as quickly as possible and labelled (name or identifying number).

3.3 Blood Film Fixation and Staining

1. MG staining: After drying (air or with hot-air blower or a fan), put the blood smears in a slides holder and plunge it in a tub containing MG during 4–5 min.
2. G staining: Drain the tub without rinsing it and plunge it in diluted G (1.3/10, vol/vol) 15 min. Drain the tub again without rinsing it and plunge it in phosphate buffer pH 6.6, 3 min.
3. Rinsing and drying: Drain the tub and rinse it with cold running water (tap). Take out the slides and place them on a drying place till evaporation (1–2 min).

3.4 Blood Film Examination Using Optic Microscope

Examining a blood film using optic microscope will start using first 10× and 40× objectives successively. Then oil immersion 60× or 100× objective may be necessary for more accurate examination of platelet morphology.

3.5 Normal Platelet Morphology (See Note 3)

Platelets are 1.5–3 μm sized small elements of round or oval shape. There is a wide heterogeneity of platelets in size (Fig. 1). Platelet cytoplasm contains small azurophilic granules either scattered throughout the cytoplasm or centrally concentrated. In this latter case, the granules group is called granulomer and corresponds

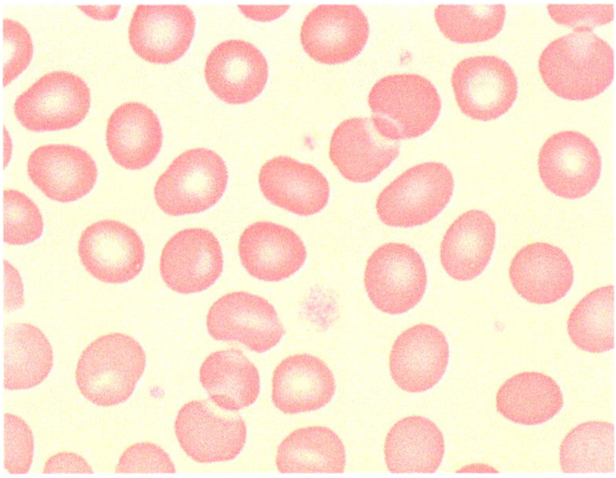

Fig. 1 Normal platelet morphology on MGG blood film stain. Physiological anisocytosis

functionally to the secretome. The thin peripheral cytoplasm is agranular and is called hyalomer. MGG-stained granules correspond to platelet α granules. By contrast, dense granules and lysosomes are not stained by MGG. Very rare megakaryocytes, the medullar precursors of platelets, are seen in blood films of healthy people. A discovery of platelet clumps or platelet satellitism onto the leukocyte membrane should lead to a control from a new blood drawing. Such analysis should include a study of the other blood cells, i.e., leukocytes and red cells.

3.6 Characteristics of Platelet Morphology in Pediatrics

Platelet anisocytosis is more pronounced in neonates than in adults due to the substantial presence of platelets with large size at birth. Platelet size varies inversely with prematurity. In neonates, small megakaryocytes with only one nucleus (Fig. 2) or bare megakaryocyte nuclei may be present (Fig. 3) (1).

3.7 Acquired Abnormalities of Platelet Morphology

3.7.1 Acquired Abnormal Platelet Morphology and Malignant Hematological Diseases

1. Myeloproliferative disorders such as essential thrombocythemia are characterized by an increase in platelet count, usually associated to some degree of platelet dystrophy (2) including marked anisocytosis and large and even giant platelets (with diameters larger than those of red cells) (Fig. 4a). Platelets may be also hypo- or agranular and some platelets appear "empty," limited by a pale pink ring (Fig. 4b). Abnormalities of α granules distribution are also observed, such as association of several granules, more intensively stained, of larger size, and having merged into a giant α granule in some cases, mimicking Paris-Trousseau aspect (Fig. 4c). In these syndromes, platelets may have acquired an increased capacity of spreading on the glass and appear of large size on blood smears. In some cases, they show distortions of cytoplasm outlines leading to vacuole formation (Fig. 4d). Megakaryocyte fragments are often present

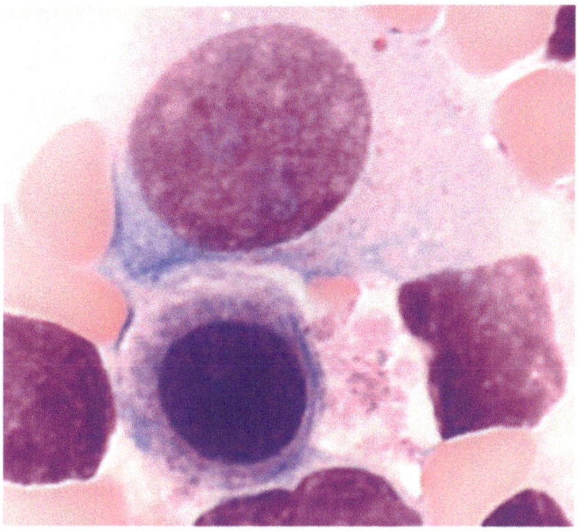

Fig. 2 Mononucleated megakaryocyte of small size in an infant on MGG blood film stain

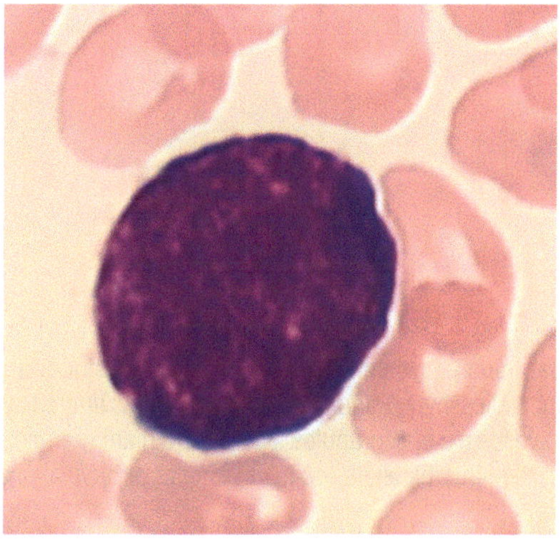

Fig. 3 Bare megakaryocyte nuclei in the peripheral blood of an infant

and numerous platelet clumps as well. These anomalies are reported to more marked in chronic idiopathic myelofibrosis.

2. It is mainly in myelodysplastic syndromes that one can find marked platelet anomalies: anisocytosis, macrocytosis, and even gigantism, which may result in an increase in the mean platelet volume (MPV) (3). Platelet anisopoïkilocytosis, loss of round shape, and heterogeneously distributed cytoplasmic blebs may be observed (Fig. 5). Several granule anomalies may be observed, either decrease in/or absence of granules—mimicking gray platelets (Fig. 6)—or presence of a unique giant α granule—mimicking Paris-Trousseau platelet. Circulating megakaryocyte

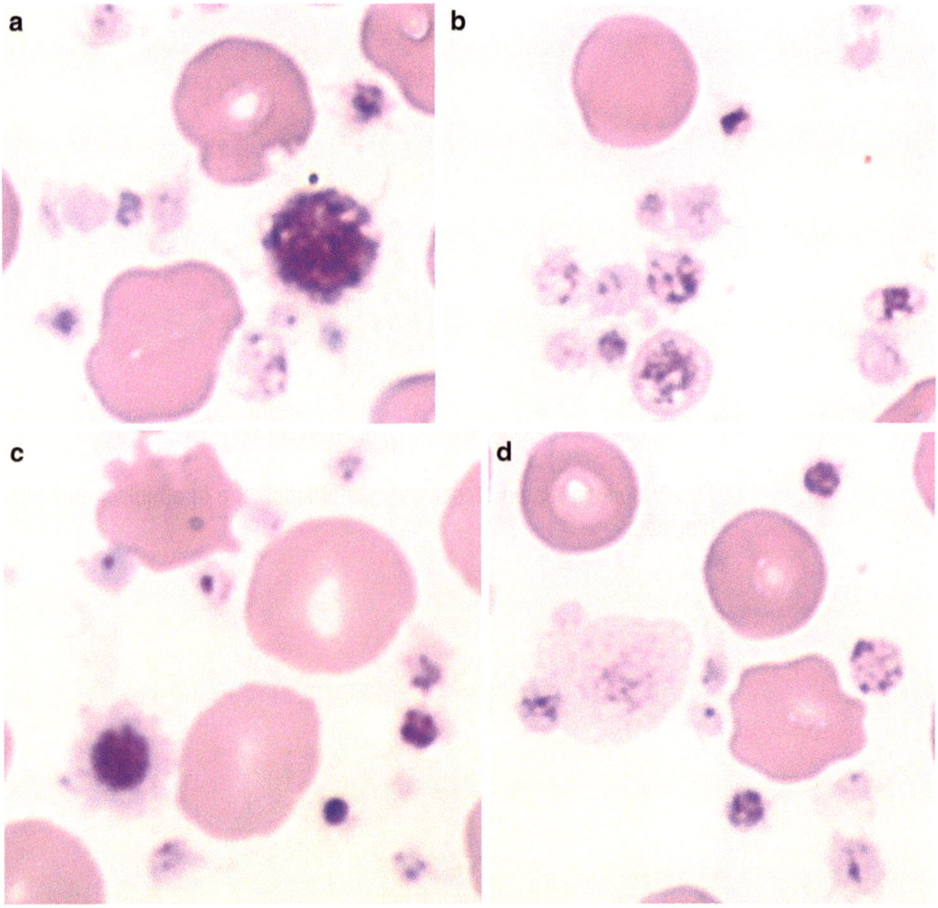

Fig. 4 Essential thrombocythemia on MGG blood film stain: (**a**) Platelet anisocytosis with a giant platelet. (**b**) Granules anomalies, hypogranular platelets, platelets limited by a *pale pink* ring. (**c**) Abnormality of granules distribution, coalescence of α granules leading to a giant granule. (**d**) One spreaded large platelet, hypogranular, vacuolated; the other platelets are hypogranular or have anomaly of α granules distribution

fragments and micromegakaryocytes are markers of medullar dysmegakaryocytopoiesis (see Note 4).

3. Acute megakaryocytoblastic leukemia (M7) is characterized by the presence of megakaryoblasts and frequent platelet dystrophy (anisocytosis, agranular macroplatelets, and micromegakaryocytes) (4). Similar platelet anomalies are also observed during transient leukemoid reactions occurring in neonates with Down's syndrome.

3.7.2 Acquired Abnormal Platelet Morphology and Drug Therapy

Drug-induced anomalies of platelet morphology have been reported in rare cases and are probably underestimated. The cases that have been published describe very large platelets during

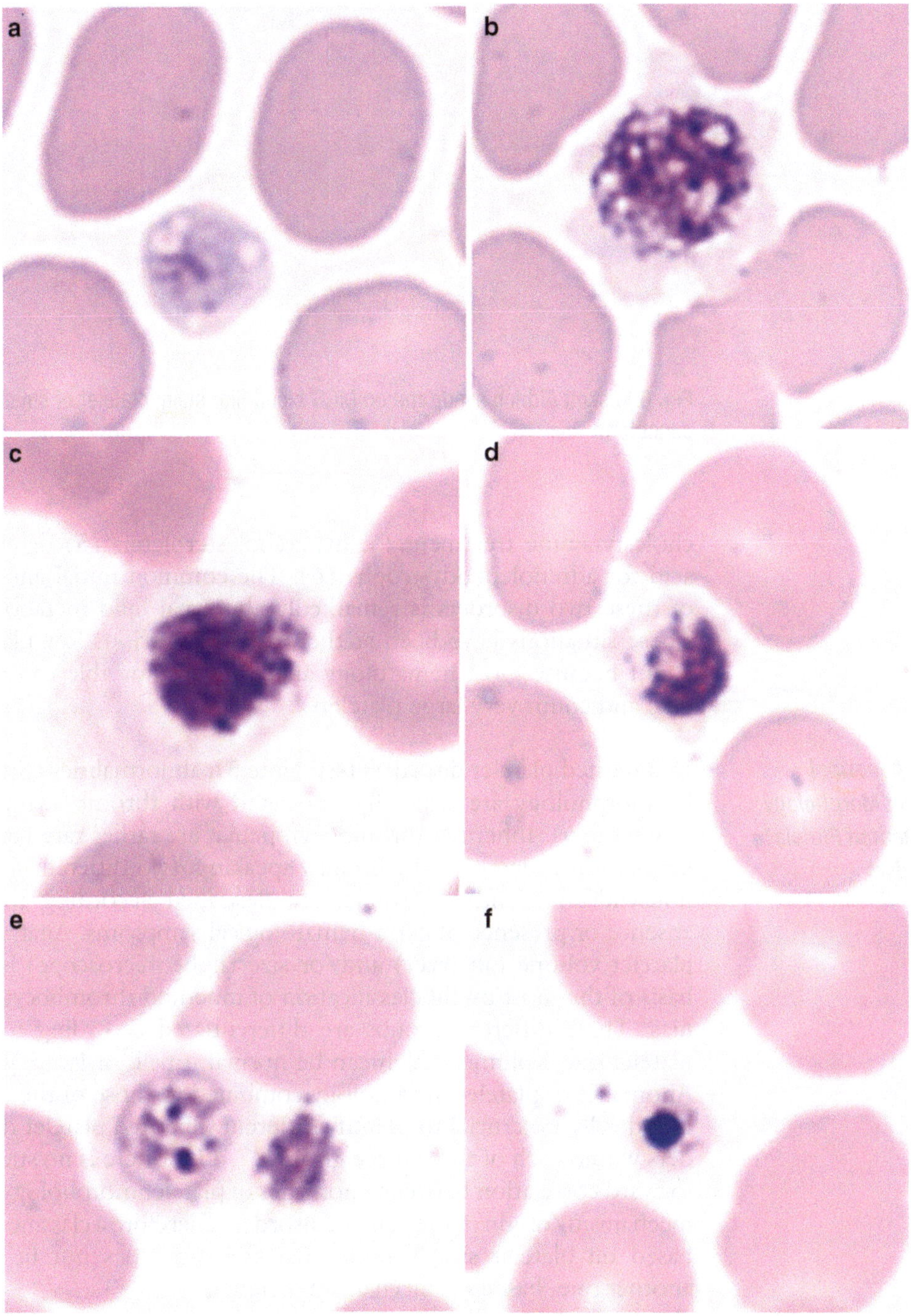

Fig. 5 Myelodysplastic syndrome on MGG blood film stain: (**a**) hypogranular platelet; (**b**) platelet with large size, cytoplasmic blebs of heterogeneous distribution; (**c**) large platelet with anomaly of α granules distribution leading to a giant α granule; (**d**) vacuolated macroplatelet and anomaly of α granules distribution: polar distribution; (**e**) large platelet, hypogranular, limited by a *pale pink* ring; (**f**) platelet of normal size, Paris-Trousseau like

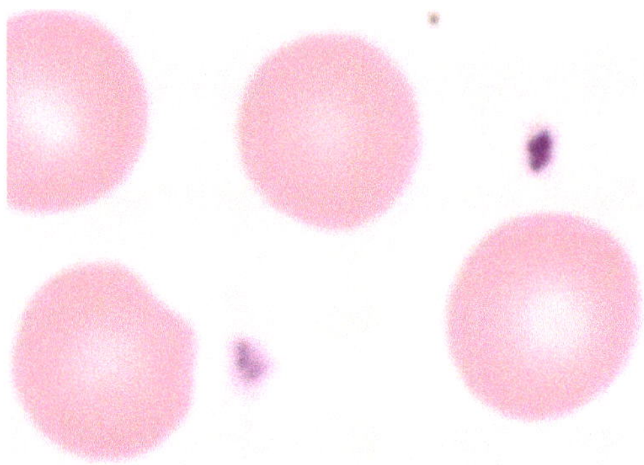

Fig. 6 Wiskott Aldrich syndrome on MGG blood film stain: platelet of small size, punctiform

cholestyramine treatment for hypercholesterolemia (5) or erucic acid for adrenoleukodystrophy (6). The common initial anomaly of these two disorders is a markedly abnormal lipid metabolism. These situations have been at the origin of spurious low platelet count because most hematology analyzers are not able to recognize and count very large platelets.

3.8 Abnormal Platelet Morphology in Inherited Platelet Disorders

In inherited platelet disorders (see Note 5), abnormalities of platelet morphology are generally associated with thrombocytopenia (see Note 6). Inherited thrombocytopenias are rather rare heterogeneous disorders (7–10). Broadly speaking, two different forms, nonsyndromic and syndromic, are described according to the absence or presence of extra-hematological symptoms. Analysis of platelet volume (analyzer) and/or size (light microscope) is the basis of the most useful classification of inherited thrombocytopenias. Three different groups are differentiated according to the platelet size/volume, which can be normal, small, or large/giant. Anomalies of platelet morphology combined to those of the other blood cells are crucial to identify different inherited platelet disorders within each of these three groups (7, 11). There is no straight forward correlation between anomalies of platelet morphology and mechanism/origin of the platelet disorder. Therefore a classification based on platelet size/volume characteristics does not fit with another one, based on mechanism/origin.

3.8.1 Platelet Anomalies According to Size/Volume

Platelets with Size/Volume Within Normal Ranges (Usual Values)

1. Autosomal-dominant (AD) familial thrombocytopenia diagnosis should be considered after exclusion of the other known rare causes of inherited thrombocytopenia with normal MPV. Bleeding is rare, and even absent. Thrombocytopenia is the only abnormality and platelet count varies between 20 and 110 G/L. Platelet volume/size and morphology are normal (12).

Very recently mutations in the 5'UTR of *ANKRD26*, the ankirin repeat domain 26 gene, have been identified in patients with AD form of inherited thrombocytopenia with platelets of normal size, THC2 (13).

2. Congenital amegakaryocytic thrombocytopenia (CAMT), an exceedingly rare disorder with autosomal recessive inheritance, is much more severe. By contrast with normal platelet morphology, bleeding manifestations are constant and occur early in life, even during the neonatal period. They can be severe (either intracerebral or digestive hemorrhage). Marked thrombocytopenia (platelet count <30 G/L) is progressively associated with macrocytic anemia and may evolve towards pancytopenia (14). Type I (60% of cases) is the most severe form characterized by a persistent and severe thrombocytopenia (7–30 G/L) and rapidly evolving towards pancytopenia. Type II has a slower evolution; thrombocytopenia is less severe (10–87 G/L), occurs later in life, and is corrected during the first year. The diagnosis is based on the identification of mutations in the *c-MPL* gene encoding the thrombopoïetin receptor.
3. Thrombocytopenia with absent radii (TAR syndrome) is readily diagnosed because of the associated malformative syndrome characterized by shortened or absent forearms due to bilateral radial aplasia in 100% of cases (15). Platelet size and morphology are normal. Thrombocytopenia is very severe (<10 G/L) at birth and at the origin of frequent and sometimes life-threatening bleeding episodes during the first months of life, such as intracerebral and gastrointestinal bleeding. Platelet count is partially corrected during the first years of life, increases during childhood, and can be normal in adulthood. Inheritance is autosomal recessive.
4. Familial thrombocytopenia with predisposition to acute myelogenous leukemia is considered to be a very rare (20 families or isolated cases reported) autosomal dominant platelet disorder associated to mutations in *RUNX1* (also called *AML1* or *CBFA2*) gene, especially if familial cases of myeloid or lymphoid hematological disorder or other neoplasia are reported (16). Platelet morphology is normal at MGG staining and numerous normal alpha granules are present. Nevertheless this syndrome is frequently associated to δ storage pool disease-like thrombocytopathy, which is a phenotypic feature of diagnostic value. Platelet count varies between 40 and 145 G/L. Diagnosis relies on a DNA analysis after informed consent.

Platelets with Small Size/Volume

The association of small platelets (Fig. 6) and thrombocytopenia, severe in most cases, is highly suggestive of X-linked thrombocytopenia (XLT) or Wiskott-Aldrich syndrome (WAS) (see Note 7).

WAS is an X-linked recessive disease characterized by moderate to severe thrombocytopenia associated with cutaneous bleeding (84% of cases), eczema (80% of cases), immune deficiency (60% of cases), autoimmune features (40% of cases), and possible EBV-associated lymphomas (13% of cases). A dense granule anomaly is sometimes evidenced and can increase bleeding symptoms. XLT phenotype is purely hematological. Platelet microcytosis is important ("dwarf platelets," MPV 5.5–6 fL) and analyzers are frequently unable to smooth the volume distribution curve (17) (cf Chapter 15).

Platelets with Large Size/Volume or Giant

Large platelets in a young patient with sustained thrombocytopenia should suggest an inherited thrombocytopenia, especially when associated with extra-hematological symptoms and/or familial cases of thrombocytopenia. As much as possible, it is desirable to differentiate large platelets from giant ones.

1. The 22q11.2 deletion syndrome includes a wide spectrum of phenotypes known as velo-cardio-facial (VCF) syndrome and DiGeorge syndrome. VCF phenotype associates cardiac, facial, and palate anomalies; hypocalcemia; and behavior and learning troubles. Thrombocytopenia is present in 35% of cases. Bleeding symptoms are not frequent and generally discovered before surgery (18, 19). Large platelets are present in 82% of cases, and MPV is moderately increased. Therefore platelet counting by analyzers is reliable but the presence of these large platelets can escape notice if blood films are not carefully examined.
2. Autosomal dominant familial macrothrombocytopenia, also referred to as Mediterranean macrothrombocytopenia, associates a moderate thrombocytopenia (platelet count >50 G/L) and a moderately increased platelet volume (10–13 fL) (20, 21). It is an exclusion diagnosis because macrothrombocytopenia is isolated, not associated to thrombocytopathy, bleeding, or malformations. The familial origin and clinical history are of high value. A mutation of GPIbα gene has been reported (variant Bolzano, which can be considered as a Bernard–Soulier syndrome (BSS variant)).
3. A very rare syndrome associating X-linked thrombocytopenia and dyserythropoiesis, linked to *GATA 1* mutations in Xp11.23, has been reported (22). Thrombocytopenia varies according to the type of mutation but may be severe (<10 G/L). Macroplatelets can be observed, but granules are normal. Anemia; erythrocytes anomalies such as anisocytosis, poïkilocytosis, and acanthocytosis; and dystrophic erythroblastemia are suggestive of the diagnosis.
4. The discovery of platelets with very large size (over erythrocyte size), called giant platelets, should suggest either two entities

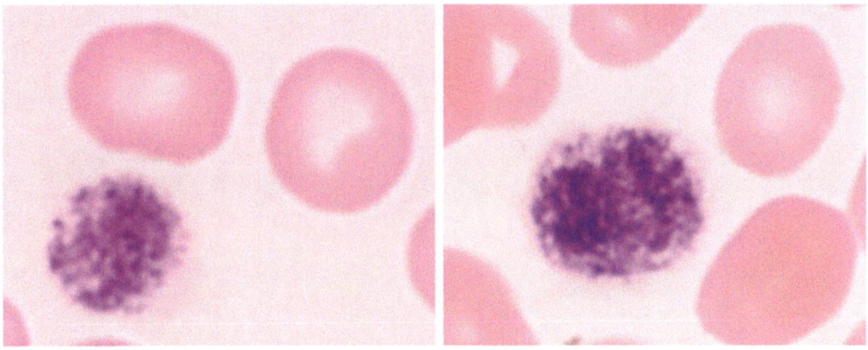

Fig. 7 Bernard–Soulier syndrome on MGG blood film stain: majority of giant platelets

thoroughly studied: Bernard–Soulier syndrome (BSS) and MYH9 syndrome, or another disorder recently discovered, the Mediterranean stomatocytosis/macrothrombocytopenia and phytosterolemia. These large/giant platelets are classical pitfalls for hematology analyzers. In such cases, the platelet count and the platelet volume (over 20 fL in a number of cases) are underestimated (cf Chapter 15). A careful analysis of the MGG-stained blood smears is crucial because it is the only reliable direct mean to detect these giant platelets, to estimate their percentage among the platelet population, and to select a reliable technique for platelet counting.

The association of thrombocytopenia and large/giant platelets in a young child, even in a neonate, and bleeding symptoms are highly suggestive of BSS, of autosomal recessive inheritance. The diagnosis of this syndrome, due to an inherited deficiency of GPIb-IX-V platelet complex, is based on the absence of ristocetin-induced platelet agglutination and deficient or absent expression of platelet GPIb-IX-V when studied by flow cytometry. MGG-stained blood smears show a majority (80%) of giant platelets (diameter >8 μm), of spherical shape, with a normal or increased number of α granules according to the platelet size (Fig. 7). Atypical forms of BSS with moderate bleeding may lead to a misdiagnosis of immune thrombocytopenic purpura (ITP) and to inappropriate and potentially deleterious treatments such as corticosteroids, IVIgs, or splenectomy. A systematic examination of the graph of the platelet distribution according to volume combined to a careful analysis of blood smears should avoid such a misdiagnosis.

MYH9 syndrome, of autosomal dominant inheritance, is a group of five syndromes associated to mutations in *MYH9* gene, which codes the nonmuscle myosin heavy chain II-A (NMMHC-IIA). They are known as May-Hegglin anomaly (MHA); Sebastian, Fechtner, or Epstein syndrome; and Alport-like

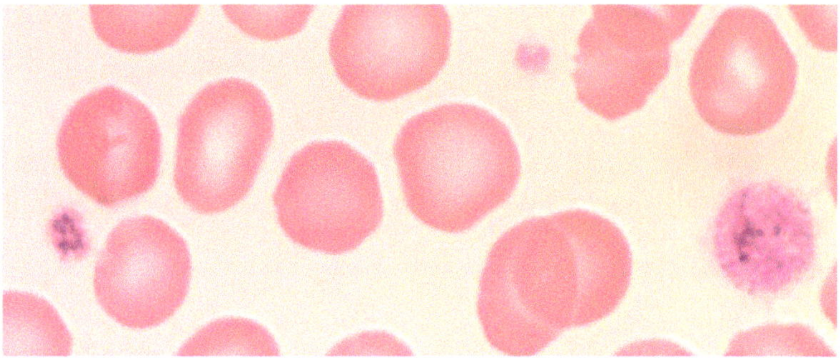

Fig. 8 MYH9 syndrome on MGG blood film stain: one giant platelet, with size similar to red blood cell

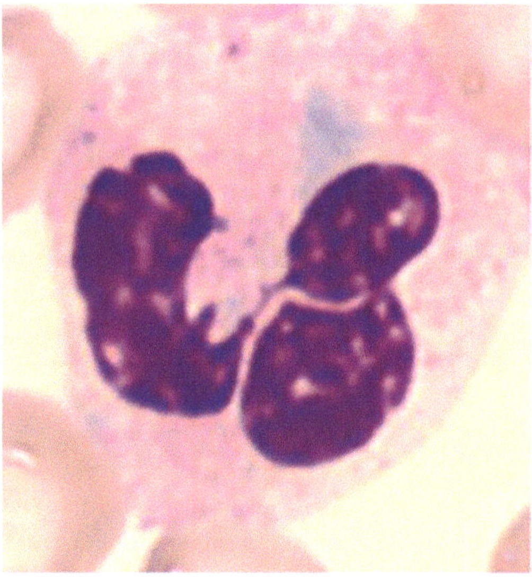

Fig. 9 May-Hegglin anomaly on MGG blood film stain: basophilic leukocyte inclusion, unique, large, and strongly stained

syndrome with macrothrombocytopenia. Thrombocytopenia and large and even giant platelets are present since birth in all these syndromes. Platelets with size larger than erythrocyte one are observed in all cases, but their percentage varies from one patient to another, and platelets of normal size are also detected on each different blood smear (Fig. 8). Besides platelet anomalies, basophilic leukocyte inclusions (Döhle-like bodies) on MGG-stained blood smears are characteristic features of MYH9 syndrome. These inclusions are aggregates of mutated NMMHC-IIA and RNA in most cases. They are generally large, strongly stained, and unique in MHA (Fig. 9), but small, pale, and more numerous in the other syndromes (Fig. 10). In Epstein cases with p.R702H mutation in the *MYH9* gene, they are invisible on usual MGG-stained films but can be seen when using immunofluorescence technique with an anti-NMMHC-IIA

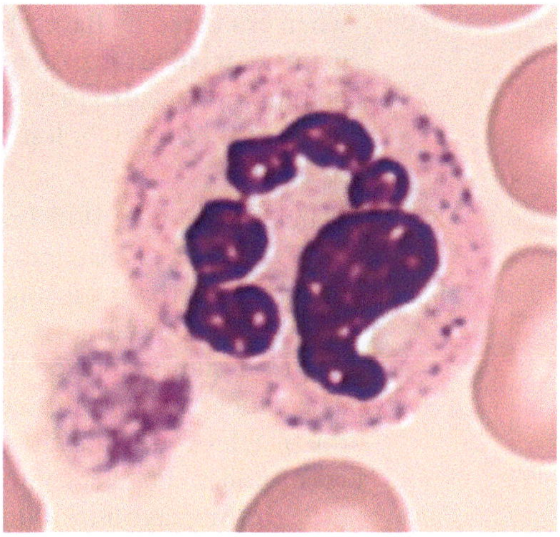

Fig. 10 Fechtner syndrome on MGG blood film stain: basophilic leukocyte inclusions of small size, and pale

only, because they contain mutated NMMHC-IIA only without RNA (23). A classification of the leukocyte inclusions (immunofluorescent technique) in three groups (I, II, and III) according to their shape, size, and number has been proposed (24). The five syndromes differ from one another by the combination of hematological features, the only manifestations observed in MHA and Sebastian syndrome, and extra-hematological features: nephropathy, sensorineural deafness and cataracts (Fechtner) or nephropathy, and deafness (Epstein and Alport-like syndromes) or nephropathy and cataract (Alport-like). They represent a wide continuum of mutated *MYH9*-related phenotypes, from the pure hematological form to the complete form including all the hematological and extra-hematological manifestations. There is no tight genotype-phenotype correlation, but mutations of the N-terminus of NMMHC-IIA are more generally associated to platelets with the largest size and to extra-hematological features as compared to those affecting the C-terminus (25, 26).

Mediterranean stomatocytosis/macrothrombocytopenia (27) is the most recently identified among inherited thrombocytopenia with giant platelets. It has been discovered in Australia in emigrates of Mediterranean origin. This thrombocytopenia of autosomal recessive transmission is the hematological presentation of phytosterolemia, an anomaly of phytosterols and cholesterol absorption able to induce hypercholesterolemia and cutaneous xanthomas (28). Hematological features encompass gather hemolysis, erythrocyte stomatocytes, and thrombocytopenia with giant platelets. Thrombocytopenia is moderate (>50 G/L), but platelet size is often higher than erythrocyte one's. Impedancemetry analyzers are unable to give values for MPV, which can reach 28.7 fL when evaluated by Bayer Advia counter. The detection of these giant platelets in a patient with hypercholesterolemia is very helpful for a reliable diagnosis and therefore an adequate treatment of this hypercholesterolemia, responding to diet but not to statins.

5. Platelet-type von Willebrand disease (VWD) and type 2B VWD. Enlarged platelets can also be found in two different disorders with confusing similar phenotype: platelet-type VWD, due to mutation in platelet GPIbα, and type 2B VWD, due to mutation in the A1 domain of VW factor (VWF) (10). The genetic origin of these two rare disorders is different, but the platelet count and the morphological aspect of platelets are very similar. Platelet clumps can be found on blood smears (29). If the diagnosis of one of these two diseases is suspected, the VWF:Co/VWF:Ag ratio is a crucial orientation criterion.
6. Amegakaryocytic thrombocytopenia with radioulnar synostosis. Thrombocytopenia may be associated to enlarged platelets. Pancytopenia may develop in some cases. This very rare disorder is also associated to malformative feature of fused radius, and incomplete range of motion. It appears to be of autosomal dominant inheritance and may be related to a *HOXA11* gene defect (30).

3.8.2 Anomalies of Platelet Alpha Granules

Gray Platelets (Gray Platelet Syndrome, GPS) (See Note 8)

GPS, also known as α-storage pool disease (α-SPD), is a very rare inherited disorder, characterized by mild to moderate thrombocytopenia and the presence of enlarged platelets (Fig. 11). Platelets have a unique ghost-like appearance on MGG-stained blood smears because α granules and their contents are absent (31). Bleeding syndrome is usually mild to moderate but can be sometimes severe. The causative

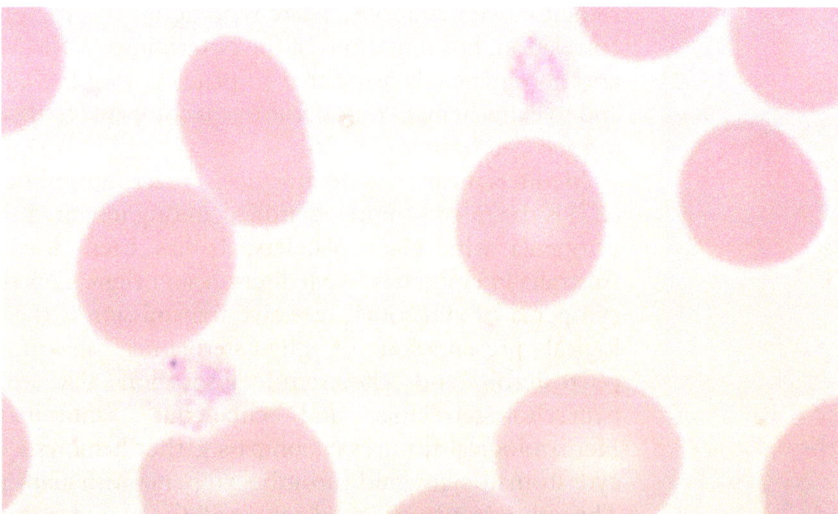

Fig. 11 Gray platelet of large size, without visible α granules

gene, *NBEAL2*, encoding a BEACH protein involved in granules development, has been identified very recently (32–34). The risk of this disorder is the development of an early myelofibrosis.

Platelets of Paris-Trousseau Syndrome/Jacobsen Syndrome (11q23 Deletion)

The initial description of Jacobsen syndrome is the association of a variable dysmorphic syndrome characterized by facial and cardiac anomalies, mental deficiency, and thrombocytopenia in approximately 50% of cases (35). Pancytopenia may occur in some cases. This syndrome is associated with 11q23 deletion. Bleeding is generally absent. Thrombocytopenia is mild (50–140 G/L), discovered between the first month of life the age to 12 (36), fluctuating with time and tendencies to decrease with aging. Spontaneous normalizations have even been reported. MPV is slightly increased in 80% of cases (about 11 fL). Blood smears show an association of homogeneously granular macroplatelets and characteristic platelets with abnormal α granules distribution leading to a unique red-stained giant granule (Fig. 12). These platelets

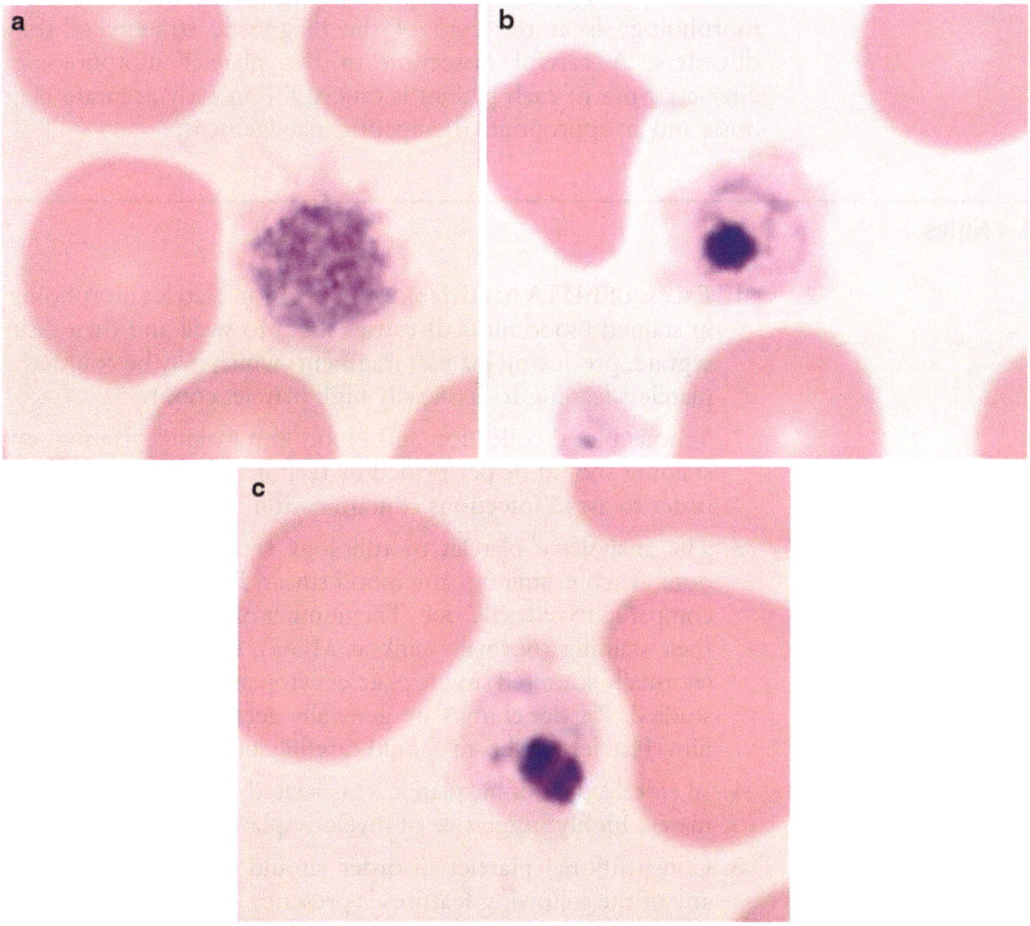

Fig. 12 Jacobsen syndrome: macroplatelet (**a**) and Paris-Trousseau platelets with giant α granule (**b, c**)

known as Paris-Trousseau platelets are the results of α granules merger, as shown by electron microscopy (37). The mild increase in MPV is due to a low percentage (mean: 10%) of macroplatelets. The percentage of Paris-Trousseau platelets varies with time in each patient, and varies from one patient to another. Platelets with giant α granules persist after normalization of platelet count. Paris-Trousseau platelets have been described in cord blood of a patient with a prenatal form associated to mosaicism of 11q region (38). Platelets with giant α granule can be found in healthy people (0.04% of platelets), in platelet concentrates, but also in other blood disorders such as myeloproliferative syndromes (see above) or Chediak-Higashi syndrome, a very rare autosomal recessive disease with platelet-dense granules deficiency and other defects such as albinism and lysosomal-related organelles anomalies. In these disorders, giant granules formation is linked to cell suffering (hypoxia, anomalies of cell regulation), cell destruction (surgical or functional asplenism), or dysmegakaryopoiesis.

In conclusion, mucocutaneous bleeding symptoms are the common features to all the platelets functional defects. Platelet morphology is at the core of the diagnostic strategy of these disorders. A careful dissection of the platelet morphological characteristics of each patient is crucial for an early accurate diagnosis and an appropriate therapeutic management.

4 Notes

1. Excess of EDTA has deleterious effects on platelet morphology in stained blood films. It causes them to swell and then disintegrate, producing platelet fragments which may be counted as platelets leading to artificially high platelet count.
2. Venous blood collection and blood film making, fixating, and staining should be performed by technicians wearing gloves in order to avoid infectious contamination.
3. The analysis of platelet morphology should systematically be done when examining any blood smear. Platelet size should be compared to red cells' one. The number of platelet granulations, their staining (normally pink at MGG), and their distribution (normally scattered) in the platelet cytoplasm should be carefully studied. Platelet clumps are generally detected in the tail of the film. Platelet satellitism should carefully be searched for.
4. In elderly, dystrophic platelets associated with thrombocytopenia are highly suggestive of myelodysplastic syndrome.
5. Constitutional platelet disorder should be considered when any of the following features is present:
   (a) Bleeding symptoms since birth
   (b) Excessive bleeding after minor trauma or surgery since childhood

(c) Familial cases of bleeding and/or thrombocytopenia and/ or hematological malignancy

(d) Chronicity of thrombocytopenia and absence of any normal platelet count in the past

(e) Lack of response to idiopathic thrombocytopenic purpura therapies

(f) No recent clinical alteration

6. Normal platelet morphology can be associated not only with inherited thrombocytopenia but also with inherited thrombocytopathia alone (without thrombocytopenia) such as Glanzmann thrombasthenia (GT). GT is the main inherited platelet aggregation deficiency due to genetic defects in GPIIb-IIIa, the platelet receptor for fibrinogen.
7. In neonates, very rare small/dwarf, punctiform platelets associated with thrombocytopenia are highly suggestive of WAS or XLT.
8. Gray platelets are not specific of GPS. Platelets can appear gray, as exhausted, because they have released the content of alpha granules. Several mechanisms can induce this release such as coagulation activation during blood drawing, thorough blood/ anticoagulant mixing, or true disseminated intravascular coagulation (DIC).

References

1. Levine RF, Olson TA, Shoff PK, Miller MK, Weisman LE (1996) Mature micromegakaryocytes: an unusual developmental pattern in term infants. Br J Haematol 94: 391–399
2. Brière J (1995) Thrombocytémie essentielle. Encycl Med Chir Hématologie 13-020-B-05, p 10.
3. Flandrin G, Lessard M (1991) Syndromes myélodysplasiques. Encycl Med Chir, (Paris-France), Hématologie, 13012 A10, p 8.
4. Benett JM, Catovsky D, Daniel MT, Flandrin G, Galton DA, Gralnick HR et al (1985) Criteria for the diagnosis of acute leukaemia of megakaryocyte lineage. A report of the French-American-British Cooperative Group, Ann Intern Med. 103:460–462.
5. Latger-Cannard V, Sommelet D, Guerci B, Tréchot P, Lecompte T (2001) Platelet gigantism associated with cholestyramine therapy. Arch Intern Med 161:2619–2620
6. Stöckler S, Molzer B, Plecko B, Zen W, Muntean W, Söling U et al (1993) Giant platelets in erucic acid therapy for adrenoleukodystrophy. Lancet 341:1414–1415
7. Balduini CL, Cattaneo M, Fabris F, Gresele P, Iolascon A, Pulcinelli FM, on behalf of the Italian "Gruppo di Studio delle Piastrine" et al (2003) Inherited thrombocytopenias: a proposed diagnostic algorithm from the Italian Gruppo di Studio delle Piastrine. Platelets 88:582–592
8. Geddis AE, Kaushansky K (2004) Inherited thrombocytopenias: towards a molecular understanding of disorders of platelet production. Curr Opin Pediatr 16:15–24
9. Nurden AT (2005) Qualitative disorders of platelets and megakaryocytes. J Thromb Haemost 3:1773–1782
10. Nurden P, Nurden AT (2008) Congenital disorders associated with platelet dysfunctions. Thromb Haemost 99:253–263
11. Latger-Cannard V, Salignac S, Salmon A, Mansuy L, de Maistre E, Botte C et al (2005) Thrombocytopenia: clinicobiologic validation and classification. Ann Biol Clin 63:1–12

12. Drachman JG, Jarvik GP, Mehaffey MG (2000) Autosomal dominant thrombocytopenia: incomplete megakaryocyte differentiation and linkage to chromosome 10. Blood 96:118–125
13. Pipucci T, Savoia A, Perrotta S, Pujol-Moix N, Noris P, Castegnaro G et al (2011) Mutations in the 5 -UTR of ANKRD26, the ankirin repeat domain 26 gene, cause an autosomal-dominant form of inherited thrombocytopenia, THC2. Am J Hum Genet 88:115–120
14. King S, Germeshausen M, Strauss G, Welte K, Ballmaier M (2005) Congenital amegakaryocytic thrombocytopenia: a retrospective clinical analysis of 20 patients. Br J Haematol 131:636–644
15. Greenhalgh K, Howell R, Bottani A, Ancliff P, Brunner H, Verschuuren-Bemelmans C et al (2002) Thrombocytopenia-absent radius syndrome: a clinical genetic study. J Med Genet 39:876–881
16. Béri-Dexheimer M, Latger-Cannard V, Philippe C, Bonnet C, Chambon P et al (2008) Clinical phenotype of germline RUNX1 haploinsufficiency: from point mutations to large genomic deletions. Eur J Hum Genet 16:1014–1018
17. Latger-Cannard V, Proust A, Devignes J, Salignac S, Bensoussan D, Salmon A et al (2008) A Wiskott-Aldrich syndrome revealed by a careful morphological examination of the platelets in a child. Hématologie 14:387–391
18. Latger-Cannard V, Bensoussan D, Grégoire MJ, Marçon F, Cloez JL, Leheup B et al (2004) Frequency of thrombocytopenia and large platelets correlate neither with conotruncal cardiac anomalies nor immunologic features in chromosome 22q11.2 deletion syndrome. Eur J Pediatrics 163:327–328
19. Liang HP, Morel-Kopp MC, Curtin J, Wilson M, Hewson J, Chen W et al (2007) Heterozygous loss of platelet glycoprotein (GP) Ib-V-IX variably affects platelet function in velocardiofacial syndrome (VCFS) patients. Thromb Haemost 98:1298–1308
20. Najean Y, Lecompte T (1990) Genetic thrombocytopenia with autosomal dominant transmission: a review of 54 cases. Br J Haematol 74:203–208
21. Savoia A, Balduini CL, Savino M, Noris P, Del Vecchio M, Perrotta S et al (2001) Autosomal dominant macrothrombocytopenia in Italy is most frequently a type of heterozygous Bernard-Soulier syndrome. Blood 97:1330–1335
22. Ciovacco W, Raskind W, Kacena M (2008) Human phenotypes associated with GATA-1 mutations. Genet 427:1–6
23. Kunishima S, Yoshinari M, Nishio H, Ida K, Miura T, Matsushita T et al (2007) Haematological characteristics of *MYH9* disorders due to *MYH9* R702 mutations. Eur J Haematol 78:220–226
24. Kunishima S, Matsushita T, Kojima T, Sako M, Kimura F, Jo E-K et al (2003) Immunofluorescence analysis of neutrophil Non Muscle Myosin Heavy Chain-A in *MYH9* disorders: association of subcellular localization with *MYH9* mutations. Lab Invest 83:115–122
25. Pecci A, Panza E, Pujol-Moix N, Klersy C, Di Bari F, Bozzi V et al (2008) Position of non-muscle myosin heavy chain IIA mutations predicts the natural history of MYH9-related disease. Hum Mutat 29:409–417
26. Pecci A, Panza E, De Rocco D, Pujol-Moix N, Girotto G, Podda L et al (2009) MYH9 related disease: four novel mutations of the tail domain of myosin-9 correlating with a mild clinical phenotype. Eur J Haematol 84:291–297
27. Stewart GW, Makris M (2008) Mediterranean macrothrombocytopenia and phytosterolaemia/sitosterolaemia. Haematologica 93:e29
28. Rees DC, Iolascon A, Carella M, O'marcaigh AS, Kendra JR, Jowitt SN et al (2005) Stomatocytic haemolysis and macrothrombocytopenia (Mediterranean stomatocytosis/macrothrombocytopenia) is the haematological presentation of phytosterolaemia. Br J Haematol 130:297–309
29. Nurden P, Debili N, Vainchenker W, Bobe R, Bredoux R, Corvazier E et al (2006) Impaired megakaryocytopoiesis in type 2B Willebrand disease with severe thrombocytopenia. Blood 108:2587–2595
30. Thompson AA, Nguyen LT (2000) Amegakaryocytic thrombocytopenia and radio-ulnar synostosis are associated with *HOXA11* mutation. Nat Genet 26:397–398
31. Nurden AT, Nurden P (2007) The gray platelet syndrome: clinical spectrum of the disease. Blood Rev 21:21–36
32. Gunay-Agun M, Falik-Zaccai TC, Vilboux T, Zivony-Elboum Y, Gumruk F, Cetin M et al (2011) *NBEAL2* is mutated in gray platelet syndrome and is required for biogenesis of platelet alpha-granules. Nat Genet 43:732–734
33. Fabbro S, Hinckley J, Li L, Schwertz H, Christensen H, Rowley JW et al (2011) Mutations in *NBEAL2*, encoding a BEACH protein, cause gray platelet syndrome. Nat Genet 43:738–740
34. Albers CA, Cvejic A, Favier R, Bouwmans EE, Alessi MC, Bertone P et al (2011) Exome sequencing identifies *NBEAL2* gene as the causative gene for gray platelet syndrome. Nat Genet 43:735–737
35. Jacobsen P, Hauge M, Henningsen K (1973) An (11;21) translocation in four generation

with chromosome 11 abnormalities in the offspring. A clinical, cytogenetical and gene marker study. Hum Hered 23:568–585
36. Favier R, Jondeau K, Boutard P, Grossfeld P, Reinert P, Jones C et al (2003) Paris-Trousseau syndrome: clinical, hematological, molecular data of ten new cases. Thromb Haemost 90:893–897
37. Breton-Gorius J, Favier R, Guichard J, Cherif D, Berger R, Debili N et al (1995) New congenital dysmegakaryopoietic thrombocytopenia (Paris-Trousseau) associated with giant platelet alpha-granules and chromosome 11 deletion at 11q23. Blood 85:1805–114
38. Valduga M, Latger-Cannard V, Philippe C, Romana S, Miton A, Droulle P et al (2007) Prenatal diagnosis of mosaïcism for 11q terminal deletion. Eur J Med Genet 50: 475–481

Chapter 17

Light Transmission Aggregometry

Juan Pablo Frontroth

Abstract

Laboratory testing of platelet function is essential for the diagnosis of several congenital and acquired platelet disorders. Moreover, it is increasingly being utilized to monitor the efficacy of antiplatelet therapy. Light transmission platelet aggregation is the most useful in vitro test of platelet function currently available, and it is still the gold standard to detect platelet disorders and to initiate a more precise characterization.

Key words Platelet aggregation, Light transmission aggregometry, Platelet function testing, Turbidimetric aggregation assays

1 Introduction

Platelets are known to aggregate under a variety of conditions and in the presence of a number of different agonists. The term "platelet aggregation" is used to stress the adherence of platelets to each other. This phenomenon can be induced in vitro by adding aggregating agents to a platelet-rich plasma (PRP), that means, to a plasma depleted of red cells and leucocytes but not of platelets. This is the basis for turbidimetric aggregometry. Laboratory testing of platelet function is fundamental for the diagnosis of several congenital and acquired platelet disorders and to monitor antiplatelet therapy (1).

Platelet aggregation is the most useful in vitro test of platelet function currently available, and it is still the gold standard to detect platelet disorders and to initiate a more precise characterization (2).

There are many plasmatic factors on which platelet aggregation depends. Moreover, the type and concentration of the stimulus will determine different patterns of response. Adenosine diphosphate (ADP), epinephrine, collagen, and ristocetin are extensively used for screening and provide the most immediate information for basic diagnostic considerations (3, 4).

Paul Monagle (ed.), *Haemostasis: Methods and Protocols*, Methods in Molecular Biology, vol. 992,
DOI 10.1007/978-1-62703-339-8_17, © Springer Science+Business Media New York 2013

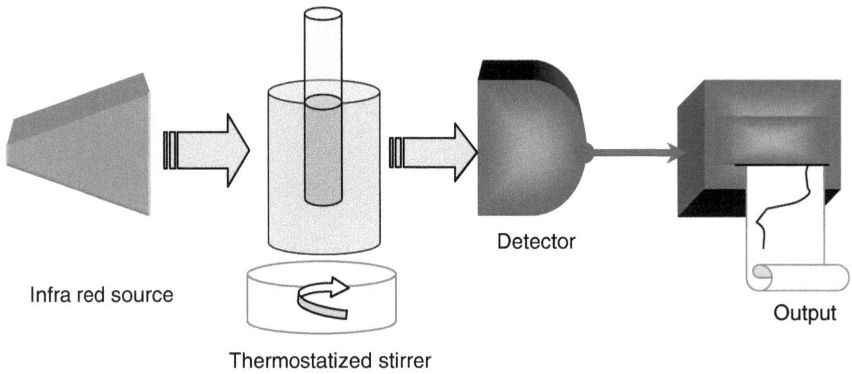

Fig. 1 Scheme of an aggregometer

Other reagents such as thrombin, arachidonic acid, and calcium ionophore A23187 have also been used to study other aspects of platelet functions.

1.1 Optical Aggregation Test Principle

First described by Born et al., this procedure is performed on a turbidimetric aggregometer.

The aggregometer is a fixed infrared wavelength spectrophotometer with a sample chamber heated to 37°C, while constantly stirring the sample. This stirring is intended to reproduce the shear stress of a vessel (Fig. 1). The change in absorbance is recorded as PRP is stirred in a cuvette with the addition of an aggregating reagent.

The sample chambers are designed so that a beam of infrared light passes through two cuvettes, one containing PRP as the sample to be analyzed, and the other containing platelet-poor plasma (PPP) as the reference. PRP is considered to be 0% light transmission or 0% aggregation whereas PPP, the corresponding reference, is 100% light transmission or 100% aggregation. The output signal is proportional to the continuously measured difference in light transmission between the analyzed and the reference samples.

2 Materials

2.1 Adenosine Diphosphate

ADP (Biopool, Ventura, USA).

Vial to be diluted with 0.5 mL of distilled water giving a stock solution of 0.2 mM.

Working solution is made diluting 1/8 the stock solution in water (i.e., 350 μL water + 50 μL ADP 0.2 mM), thus obtaining a working solution of 25 μM. Aliquot and store at −70°C.

Test	450 μL PRP + 50 μL ADP 25 μM (Final concentration: 2.5 μM)

2.2 Epinephrine

Epinephrine (Biopool, Ventura, USA).

Vial to be diluted with 0.5 mL of distilled water giving a stock solution of 1.0 mM. Make a 1/10 dilution of the former stock solution with normal saline to make a working solution of 100 μM. Aliquot and store at −70°C.

Test	450 μL PRP + 25 μL epinephrine 100 μM
	(Final concentration: 5 μM)

2.3 Collagen (Equine Tendon)

Collagent reagent (Helena Laboratories, Beaumont, Texas, USA).

Vial with 1.0 mL (stock solution: 100 μg/mL).

Keep at 4–8°C, never freeze.

Before start assaying collagen, allow the vial to reach room temperature. A few minutes at 37°C may accelerate this process. The reagent should appear as a uniform clear suspension once it has been swirled. Avoid using the reagent if suspension is not uniform.

Collagen 10 μg/mL

Test	450 μL PRP + 50 μL collagen 100 μg/mL
	(Final concentration: 10 μg/mL)

Collagen 1 μg/mL

Make a 1/10 dilution in distilled water to the former solution, thus obtaining a working solution of 10 μg/mL. Dilution can be kept at 4–8°C for up to 1 week.

Test	450 μL PRP + 50 μL collagen 10 μg/mL
	(Final concentration: 1 μg/mL)

2.4 Arachidonic Acid

Arachidonic acid (Biopool, Ventura, USA).

Vial to be diluted with 0.5 mL of distilled water giving a stock solution of 15 mM.

Test	450 μL PRP + 28 μL arachidonic acid 15 mM
	(Final concentration: 1 μg/mL)

2.5 Ristocetin

Ristocetin (Biopool, Wicklow, Ireland).

Manufacturer recommends to dilute the vial with 0.5 mL of high-purity water to obtain a working solution of 15 mg/mL. In our experience, we obtain better results when reconstituting the former vial with 0.75 mL of normal saline, thus obtaining a working solution of 10 mg/mL. Aliquot and store at −70°C.

Ristocetin 0.5 mg/mL

Test	450 μL PRP + 25 μL ristocetin 10 mg/mL
	(Final concentration: 0.5 mg/mL)

Ristocetin 1.0 mg/mL

Test	450 μL PRP + 50 μL ristocetin 10 mg/mL (Final concentration: 1.0 mg/mL)

2.6 Calcium Ionophore (A23187)

SIGMA (Cat # C-7522): 50 mg.

Dissolve 1 mg of calcium ionophore in 10 mL absolute ethanol. This solution may be kept aliquoted at −70°C. At the time of the test, make a 1/10 dilution in Tris buffer (pH: 7.4) to obtain a working solution of 10 μg/mL.

Test	450 μL PRP + 50 μL calcium ionophore A-23187 10 μg/mL (Final concentration: 1 μg/mL)

2.7 Bovine Plasma

(Homemade). Keep frozen at −70°C.

Obtained from cow blood collected in 3.13% citrate in a 9 to 1 proportion. The optimal dilution of bovine plasma may vary, depending on the response over normal PRP. At least ten normal PRPs should be tested to ensure that a biphasic curve is obtained. Commonly, a 1/5 to 1/10 dilution in normal saline works well.

Test: 450 μL PRP + 50 μL bovine plasma (1/5)

3 Methods

3.1 Quality Assurance

Platelet function testing presents many challenges in ensuring that accurate and meaningful results are obtained. Firstly, unlike other tests, there are no widely available internal or external quality control materials available. Quality assurance requires that platelet function assays be carefully designed, developed, and implemented. Platelets are inherently prone to artifactual activation but also to desensitization. To minimize the potential artifact occurrence, it is important to control preanalytical variables, including drug therapy, improper sample collection, sample handling, transit, age of the sample, and test procedures (5).

3.2 Obtaining the Samples

Each laboratory should define its own procedure to obtain the samples but some details should be taken into account. Over the previous 4 h to the procedure, subjects should have rested, fasted, and avoided smoking. They should also avoid taking any drugs known to affect platelet function for 10 days prior to the test (see Note 1).

3.3 Specimen Collection

Blood samples should be drawn with a minimum of trauma or stasis at the venipuncture site and anticoagulated with 3.2 % sodium citrate, in a ratio of 1 part anticoagulant to 9 parts of blood. Plastic material should be used in order to minimize activation of platelets during sample preparation. The samples should be mixed by various gentle inversions but should not be shaken (see Notes 2 and 3).

3.4 Preparation of Platelet-Rich Plasma

Platelets in a suspension of plasma are isolated from an anticoagulated blood sample by a relatively low-force centrifugation. This material is known as PRP. Many ways to obtain this material have been described. Some were prepared by centrifugation of anticoagulated blood at 180 × *g* for 10 min at room temperature. However, by using the following scheme for only a fraction of the time, very similar results are achieved (see Notes 4 and 5).

1. Centrifuge sample at 720 × *g* for 1.5 min.
2. Remove the cloudy yellow supernatant containing the platelets with a plastic transfer pipette and put it into a plastic tube.
3. Centrifuge sample again at 720 × *g* for 1.5 min.
4. Take off the PRP with a plastic transfer pipette and put it into the former plastic tube.
5. Label the tube properly, including patient's name and sample type (PRP). Cap the tube (see Note 6).

3.4.1 Preparation of Platelet-Poor Plasma

1. Centrifuge sample at 2,400 × *g* for 10 min.
2. Take off the PRP with a polypropylene transfer pipette and put it into a polypropylene plastic tube.
3. Label the tube properly, including patient's name and sample type (PPP). Cap the tube.

A single sample of PPP can be used as the reference sample for all the tests of the same patient, so the amount of PPP required is only 500 μL per sample channel.

3.5 Adjusting the Platelet Count of the Working PRP

In order to maintain standardized procedures, the working PRP should be kept at certain values: between 200,000 and 300,000 platelets/μL are acceptable for routine practice. If PRP has higher counts, adjust it with the addition of its own PPP.

Example
Sample: 2,000 μL of a PRP with a platelet count of 310,000 platelet/μL:

$$\frac{310{,}000\ \text{platelet}/\mu\text{L} \times 2{,}000\ \mu\text{L}}{250{,}000\ \text{platelet}/\mu\text{L}} = 2{,}480\ \mu\text{L}$$

$$2{,}480\ \mu\text{L} - 2{,}000\ \mu\text{L} = 480\ \mu\text{L}$$

This means that we should add 480 μL of PPP to the 2,000 μL of PRP, to obtain 2,480 μL of PRP with a platelet count of 250,000 platelet/μL.

3.6 Basic Procedure of Light Transmission Aggregometry

This instruction assumes the use of a Chrono-Log lumi-aggregometer (model 500) and a Chrono-Log dual channel recorder (model 707). This procedure is intended for an aggregometer with a graphic readout. Computerized interface devices are also available which facilitate graphics, calculation, and data handling.

1. Turn on the aggregometer and wait at least 30 min to allow temperature stability of the thermostated block.
2. Thaw the required agonists at 37°C for 2 min.
3. Prepare two microtubes with PPP, one for the patient's sample and the other as control. This latter tube acts as a blank for each sample, giving the signal of the maximum aggregation possible.
4. Pipette 450 μL of PRP in a microtube and put it to reach a temperature of 37°C in the corresponding incubation well for at least 2 min.
5. Put the PRP microtube with the stirring bar in the sample well (see Note 7). Verify that PPP tube is settled in the corresponding well and that the PPP belongs to the sample to be analyzed.
6. Lower the recording pen and start running the paper.
7. Set baselines. At this point, the maximum value of transmittance for the system PRP–PPP will be recorded allowing postcalculations.
8. Allow the pen to record for at least 2 min.
9. Test the desired agonist following the corresponding procedure (see Notes 8–10).
10. Raise the recording pen and stop the paper after at least 6 min.
11. Remove the magnet from the microtube and rinse it thoroughly in 10 mL of distilled water. Dry it with filter paper.
12. Put the assayed microtube in a solution of sodium hypochloride at 1%.
13. The contents of this tube may be saved to measure products which are derived from platelet activation like serotonin and thromboxane.

3.7 Changes in Light Transmission During Normal Platelet Aggregation

Once a stimulus is added into the test tube, changes in the curve tracing may be observed.

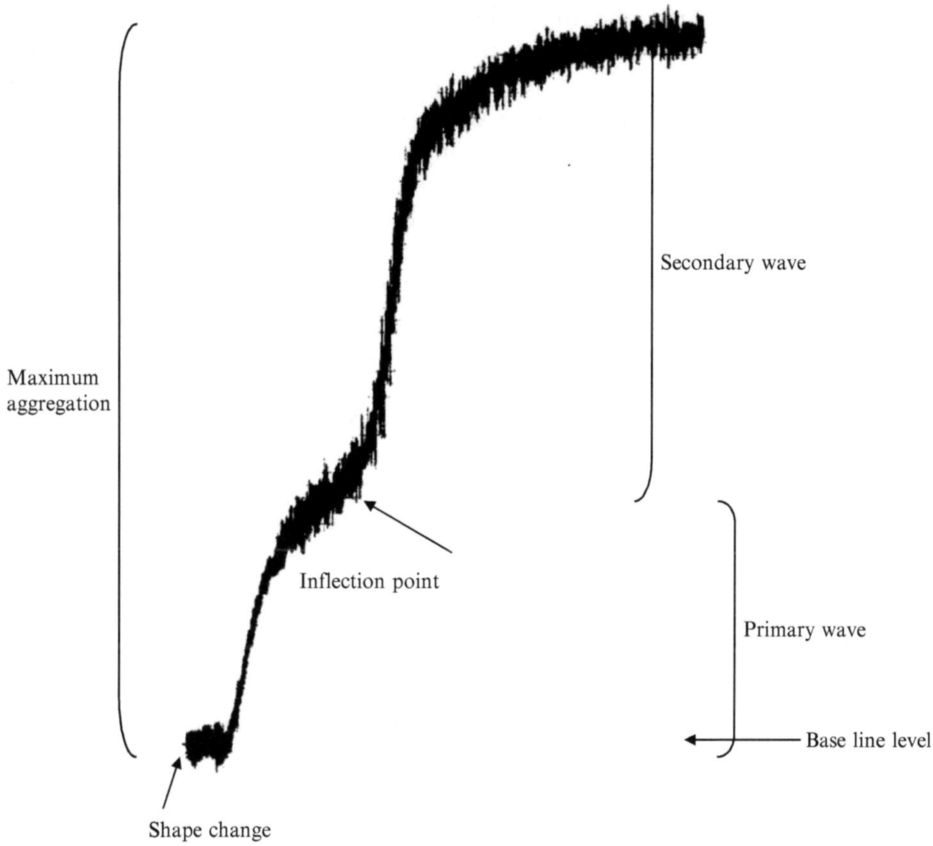

Fig. 2 Normal platelet aggregometry response

3.7.1 Shape Change

When platelets undergo a stimulus (agonist or aggregating agent), a shape change occurs, from discoid to spherical. As a result of this, platelets change to a larger size and allow less light to pass through the PRP, recorded as less light transmission through the sample relative to the reference (Fig. 2).

3.7.2 First Wave of Aggregation (or Primary Aggregation)

If the dose of aggregating agent is strong enough to cause the platelets to adhere each other and form aggregates, more light is able to pass through the PRP sample. The change in light transmission recorded, over time, shows a trend towards the PPP level (100% aggregation or 100% light transmission) (Fig. 2).

3.7.3 Inflection Point

If the stimulus is strong enough, a change in the curve slope can be observed, usually noted as a brief "lag" phase of the trace. In case the stimululs is not sufficient, the platelets will disaggregate turning the trace towards the PRP level (0% aggregation). It is thought that this point is the beginning of the process of "release" and is coincident with the start of the ATP-release signal increase detected with luciferin–luciferase. Granule content release is necessary to promote the "secondary wave of aggregation."

3.7.4 Secondary Wave of Aggregation (or Secondary Aggregation)

When the stimulus is adequate, platelets release their granule contents and the trace continues aggregating to a maximum extent giving a secondary wave of aggregation.

When a strong agonist such as thrombin, arachidonic acid, calcium ionophore, or collagen is used, only one trace is obtained and inflection point is indistinguishable.

As the aggregation trace is obtained, a number of parameters can be calculated for further analysis.

Slope or Rate of Aggregation

The rate of change (in % aggregation per minute) in the output device.

Maximum Change in Light Transmission (Percent of Aggregation)

The maximum deflection of the registered trace starting at the basal level. This parameter may be measured at a fixed time (usually 6 min) or when the trace reaches a *plateau* (see Notes 11 and 12).

3.8 Interpretation of Results

3.8.1 Threshold Concentration

For all agonists, the lowest concentration of stimulus giving a full tracing, both primary and secondary wave of aggregation, is the threshold concentration. Tracings at this concentration should be impaired while in aspirin treatment.

3.8.2 ADP-Induced Aggregation

After agonist is added there is an initial shape change resulting in a decrease in light transmittance followed by a primary wave of aggregation. If the stimulus is not sufficient, or an inhibitory effect is present (i.e., aspirin), platelets will disaggregate. If the stimulus is strong enough, the secondary wave of ADP-induced aggregation arises. It is this moment when there is a release of platelet granule contents that include fibrinogen, serotonin, thromboxane, and ADP that potentiates the primary aggregation response. Our threshold concentration for ADP starts at 2.5 μM of ADP in testing aggregation. If no response is seen, higher concentrations (5.0 and 10 μM) are tested (see Fig. 3).

3.8.3 Epinephrine-Induced Aggregation

Epinephrine induces a slight change of shape whilst added, and the primary wave begins soon after the instillation of the agonist, followed by the secondary wave. Our threshold concentration for epinephrine starts at 5.0 μM. If no response is seen, 10 μM are tested (see Fig. 4).

3.8.4 Collagen-Induced Aggregation

Platelet aggregation in response to collagen typically displays a lag phase between the addition of the agonist and the shape change. This agonist does not induce a biphasic change in tracings as does ADP. Threshold concentration for collagen begins at 2.0 μg/mL that should induce platelet activation in normal platelets and is impaired in the presence of aspirin. Higher concentration (10 μg/mL) is used

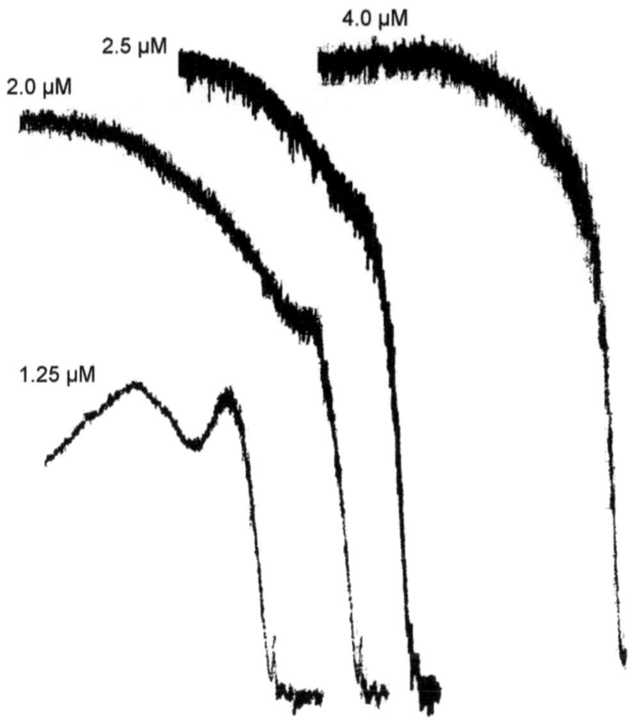

Fig. 3 Patterns of aggregation at different ADP concentrations

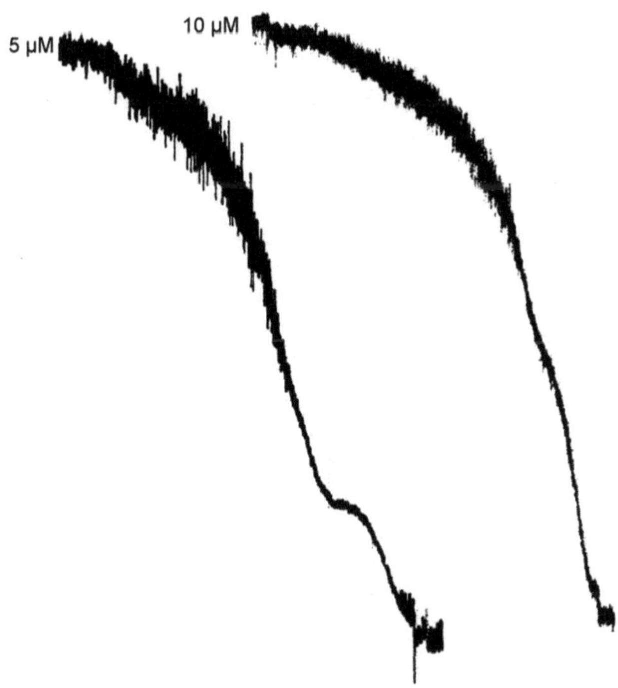

Fig. 4 Patterns of aggregation at different epinephrine concentrations

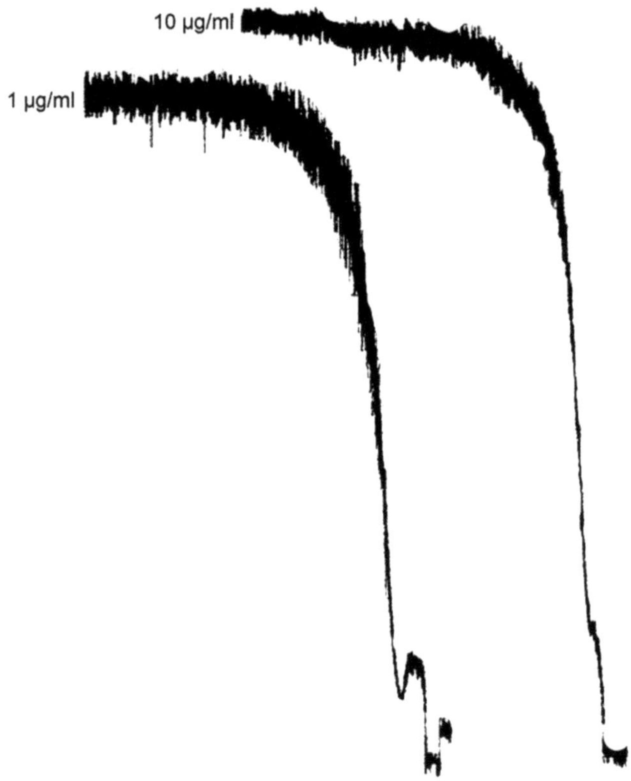

Fig. 5 Patterns of aggregation at different collagen concentrations

when impaired tracings are obtained with the former amount of agonist (see Fig. 5).

3.8.5 Arachidonic Acid-Induced Aggregation

The addition of arachidonic acid induces a shape change followed by a single response wave which is blocked by aspirin treatment. Alternatively, thromboxane analogue can help distinguish defective thromboxane generation (e.g., from COX-1 inhibition or a congenital defect in COX-1 or thromboxane synthetase) from defects in thromboxane responses (e.g., due to receptor defects or other signaling abnormalities) (see Fig. 6).

3.8.6 Ristocetin-Induced Aggregation

Ristocetin-induced platelet aggregation is used to determine the presence and integrity of GP Ibα–V–IX complex on platelets and von Willebrand factor in the PRP. Trace patterns in normal platelets are dose dependent and go from nil aggregation (0.5 mg/mL) and a biphasic curve (1.0 mg/mL) to a single trace curve (1.5 mg/mL). Normal platelets should respond to 1.0 mg/mL of ristocetin but not to 0.5 mg/mL. Impairment to respond to 1.0 mg/mL concentrations may indicate defects whether in von Willebrand

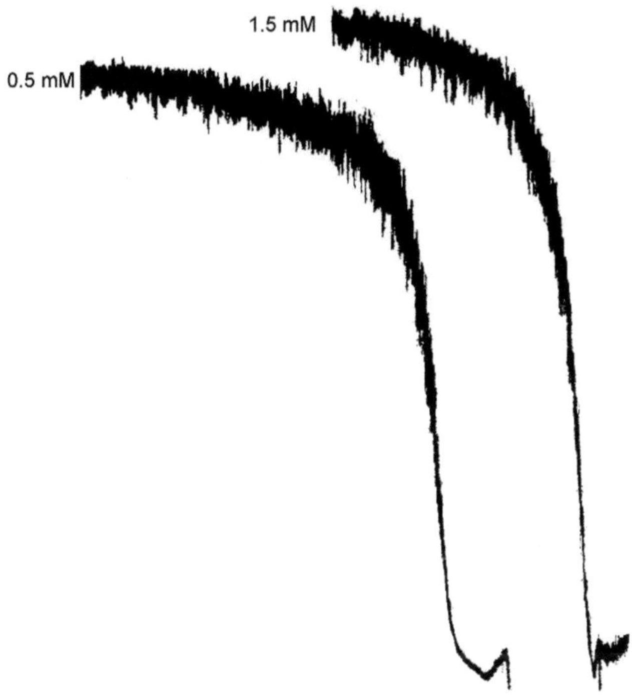

Fig. 6 Patterns of aggregation at different arachidonic acid concentrations

factor function/quantity or in GP Ibα–V–IX function/quantity (see Fig. 7).

3.8.7 Bovine Plasma-Induced Aggregation

Bovine plasma-induced platelet aggregation is used to determine the presence and integrity of GP Ibα–V–IX complex on platelets independently of the von Willebrand factor present in PRP. Typically present as a biphasic curve, it is a useful tool to distinguish impaired ristocetin-induced platelet aggregation due to von Willebrand factor defects from platelet receptor impairment (i.e., Bernard–Soulier syndrome).

3.9 Normal Reference Ranges

Non-parametrical tests are recommended to obtain normal reference ranges, since they are more descriptive of the population studied.

As the result of our experience, data from 77 healthy children and 162 healthy adults are reported, considering children aged from 1 to 5 years, 6 to 10 years, and 11 to 18 years and adults (Table 1). Results were expressed as median together with intervals covering 95% (between the 2.5th to 97.5th centiles) of the population. Tukey's testing was performed to detect differences between the age groups. This test is based on comparison of the medians and estimates of variances among the groups. A P-value <0.05 was considered statistically significant. Statistical software package STATA, Release 8.0 (Stata Corporation, College Station, USA), was used for analysis. No statistical differences were observed between age groups.

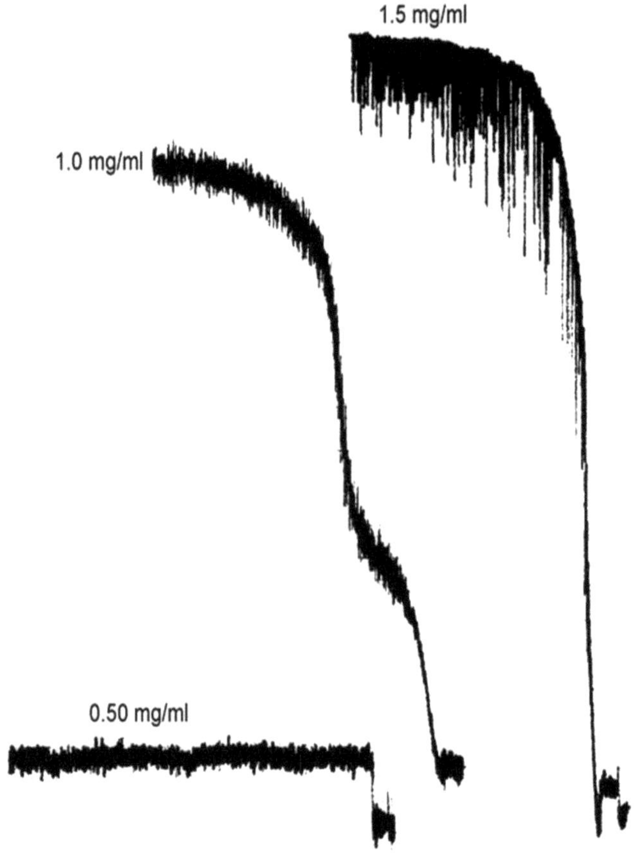

Fig. 7 Patterns of aggregation at different ristocetin concentrations

4 Notes

1. Drug and food intake before a platelet study is a main point to be considered. Although it is well known that several drugs influence platelet responses, many foods (over 90) that usually are not included in the previous questionnaire are described to modify platelet response as well.
2. Delayed sample handling may induce plasma activation followed by thrombin generation that is a strong platelet stimulus.
3. The use of an inappropriate anticoagulant ratio for sample collection may lead to abnormal aggregation patterns due to impaired calcium chelation. Moreover, the use of the wrong anticoagulant (i.e., EDTA instead of citrate) may give patterns that mimic Glanzmann thrombasthenia.
4. When thrombocytopenia is present or suspected such as in Bernard–Soulier syndrome, allow the blood to spontaneously

Table 1
Reference ranges for platelet aggregometry in healthy children

Group	1–5 years	6–10 years	11–18 years	Adults	*P*-value
n (gender)	21 (8F/13M)	26 (11F/15M)	30 (16F/14M)	162 (66F/74M)	–
Age (years)	4.1 (1.9–5.9)	7.7 (6.2–9.8)	14.3 (10.6–17.9)	33 (22.0–45.3)	–
Ristocetin (1.5 mg/mL) (%)	91 (87–93)	85 (78–99)	85 (72–95)	84 (72–100)	0.9590
ADP (2.5 μM) (%)	76 (69–91)	77 (68–90)	81 (66–104)	80 (69–101)	0.0935
Collagen (2 μg/mL) (%)	75 (64–84)	81(66–90)	86 (71–100)	81 (69–101)	0.1594
Collagen (10 μg/mL) (%)	83 (74–97)	84 (68–99)	85 (71–102)	86 (73–105)	0.4043
Epinephrine (10 μM) (%)	80 (70–91)	81 (73–96)	82 (74–105)	84 (71–100)	0.1772
Arachidonic acid (1 mM) (%)	79 (73–92)	84 (75–95)	80 (74–102)	84 (73–101)	0.3312
A 23187 (1 μg/mL) (%)	85 (79–88)	74 (68–83)	80 (71–90)	78 (69–99)	0.079

Values are expressed as median with the interval covering 95% of the population studied (between 2.5th and 97.5th centiles)

sediment for 1 h. Care must be taken to make cell count after harvesting the supernatant PRP.

5. Red cells and leukocytes can interfere in platelet response, so cell contamination should be kept at the lowest counts. For routine analysis, below 9,000/μL for red cells and below 200/μL for leukocytes which is achievable using the centrifugation procedure described to obtain PRP.
6. Uncapped sample can change pH, leading to platelet activation.
7. A Teflon-coated magnetic stirrer is recommended. Precut disposable stirrers are also available but these have proved to give a higher CV% while testing the same PRP in two different channels at the same time. The stirring speed and the nature of

the stirrer might vary according to the different manufacturers. A speed of 1,200 rpm is recommended.

8. It is useful to work with agonist concentrations which allow the use of a single set volume in a pipette. This minimizes the chance of making mistakes by having different volume settings.
9. Try to avoid the use of very small volumes (i.e., 2–5 μL) of highly concentrated agonists. Small variations in these volumes will produce great changes in the final concentration of the agonist. Volumes between 25 and 50 μL proved to be very useful for our routine.
10. Try not to use wide tips since they can stack in the mouth of the test tube and when trying to lift the pipette, you will lift the test tube as well. If they are too thin and long, they may touch the stirring bar and will make it to give a big noise in the output signal. Always verify that the desired amount of agonist is within the tip before adding it into the test tube.
11. Unless set automatically, aggregometers need that once reference and test tubes are in position, a baseline must be done in order to establish the scale between 0% aggregation (PRP signal) and 100% aggregation (PPP signal).
12. If the curve that you expect is not achieved, many problems should be discarded before assigning a pathological response to a given PRP.
    (a) Absence of the reference tube, if you are using one, or a variation in the position of it may lead to a trace problem such as shallow curves, or even absence of one.
    (b) Absence or insufficient agonist volume due to a pipette "mistake."
    (c) Missing to put the stirrer into the test tube.
    (d) Connection problems between aggregometer and output device.
    (e) Avoidance to set baseline before the run.

References

1. Harrison P (2005) Platelet function analysis. Blood Rev 19:111–123
2. Zhou L, Schmaier AH (2005) Platlet aggregation testing in platelet-rich plasma. Am J Clin Pathol 123:172–183
3. Harrison P, Frelinger AL III, Furman MI, Michelson AD (2007) Measuring antiplatelet drug effects in the laboratory. Thromb Res 120:323–336
4. Hayward CPM, Rao KA, Cattaneo M (2006) Congenital platelet disorders: overview of their mechanisms, diagnostic evaluation and treatment. Haemophilia 12:128–136
5. Hayward CPM, Eikelboom J (2007) Platelet function testing: quality assurance. Semin Thromb Hemost 33:273–282

Chapter 18

Platelet Flow Cytometry

Matthew D. Linden

Abstract

Flow cytometry is a powerful and versatile tool which can be used to provide substantial phenotypic data on platelets by yielding quantitative information of their physical and antigenic properties. This includes surface expression of functional receptors, bound ligands, expression of granule components, interaction of platelets with other platelets via aggregation, or interaction with other blood components, such as leukocytes or the plasma coagulation system. Quantitative assessment of these parameters may facilitate the diagnosis of inherited or acquired platelet disorders, assist in the diagnosis of diseases associated with platelet activation, or assist in the monitoring of safety and efficacy of antiplatelet therapy.

Key words Platelet activation, Flow cytometry, Heterotypic aggregates, Platelet immunophenotyping, Platelet disorders, Monoclonal antibodies, Fluorescence

1 Introduction

Flow cytometry rapidly measures the physical and antigenic characteristics of a large number of cells in suspension (1, 2). Typically, cells are labelled with fluorescently conjugated monoclonal antibodies (mAbs) and passed single file through the beam of a laser, causing fluorescent activation of the fluorophore at the excitation wavelength. The emitted fluorescence and light scattering properties of the cell are measured by several detectors (2). Thus, the number of surface epitopes for which the labelled mAbs specifically bind can be determined for thousands of cells in suspension by measuring the emitted fluorescence. Meanwhile, cells may be categorized according to their light scatter properties which generally reflect the size and granularity of the cell. Platelets are particularly amenable to analysis by flow cytometry because they are already suspended in blood, and undergo a number of changes in antigenic expression on the cell surface with activation or in association with disease states (3).

Interrogation of platelet phenotype by flow cytometry has been successfully used to assist the diagnosis of many disease

Paul Monagle (ed.), *Haemostasis: Methods and Protocols*, Methods in Molecular Biology, vol. 992,
DOI 10.1007/978-1-62703-339-8_18, © Springer Science+Business Media New York 2013

states, including inherited platelet defects such as Bernard–Soulier syndrome, Glanzmann thrombasthenia, or storage pool disease (3). These techniques have also been employed in blood bank applications for immunophenotyping surface receptor polymorphisms and platelet crossmatching (4) and the investigation of hemorrhage associated with platelet hyporeactivity or intravascular thrombotic and cardiovascular disorders associated with platelet hyperreactivity (4, 5). A more complete list of applications for flow cytometric analysis of platelets is shown in Table 1.

Resting platelets constitutively express many surface glycoproteins that are easily identifiable by flow cytometry. Platelets undergo changes in antigenic expression on the cell surface with activation (6–8). One of the major benefits of flow cytometry is that it has the ability to quantitatively and mechanistically measure both the activation state of circulating platelets and the function of different pathways of platelet activation by stimulation with specific agonists and measuring changes in antigenic characteristics. This allows a far more specific, mechanistic, and molecular measure of platelet function than can be obtained by functional platelet aggregometry.

Immunophenotyping of platelets by flow cytometry may be performed on platelets in whole blood, on washed platelets, or in platelet-rich plasma (PRP). The additional sample preparation required for PRP or washed platelet may result in unintended platelet alteration, activation, or loss of platelet subpopulations, confounding results (9). Other advantages of whole blood analysis include the minimal required sample volume (10), and a more physiologically relevant assessment of haemostasis, which includes interactions of platelets with erythrocytes, leukocytes, and the coagulation system (11–14).

There are, however, several disadvantages to the use of flow cytometry for immunophenotyping platelets. These include the high instrument expense both for purchase and maintenance; some lack of consistency among different cytometer models (3, 15); the possibility of subpopulations which, due to size and low copy number of the epitope being measured, may fall below the detectible threshold of the instrument or software; and the need for rapid and relatively complicated sample preparation to ameliorate artificial platelet activation/phenotypic change.

2 Materials

2.1 Blood Collection and Sample Preparation

1. 21 G (or larger bore) needle.
2. Choice of anticoagulant blood collection tube (see Note 1).

Table 1
Common applications for flow cytometry for the study of platelet-related disorders

Application of flow cytometry	Disorders
Measurement of increased platelet activation and heterotypic aggregation	Atherothrombotic disease, chest pain, unstable angina, myocardial infarction (41, 69) Ischemic stroke (92–94) Diabetes mellitus (95, 96) Haemodialysis (97) Monitoring percutaneous coronary intervention (11, 40, 70, 98–100) Monitoring antiplatelet therapy (71, 85, 101–103) Peripheral arterial occlusive disease (104) Chronic venous stasis ulceration (105) and insufficiency (106) Uremia (107) Cystic fibrosis (108, 109) Systemic inflammation and sepsis (110, 111) Alzheimer's disease (112) Heart transplant vasculopathy (113) Preeclampsia (both mother and neonate) (114, 115) Myeloproliferative disorders (116)
Measurement of impaired platelet reactivity	Cardiopulmonary bypass (46–49) Monitoring antiplatelet therapy (71, 85, 101–103, 117–123) Low birth weight neonates (10, 79) Hemorrhagic stroke (1)
Measurement of GPIb–IX–V expression	Bernard–Soulier syndrome (18, 19)
Measurement of GPIIb–IIIa expression	Glanzmann thrombasthenia (20, 21)
Measurement of granule components	Dense granule storage pool deficiency (24, 25) Myeloproliferative disorders (24) Renal failure (26)
Formation of a procoagulant platelet surface	Heparin-induced thrombocytopenia (124) von Willebrand disease (31)
Detection of platelet autoantibodies	Immune thrombocytopaenic purpura (30) Fibrinogen receptor-induced thrombocytopenia and thrombosis (125, 126)

3. Citrate wash buffer: 11 mM glucose, 128 mM NaCl, 4.3 mM NaH_2PO_4, 7.5 mM Na_2HPO_4, 4.8 mM $Na_3C_6H_5O_7$, 2.4 mM $C_6H_8O_7$, 0.35% BSA, 50 ng/mL prostaglandin PGE_1, pH 6.5.
4. Sepharose 2B beads (Pharmacia).

5. HEPES-buffered saline: 10 mM HEPES, 0.15 mM NaCl, pH 7.4 is required.

2.2 Diagnosis of Specific Platelet Disorders

1. HEPES-buffered saline (HBS) (see Subheading 2.1, item 5).
2. Platelet-specific identifier antibody titrated in HEPES-buffered saline conjugated to a fluorochrome (e.g., monoclonal anti-CD41, anti-CD61, anti-CD42a, anti-CD42b) (see Note 2).
3. Platelet phenotypic marker antibody (see Note 3).
4. Negative controls: antibody isotype, concentration, fluorochrome, and F:P ratio matched to the specific platelet marker antibody, or a blocking agent that inhibits specific antibody binding to the epitope.
5. 1% formalin fixative in HBS.

2.3 Measurement of Platelet Activation and Degranulation

1. HBS.
2. Siliconized microcentrifuge tubes (Corning) (see Note 4).
3. Fluorophore-conjugated platelet-specific identifier (see Subheading 2.2 above).
4. Platelet activation/degranulation marker (e.g., monoclonal anti-CD62P or PAC1). See Table 2 for a comprehensive list of platelet activation and degranulation markers.
5. Platelet agonist, e.g., ADP, epinephrine, thrombin receptor-activating peptide (TRAP) (see Note 5). See Table 3.
6. Negative controls: antibody isotype, concentration, fluorochrome, and F:P ratio matched to the platelet activation marker (see Note 6).
7. 1% formalin fixative in HBS.
8. If using thrombin as an agonist, 10 mM Gly–Pro–Arg–Pro (GPRP) in HEPES saline is required to prevent fibrin polymerization.

2.4 Measurement of Heterotypic Aggregates

1. HBS.
2. Siliconized microcentrifuge tubes.
3. Fluorophore-conjugated anti-CD14 mAb.
4. Platelet-specific identifier (see Subheading 2.2 above) (see Note 7).
5. Platelet agonist.
6. Negative controls: antibody isotype, concentration, fluorochrome, and F:P ratio matched to the platelet-specific identifier.
7. FACSLyse solution (Becton Dickinson).

Table 2
Activation-dependent platelet markers

Activation-dependent platelet surface change	Prototypic antibodies	References
Conformational changes in integrin $\alpha_{IIb}\beta_3$		
– Activation-induced conformational change in $\alpha_{IIb}\beta_3$ resulting in exposure of the fibrinogen binding site	PAC1	(7)
– Ligand-induced conformational change in $\alpha_{IIb}\beta_3$	PM 1.1, LIBS1, LIBS6, D3	(127–130)
– Receptor-induced conformational change in bound ligand (fibrinogen)	2G5, 9F9, F26	(131–133)
Exposure of granule membrane proteins		
– P-selectin (α-granules)	S12, AC1.2, 1E3	(76, 134, 135)
– CD63 (lysosomes)	CLB-gran/12	(136)
– LAMP-1 (lysosomes)	H5G11	(137)
– LAMP-2 (lysosomes)	H4B4	(138)
– CD40L	TRAP1	(139)
– Lectin-like oxidized LDL receptor-1 (LOX-1)	JTX68	(140)
Platelet surface binding of secreted proteins		
– Thrombospondin	P8, TSP-1	(141, 142)
– Multimerin	JS-1	(143, 144)
Development of a procoagulant surface[a]		
– Factor V/Va binding	V237	(145)
– Factor X/Xa binding	5224	(81)
– Factor VIII binding	1B3	(80)
– Phosphatidylserine	Annexin V[a]	(14)

[a]Annexin V is not a monoclonal antibody, but may be used as one for its ability to specifically bind to membrane phosphatidylserine

2.5 Measurement of Procoagulant Platelets and the Formation of the Prothrombinase Complex

1. Modified HEPES Tyrodes (HT) buffer (10 mM HEPES, 137 mM NaCl, 2.8 mM KCl, 1 mM $MgCl_2$, 12 mM $NaHCO_3$, 0.4 mM Na_2HPO_4, 5.5 mM glucose, 0.35% BSA, pH 7.4).
2. 5 mM GPRP.
3. Siliconized microcentrifuge tubes.
4. Coagulation factor V/Va or X/Xa (Stago).
5. Platelet agonist in 6 mM $CaCl_2$.
6. Platelet-specific identifier mAb.
7. Marker of platelet procoagulant activity, e.g., annexin V, antico-agulation factor V/Va, or X/Xa mAb.
8. 1% formalin fixative.

Table 3
Commonly used platelet agonists for flow cytometric analysis

Agonist	Mechanism	References
Adenosine diphosphate (ADP)	Binds to purinergic G-protein-coupled receptors $P2Y_1$, which activates phospholipase C, and $P2Y_{12}$, which activates phospholipase C and suppresses cyclic adenosine monophosphate (cAMP)	(146–152)
Arachidonic acid	Converted to prostaglandin G_2 and then to H_2 by cyclooxygenase, then to thromboxane A_2 by thromboxane A synthase	(153)
Collagen	(1) Binds to GPIb–IX–V complex and GPIIbIIIa via von Willebrand factor, (2) directly binds to and activates GPIaIIa, and (3) directly binds to, and causes clustering of, GPVI	(154–158)
Epinephrine	Binds to the G_z-coupled α_{2A}-adrenergic receptor, which inhibits cAMP	(152, 159–161)
Thrombin	Cleaves the extended N-terminus of G-protein-coupled protease-activated receptor (PAR)1 and PAR4, which exposes a tethered ligand. This leads to increased cytosolic Ca^{2+}, activation of protein kinase C, reorganization of the actin cytoskeleton, and suppression of cAMP	(152, 162–164)
Thrombin receptor-activating peptide (TRAP)	Directly binds the PAR1 tethered ligand recognition site	(152, 162, 163, 165)
Thromboxane A_2 analogues (e.g., U44619)	Bind to G-protein-coupled TPα and TPβ receptors, which cause phosphoinositide hydrolysis, protein phosphorylation, and increased cytosolic Ca^{2+}	(152, 166, 167)

3 Methods

The concentration of monoclonal antibody reagents for platelet immunophenotyping must be determined by titration and will vary between instrument, manufacturers, and F:P ratio. Usually two different antibodies are used, each conjugated to a different fluorochrome, usually fluorescein isothiocyanate (FITC) or phycoerythrin (PE). In general, one antibody is used to identify the platelets in whole blood and a threshold is set to this parameter to exclude non-platelet cells from analysis, while the other is used to measure the phenotype of the platelets.

3.1 Blood Collection and Sample Preparation

1. Blood is usually drawn from either a vein or artery into anticoagulant (16) (see Note 8).
2. Light tourniquet only or no tourniquet should be used. A 21 G or larger bore needle and technique to ensure good blood flow and a smooth draw are essential.
3. Discard the first ~2 mL of blood drawn to minimize tissue factor or red cell hemolysis that may lead to platelet activation (12, 16).
4. Blood samples should be processed within 15 min of collection. In the interim blood should be kept at room temperature, because refrigeration may lead to cold-induced platelet activation (17).
5. Artifact platelet aggregation/agglutination may be minimized by dilution of the blood in buffered saline and by gentle mixing of reagents followed by undisturbed incubation.
6. Some studies may require the isolation of platelets from other cellular components of the blood by centrifugation to form PRP, or even isolation from the plasma itself by gel filtration or washing.

3.1.1 Preparation of Platelet-Rich Plasma

1. Centrifuge anticoagulated whole blood for 10–15 min at 150–200 × g. Care must be taken to ensure platelets remain at room temperature as heat or cold may affect platelet function.
2. Remove the PRP to a clean test tube, being careful not to disturb the buffy coat or red cell layers.

3.1.2 Isolation of Platelets by Gel Filtration

1. Pack a 10 mL syringe with Sepharose 2B beads.
2. Equilibrate the column with water followed by HBS.
3. Layer PRP on the top of the column, allow it to fully enter the column, and then follow with 30 mL HBS.
4. The eluent will contain gel-filtered platelets.

3.1.3 Isolation of Platelets by Washing

1. Dilute PRP 1:8 with citrate wash buffer.
2. Centrifuge for 10 min at 1,200 × *g* at room temperature.
3. Aspirate the supernatant and gently resuspend the pellet in citrate wash buffer (do not vortex).
4. Repeat wash, after final wash resuspend in HBS.

3.2 Diagnosis of Specific Platelet Disorders

Bernard–Soulier syndrome is an inherited deficiency of the GPIb–IX–V complex, resulting in giant platelets, mild thrombocytopenia, and bleeding (18, 19). Measurement of platelet GPIb (CD42b), GPIX (CD42a), and GPV (CD42d) expression by flow cytometry can assist in the diagnosis of this disorder (20). Similarly, Glanzmann thrombasthenia is an inherited deficiency of integrin $\alpha_{IIb}\beta_3$, which can be measured using flow cytometry (20, 21). The method for measuring these and other such disorders of platelet function is given below. However, there are a multitude of variations on this protocol for measuring other disorders such as dense granule storage pool deficiency (22–26), heparin-induced thrombocytopenia (HIT) (27–29), immune thrombocytopenic purpura (30), and von Willebrand disease (31).

1. Dilute anticoagulated whole blood 1:10 in HBS. Normal control blood from a healthy volunteer should be used as a control.
2. Mix diluted blood with appropriately titrated mixture of platelet-specific identifier mAb and platelet phenotypic marker mAb in HBS (see Note 9). The ratio of antibody mixture to blood should be about 3:1.
3. Incubate for 20 min at room temperature.
4. Fix labelled cells by diluting 15:1 in 1% formalin solution and incubating for 15 min. After fixation, samples may be stored at 4°C for up to 24 h before analysis.
5. Using a flow cytometer, identify platelets by characteristic forward and size light scatter and expression of the platelet identifier. A threshold on the identifier fluorochrome may be used to prevent display of non-platelet events (Fig. 1).
6. Collect light scatter parameters in logarithmic mode at ~200 platelet events/second and measure the platelet phenotypic

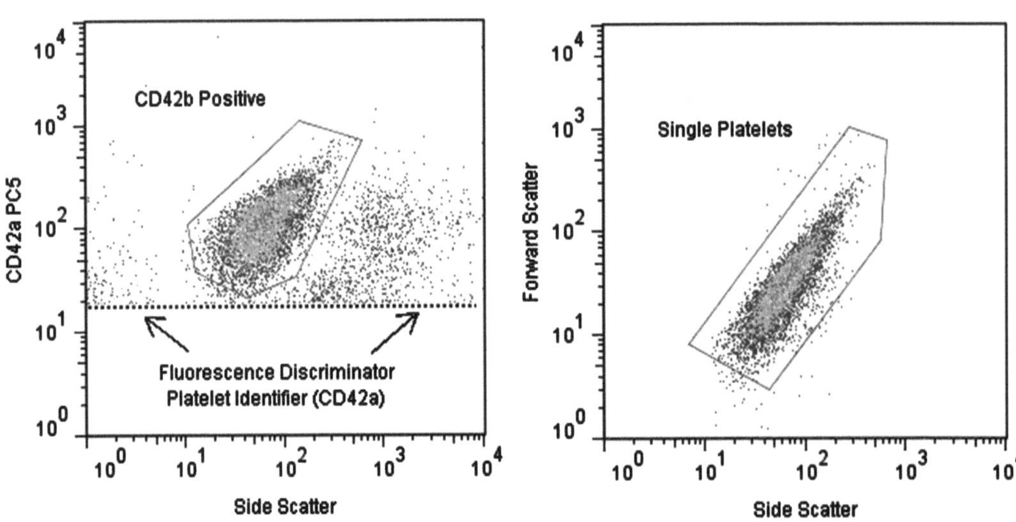

Fig. 1 Identification of platelets by whole blood flow cytometry. A discriminator is set to only record events that express a platelet-specific marker (e.g., CD42a). Events are double gated for platelet-specific marker expression and characteristic light scatter

marker of interest by fluorescent intensity of the associated fluorophore. Alternatively, an isotypic control can be used to mark a region to identify the proportion of platelets with and without the marker of interest (% positive). Platelets lacking the receptor of interest will also lack the corresponding fluorescence, relative to the normal control.

3.3 Measurement of Platelet Activation and Degranulation

Platelet hyperreactivity and/or circulating activated platelets play a role in atherothrombotic and peripheral arterial diseases (32–38) and may play a role in the pathogenesis of atherosclerosis (39). In addition, percutaneous coronary intervention (PCI) results in platelet activation as demonstrated by whole blood flow cytometry (40) and the degree of platelet activation correlates to both acuity of disease (41) and cardiovascular outcome (42–44).

Conversely, measuring platelet activation by flow cytometry may be useful in the clinical assessment of disorders associated with platelet hyporeactivity and hemorrhage, such as intracranial hemorrhage in very low birth weight neonates (10, 45), the hemostatic defect of cardiopulmonary bypass (46–49) or drug-associated platelet disorders (50–58), dietary and lifestyle effects (58–67), and antiplatelet therapy (68).

Therefore flow cytometric measurement of platelet activation may assist in the diagnosis of angina (69, 70), guiding optimal antiplatelet therapy (71, 72).

1. Mix platelet identifier antibody, platelet activation marker, and agonist at appropriately titrated concentrations (see Notes 10–12).
2. Dilute anticoagulated whole blood 1:10 in HBS.
3. Mix diluted whole blood with the antibody–agonist cocktail at a 1:2 ratio.
4. Incubate at room temperature for exactly 5 min (see Notes 13 and 14).
5. Stop the activation and labelling reactions by diluting 15:1 in 1% formalin fixative and allow to fix for 15 min. After fixation, samples may be stored at 4°C for up to 24 h before analysis.
6. Identify platelets by light scatter and platelet-specific marker expression as described in Subheading 3.2 and Fig. 1 (see Note 15) and measure the fluorescence intensity or proportion of platelets expressing the platelet activation marker (see Fig. 2).

3.4 Measurement of Heterotypic Aggregates

Upon activation, platelet α-granules are released and P-selectin, a component of the granule membrane, becomes expressed on the platelet surface (73–76). Surface P-selectin mediates adhesion of activated platelets to leukocytes via P-selectin glycoprotein ligand

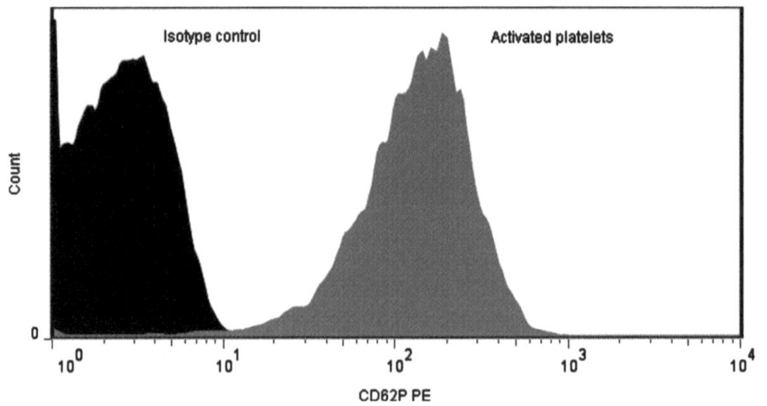

Fig. 2 Platelet activation is determined by fluorescence of a platelet activation-specific antibody (e.g., P-selectin) against an isotypic control

1 (PSGL1), which is constitutively expressed on the leukocyte surface (74).

Methodologically, it is much easier to detect one or more platelets adhered to a leukocyte than it is to identify P-selectin molecules on the surface of a platelet (12). Therefore, leukocyte–platelet aggregates, and monocyte–platelet aggregates in particular, are a more sensitive and earlier marker of platelet activation than P-selectin expression (5, 69, 77, 78).

1. Mix appropriately titrated concentrations of anti-CD14 and platelet-specific marker antibodies and agonist (see Note 16).
2. Add undiluted whole blood to the mix at a 1:3 ratio.
3. Incubate at room temperature for exactly 15 min (see Notes 13 and 14).
4. Stop the activation and labelling reactions by diluting 30:1 in FACSLyse and allow 10 min for red cell lysis to occur. After lysis, samples should be run on the same day.
5. Identify neutrophils and monocytes by characteristic light scatter and differential CD14 expression. Determine the proportion of leukocyte events which express platelet-specific markers. These are leukocytes–platelet heterotypic aggregates (Fig. 3) (see Note 17).

3.5 Measurement of Procoagulant Platelets and the Formation of the Prothrombinase Complex

Activation of platelets can lead to vesiculation of the platelet membrane, leading to a procoagulant phosphatidylserine expressing membrane which binds coagulation proteins (14, 16, 79). This plays an important role in the assembly of the tenase and prothrombinase components of the coagulation cascade in vivo. Expression of

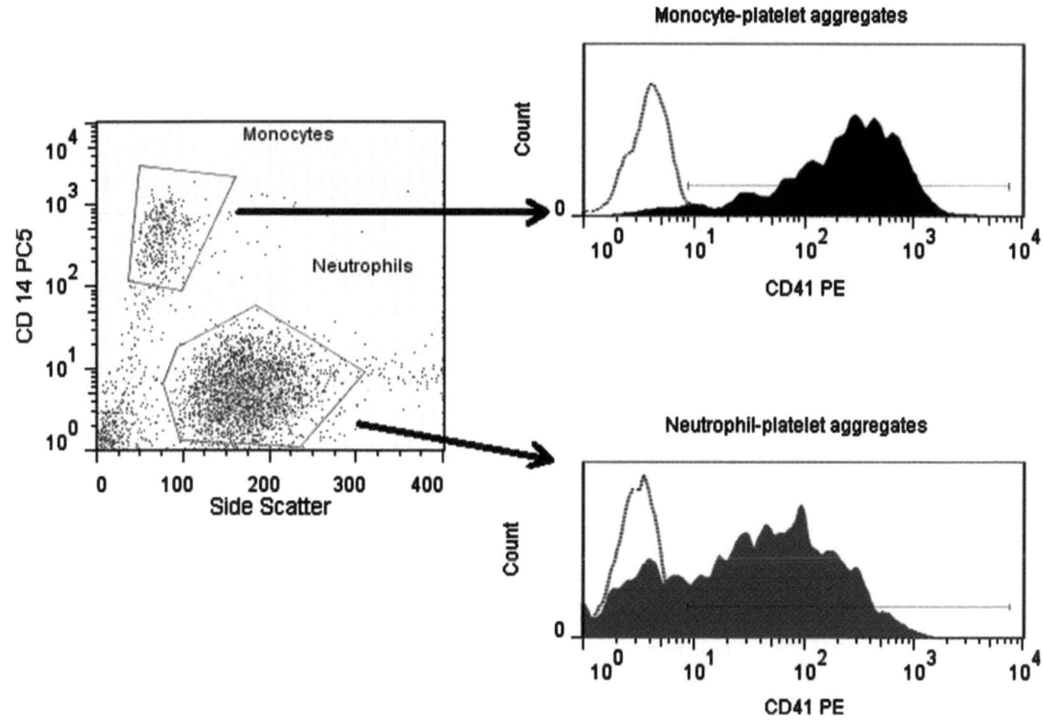

Fig. 3 Identification of heterotypic aggregates by flow cytometry. Monocytes and neutrophils are identified by characteristic light scatter and differential expression of CD14. Leukocytes with aggregated platelets are identified by expression of a platelet-specific marker (e.g., CD41)

phosphatidylserine on the membrane surface can be detected by flow cytometry with fluorescently labelled annexin V, and binding of activated coagulation factors can be detected by specific monoclonal antibodies (80, 81).

1. Dilute blood 1:10 in modified HT buffer containing 5 mM GPRP.
2. Sources of coagulation factors for platelet binding may either be from autologous plasma or addition of exogenous purified coagulation factors V/Va or X/Xa (see Note 18). These can be added directly to the HT/GPRP mix.
3. Add an appropriate concentration of platelet agonist in 6 mM $CaCl_2$ (see Note 19) at a 1:1 ratio with the buffered blood mix.
4. Incubate for exactly 20 min at 37°C.
5. Add the platelet identifier antibody at 1:3 ratio to the mix for a final concentration of 1 μg/mL and the fluorescently conjugated annexin V, anti-factor Va, and anti-factor Xa antibodies (see Note 20).

6. Incubate for exactly 20 min at room temperature.
7. Fix the samples by adding 20:1 volume of 1% formalin fixative.
8. Identify platelets by flow cytometry (see Note 21) and analyze for annexin V, factor V/Va, and X/Xa expression.

4 Notes

1. Sodium citrate, a weak calcium chelator, is the most common anticoagulant used for platelet studies. However, other weak calcium chelators such as corn trypsin inhibitor, or non-chelating anticoagulant such as hirudin or d-phenylalanyl-l-prolyl-l-arginine chloromethyl ketone (P-PACK) may also be employed (82). EDTA, a very strong calcium chelator, should be avoided because it prevents binding of natural ligands and dissociates the GPIIb–IIIa complex (83). Likewise heparin should be avoided because it binds to and activates platelets (54).
2. Note that the epitope must be constitutively expressed on platelets and different to the marker antibody for the platelet disorder that is being assayed (e.g., Bernard–Soulier platelets lack GPIb–IX–V complex, thus cannot be identified by flow cytometry using anti-CD42a, anti-42b, or anti-42d antibodies).
3. This is a monoclonal antibody specific for the epitope whose phenotype is altered in the specific disease state being assayed. Table 1 lists examples. This antibody must have a different fluorophore to the platelet-specific identifier in step 2.
4. Siliconized or pre-lubricated microfuge tubes minimize in vitro platelet activation during the incubation.
5. This must be conjugated to a different fluorophore than the platelet-specific identifier.
6. Alternatively a blocking agent that inhibits specific antibody binding to the epitope (e.g., eptifibatide will block PAC1 binding to activated GPIIb–IIIa).
7. Must be conjugated to a different fluorophore than the CD14 mAb.
8. The act of drawing blood itself is capable of causing platelet activation and thus affects expression of phenotype. Care must taken to minimize artificial platelet activation while drawing the sample. If drawing from a catheter, it must be completely flushed clear of heparin prior to drawing the sample.
9. The choice of platelet identifier is determined by the analysis being performed. For example, anti-CD42a or anti-CD42b are used as platelet identifiers when measuring expression of GPIIb–IIIa in the investigation of Glanzmann thrombasthenia.

Anti-CD41 or anti-CD61 may be used as platelet identifiers when investigating Bernard–Soulier syndrome.

10. Concentration of antibody should be determined by titration within the laboratory and will vary depending on the expression of the epitope, the fluorophore being used, the F:P ratio, and the flow cytometer model, age, and laser type. In general a concentration of between 0.5 and 1 μg/mL is sufficient for platelet identifiers, and a high concentration of platelet activation marker. An isotypic control should be prepared in parallel.
11. The concentration and type of agonist depend on the type of assay being performed. Submaximal concentrations of platelet agonists are often used to detect subtle variations in platelet reactivity via a specific activation pathway, or receptor function. For example if assessing the effectiveness of aspirin therapy, high concentration arachidonic acid (e.g., 250 μg/mL) may be used (84), while for assessing the effectiveness of clopidogrel or other P_2Y_{12} receptor antagonists, a more moderate dose ADP may be used (85–89). See Table 3 for some commonly used platelet agonists.
12. If thrombin is used as an agonist, 2.5 μM GPRP must be added to prevent fibrin polymerization and clot formation (90).
13. For certain agonists, such as arachidonic acid, the incubation temperature must be 37°C, while the majority of agonists give best results at room temperature. The incubation should never be performed cold.
14. The incubation time must be exactly measured using a stopwatch and be consistent between samples.
15. Surface expression of the common platelet-specific identifiers GPIIb–IIIa and GPIb–IX–V is modulated by platelet activation (6, 91). This must be considered when setting the threshold and gates.
16. Antibody concentrations should be titrated for individual laboratories. However, as a general guide, anti-CD14 FITC (Beckton Dickinson cat# 347493) should be between 0.5 and 1 μg/mL and a CD42a-PE (Pharmingen cat# 558819) should be 1–1.6 μg/mL. An appropriate isotypic control for the platelet identifier should be run in parallel.
17. Depending on the instrumentation and the characteristics of the flow cell, there is a possibility of coincidence of leukocyte and platelet passing through the flow cell at the same time, without being aggregated. This will cause a false-positive result, which may be observed as a high "background" level of heterotypic aggregates. This is particularly a problem with instruments with a wide aperture, such as the Cell Lab Quanta™ SC (Beckman Coulter).

18. Each laboratory must titrate the optimal concentration of autologous plasma or purified coagulation proteins for optimal platelet surface detection.
19. Ideal agonists to induce formation of procoagulant platelets or platelet-derived microparticles include collagen, collagen plus thrombin, C5b-9, or calcium ionophore A23187.
20. This can be done in the same tube if different fluorophores are used and appropriate fluorescent compensation parameters are set; otherwise each marker may be added to a separate mix.
21. The light scatter properties of platelets will change with vesiculation of the membrane and formation of a procoagulant surface. This must be accounted for when setting threshold and gating parameters to identify the platelets.

Acknowledgements

The author would like to thank Professor Alan D. Michelson, Asst. Prof. Andrew L. Frelinger III, and Marc R. Barnard from The Center for Platelet Research Studies at Children's Hospital Boston for their role in the development and optimization of many of these protocols.

References

1. Michelson AD, Linden MD, Barnard MR, Furman MI, Frelinger AL (2006) Flow Cytometry. In: Michelson AD (ed) Platelets. Academic Press, San Diego, CA, pp 545–565
2. Shapiro HM (2003) Practical flow cytometry. Wiley-Liss, New York
3. Linden MD, Frelinger AL III, Barnard MR, Przyklenk K, Furman MI, Michelson AD (2004) Application of flow cytometry to platelet disorders. Semin Thromb Hemost 30:501–511
4. Krueger LA, Barnard MR, Frelinger AL III, Furman MI, Michelson AD (2002) Immunophenotyping analysis of platelets. Curr Protoc Cytom 6:1–17
5. Linden MD, Furman MI (2005) Monocyte-platelet aggregates in patients with ischemic heart disease. In: Morrow DA, Cannon C (eds) Cardiovascular biomarkers: pathophysiology and disease management. Humana, Totowa, NJ, p 487–493
6. Michelson AD, Benoit SE, Kroll MH, Li JM, Rohrer MJ, Kestin AS, Barnard MR (1994) The activation-induced decrease in the platelet surface expression of the glycoprotein Ib-IX complex is reversible. Blood 83:3562–3573
7. Shattil SJ, Hoxie JA, Cunningham M, Brass LF (1985) Changes in the platelet membrane glycoprotein IIb.IIIa complex during platelet activation. J Biol Chem 260:11107–11114
8. Michelson AD, Furman MI (1999) Laboratory markers of platelet activation and their clinical significance. Curr Opin Hematol 6:342–348
9. Abrams C, Shattil SJ (1991) Immunological detection of activated platelets in clinical disorders. Thromb Haemost 65:467–473
10. Rajasekhar D, Barnard MR, Bednarek FJ, Michelson AD (1997) Platelet hyporeactivity in very low birth weight neonates. Thromb Haemost 77:1002–1007
11. Michelson AD, Barnard MR, Krueger LA, Valeri CR, Furman MI (2001) Circulating monocyte-platelet aggregates are a more sensitive marker of in vivo platelet activation than platelet surface P-selectin: studies in baboons, human coronary intervention, and human acute myocardial infarction. Circulation 104:1533–1537
12. Barnard MR, Krueger LA, Frelinger AL, Furman MI, Michelson AD (2003) Whole blood analysis of leukocyte-platelet aggregates. In: Robinson JP, Darzynkiewicz Z,

Dean PN, Hibbs AR, Orfao A, Rabinovitch PS, Wheeless LL (eds) Current protocols in cytometry, vol 1. Wiley, New York, pp 06.15.01–06.15.08

13. Barnard MR, Linden MD, Frelinger AL III, Li Y, Fox ML, Furman MI, Michelson AD (2005) Effects of platelet binding on whole blood flow cytometry assays of monocyte and neutrophil procoagulant activity. J Thromb Haemost 3:2563–2570
14. Furman MI, Krueger LA, Frelinger AL III, Barnard MR, Mascelli MA, Nakada MT, Michelson AD (2000) GPIIb-IIIa antagonist-induced reduction in platelet surface factor V/Va binding and phosphatidylserine expression in whole blood. Thromb Haemost 84:492–498
15. Serebruany VL, Kereiakes DJ, Dalesandro MR, Gurbel PA (1999) The flow cytometer model markedly affects measurement of ex vivo whole blood platelet-bound P-selectin expression in patients with chest pain: are we comparing apples with oranges. Thromb Res 96:51–56
16. Krueger LA, Barnard MR, Frelinger AL III, Furman MI, Michelson AD (2002) Immunophenotypic analysis of platelets. In: Robinson JP, Darzynkiewicz Z, Dean PN, Hibbs AR, Orfao A, Rabinovitch PS, Wheeless LL (eds) Current protocols in cytometry, vol 1. Wiley, New York, pp 06.10.01–06.10.17
17. Filip DJ, Aster RH (1978) Relative hemostatic effectiveness of platelets stored at 4° and 22°C. J Lab Clin Med 91:618–624
18. Nurden AT, Nurden P (2002) Inherited disorders of platelet function. In: Michelson AD (ed) Platelets. Academic, San Diego, CA, pp 681–700
19. Lopez JA, Andrews RK, Afshar-Kharghan V, Berndt MC (1998) Bernard-Soulier syndrome. Blood 91:4397–4418
20. Michelson AD (1987) Flow cytometric analysis of platelet surface glycoproteins: phenotypically distinct subpopulations of platelets in children with chronic myeloid leukemia. J Lab Clin Med 110:346–354
21. Jennings LK, Ashmun RA, Wang WC, Dockter ME (1986) Analysis of human platelet glycoproteins IIb-IIIa and Glanzmann's thrombasthenia in whole blood by flow cytometry. Blood 68:173–179
22. Rao AK, Gabbeta J (2000) Congenital disorders of platelet signal transduction. Arterioscler Thromb Vasc Biol 20:285–289
23. Reed GL (2002) Platelet secretion. In: Michelson AD (ed) Platelets. Academic, San Diego, CA, pp 181–195
24. Gordon N, Thom J, Cole C, Baker R (1995) Rapid detection of hereditary and acquired storage pool deficiency by flow cytometry. Br J Haematol 89:117–123
25. Wall JE, Buijs-Wilts M, Arnold JT, Wang W, White MM, Jennings LK, Jackson CW (1995) A flow cytometric assay using mepacrine for study of uptake and release of platelet dense granule contents. Br J Haematol 89:380–385
26. Gawaz MP, Bogner C, Gurland HJ (1993) Flow-cytometric analysis of mepacrine-labelled platelets in patients with end-stage renal failure. Haemostasis 23:284–292
27. Chong BH, Pitney WR, Castaldi PA (1982) Heparin-induced thrombocytopenia: association of thrombotic complications with heparin-dependent IgG antibody that induces thromboxane synthesis in platelet aggregation. Lancet 2:1246–1249
28. Chong BH (2002) Heparin-induced thrombocytopenia. In: Michelson AD (ed) Platelets. Academic, San Diego, CA, pp 571–591
29. Tomer A (1997) A sensitive and specific functional flow cytometric assay for the diagnosis of heparin-induced thrombocytopenia. Br J Haematol 98:648–656
30. Fabris F, Scandellari R, Randi ML, Carraro G, Luzzatto G, Girolami A (2002) Attempt to improve the diagnosis of immune thrombocytopenia by combined use of two different platelet autoantibodies assays (PAIgG and MACE). Haematologica 87:1046–1052
31. Lindahl TL, Fagerberg IH, Larsson A (2003) A new flow cytometric method for measurement of von Willebrand factor activity. Scand J Clin Lab Invest 63:217–223
32. Flores NA, Sheridan DJ (1994) The pathophysiological role of platelets during myocardial ischaemia. Cardiovasc Res 28:295–302
33. Fuster V, Badimon L, Badinon JJ, Chesebro JH (1992) The pathogenesis of coronary artery disease and acute coronary syndromes. N Engl J Med 326:310–318
34. deWood MA, Spores J, Notske R, Mouser LT, Burroughs R, Golden MS, Lang HT (1980) Prevalence of total coronary occlusion during the early hours of transmural myocardial infarction. N Engl J Med 315:897–902
35. Antithrombotic Trialist's Collaboration (2002) Collaborative meta-analysis of randomised trials of antiplatelet therapy for prevention of death, myocardial infarction, and stroke in high risk patients. Br Med J 324:71–86
36. Peripheral Arterial Diseases Antiplatelet Consensus Group (2003) Antiplatelet therapy

in peripheral arterial disease. Consensus statement. Eur J Vasc Endovasc Surg 26:1–16

37. Schultheiss HP, Tschoepe D, Esser J, Schwippert B, Roesen P, Nieuwenhuis HK, Schmidt-Soltau C, Strauer B (1994) Large platelets continue to circulate in an activated states after myocardial infarction. Eur J Clin Invest 24:243–247
38. Lee Y, Lee WH, Lee SC, Ahn KJ, Choi YH, Park SW, Seo JD, Park JE (1999) CD40L activation in circulating platelets in patients with acute coronary syndrome. Cardiology 92:11–16
39. Koyama H, Maeno T, Fukumoto S, Shoji T, Yamane T, Yokoyama H, Emoto M, Shoji T, Tahara H, Inaba M, Hino M, Shioi A, Miki T, Nishizawa Y (2003) Platelet P-selectin expression is associated with atherosclerotic wall thickness in carotid artery in humans. Circulation 105:524–529
40. Scharf RE, Tomer A, Marzec UM, Teirstein PS, Ruggeri ZM, Harker LA (1992) Activation of platelets in blood perfusing angioplasty-damaged coronary arteries. Flow cytometric detection. Arterioscler Thromb 12: 1475–1487
41. Linden MD, Furman MI, Frelinger AL III, Fox ML, Barnard MR, Li Y, Przyklenk K, Michelson AD (2007) Indices of platelet activation and the stability of coronary artery disease. J Thromb Haemost 5:761–765
42. Linden MD, Furman MI, Michelson AD, Fox ML, Barnard MR, Li Y, Barringhaus KG, Przyklenk K, Frelinger AL III (2004) Indices of platelet activation as markers of recent myocardial infarction. Circulation 110(Suppl III)
43. Frelinger AL III, Linden MD, Furman MI, Li Y, Fox ML, Barnard MR, Barringhaus KG, Przyklenk K, Michelson AD (2004) Aspirin resistance is associated with markers of platelet activation and is not accounted for by non-compliance or aspirin underdosing. Circulation 110(Suppl III):216
44. Frelinger AL III, Li Y, Linden MD, Barnard MR, Fox ML, Christie DJ, Furman MI, Michelson AD (2009) Association of cyclooxygenase-1-dependent and -independent platelet function assays with adverse clinical outcomes in aspirin-treated patients presenting for cardiac catheterization. Circulation 120:2586–2596
45. Nieuwland R, Sturk A (2002) Platelet-derived microparticles. In: Michelson AD (ed) Platelets. Academic, San Diego, CA, pp 255–265
46. Linden MD (2003) The hemostatic defect of cardiopulmonary bypass. J Thromb Thrombolysis 16:129–147
47. Zilla P, Fasol R, Groscurth P, Klepethkow A, Reichenspurner H, Wolner E (1989) Blood platelets in cardiopulmonary bypass operations. J Thorac Cardiovasc Surg 97:379–388
48. Smith BR, Rinder HM, Rinder CS (2002) Cardiopulmonary bypass. In: Michelson AD (ed) Platelets. Academic, San Diego, CA, pp 727–741
49. Michelson AD (1994). Manipulation of haemostasis during paediatric cardiopulmonary bypass. In: Jonas R, Elliott M (eds) Cardiopulmonary bypass in neonates, infants and young children. Butterworth-Heinemann, Oxford, pp 110–123
50. de Rossi L, Wessiepe M, Buhre W, Kuhlen R, Hutschenreuter G, Rossaint R (2003) Effect of propofol on adhesion of activated platelets to leukocytes in human whole blood. Intensive Care Med 29:1157–1163
51. Hu H, Hjemdahl P, Li N (2002) Effects of insulin on platelet and leukocyte activity in whole blood. Thromb Res 107:209–215
52. Keha D, Thieme A, Kurer I, Falke KJ, Gerlach H (2003) Inactivation of platelet glycoprotein IIb/IIIa receptor by nitric oxide donor 3-morpholino-sydnonimine. Blood Coagul Fibrinolysis 14:327–334
53. Kozek-Langenecker SA, Mohammad SF, Masaki T, Green W, Kamerath C, Cheung AK (2000) The effects of aprotinin on platelets in vitro using whole blood flow cytometry. Anesth Analg 90:12–16
54. Kozek-Langenecker SA, Mohammad SF, Masaki T, Kamerath C, Cheung AK (2000) The effects of heparin, protamine, and heparinase 1 on platelets in vitro using whole blood flow cytometry. Anesth Analg 90: 808–812
55. Heesch CM, Wilhelm CR, Ristich J, Adnane J, Bontempo FA, Wagner WR (2000) Cocaine activates platelets and increases the formation of circulating platelet containing microaggregates in humans. Heart 83:688–695
56. Horn NA, de Rossi L, Robitzsch T, Hecker KE, Hutschenreuter G, Rossaint R (2003) The effects of sevoflurane and desflurane in vitro on platelet-leukocyte adhesion in whole blood. Anaesthesia 58:312–319
57. Michelson AD, Benoit SE, Furman MI, Breckwoldt WL, Rohrer MJ, Barnard MR, Loscalzo J (1996) Effects of nitric oxide/EDRF on platelet surface glycoproteins. Am J Physiol 270:H1640–H1648
58. Michelson AD, Barnard MR, Khuri SF, Rohrer MJ, MacGregor H, Valeri CR (1999) The effects of aspirin and hypothermia on platelet function in vivo. Br J Haematol 104:64–68

59. Perneby C, Wallen NH, Hofman-Bang C, Tornvall P, Ivert T, Li N, Hjemdahl P (2007) Effect of clopidogrel treatment on stress-induced platelet activation and myocardial ischemia in aspirin-treated patients with stable coronary artery disease. Thromb Haemost 98:1316–1322
60. Egan BM, Papademetriou V, Wofford M, Calhoun D, Fernandes J, Riehle JE, Nesbitt S, Michelson E, Julius S (2005) Metabolic syndrome and insulin resistance in the TROPHY sub-study: contrasting views in patients with high-normal blood pressure. Am J Hypertens 18:3–12
61. Murphy KJ, Chronopoulos AK, Singh I, Francis MA, Moriarty H, Pike MJ, Turner AH, Mann NJ, Sinclair AJ (2003) Dietary flavanols and procyanidin oligomers from cocoa (Theobroma cacao) inhibit platelet function. Am J Clin Nutr 77:1466–1473
62. Michelson AD, MacGregor H, Barnard MR, Kestin AS, Rohrer MJ, Valeri CR (1994) Reversible inhibition of human platelet activation by hypothermia in vivo and in vitro. Thromb Haemost 71:633–640
63. Lekakis J, Triantafyllidi H, Galea V, Koutroumbi M, Theodoridis T, Komporozos C, Ikonomidis I, Christopoulou-Cokkinou V, Kremastinos DT (2008) The immediate effect of aerobic exercise on haemostatic parameters in patients with recently diagnosed mild to moderate essential hypertension. J Thromb Thrombolysis 25:179–184
64. Singh I, Turner AH, Sinclair AJ, Li D, Hawley JA (2007) Effects of gamma-tocopherol supplementation on thrombotic risk factors. Asia Pac J Clin Nutr 16:422–428
65. Singh I, Mok M, Christensen AM, Turner AH, Hawley JA (2008) The effects of polyphenols in olive leaves on platelet function. Nutr Metab Cardiovasc Dis 18:127–132
66. Singh I, Quinn H, Mok M, Southgate RJ, Turner AH, Li D, Sinclair AJ, Hawley JA (2006) The effect of exercise and training status on platelet activation: do cocoa polyphenols play a role? Platelets 17:361–367
67. Kestin AS, Ellis PA, Barnard MR, Errichetti A, Rosner BA, Michelson AD (1993) Effect of strenuous exercise on platelet activation state and reactivity. Circulation 88:1502–1511
68. Furman MI, Krueger LA, Linden MD, Barnard MR, Frelinger AL III, Michelson AD (2004) Release of soluble CD40L from platelets is regulated by glycoprotein IIb/IIIa and actin polymerization. J Am Coll Cardiol 43:2319–2325
69. Furman MI, Barnard MR, Krueger LA, Fox ML, Shilale EA, Lessard DM, Marchese PJ, Frelinger AL III, Goldberg R, Michelson AD (2001) Circulating monocyte-platelet aggregates are an early marker of acute myocardial infarction. J Am Coll Cardiol 38:1002–1006
70. Gurbel PA, Kereiakes DJ, Dalesandro MR, Bahr RD, O'Connor CM, Serebruany VL (2000) Role of soluble and platelet-bound P-selectin in discriminating cardiac from noncardiac chest pain at presentation in the emergency department. Am Heart J 139: 320–328
71. Langford EJ, Wainwright RJ, Martin JF (1996) Platelet activation in acute myocardial infarction and unstable angina is inhibited by nitric oxide donors. Arterioscler Thromb Vasc Biol 16:51–55
72. Wiviott SD, Trenk D, Frelinger AL, O'Donoghue M, Neumann FJ, Michelson AD, Angiolillo DJ, Hod H, Montalescot G, Miller DL, Jakubowski JA, Cairns R, Murphy SA, McCabe CH, Antman EM, Braunwald E (2007) Prasugrel compared with high loading- and maintenance-dose clopidogrel in patients with planned percutaneous coronary intervention: the Prasugrel in Comparison to Clopidogrel for Inhibition of Platelet Activation and Aggregation-Thrombolysis in Myocardial Infarction 44 trial. Circulation 116:2923–2932
73. McEver RP (1990) Properties of GMP-140, an inducible granule membrane protein of platelets and endothelium. Blood Cells 16:73–80
74. McEver RP (2006). P-Selectin/PSGL-1 and other interactions between platelets, leukocytes and endothelium. In: Michelson AD (ed) Platelets. Academic, San Diego, CA, p 231–250
75. Hsu-Lin SC, Berman CL, Furie BC, August D, Furie B (1984) A platelet membrane protein expressed during platelet activation and secretion: studies using a monoclonal antibody specific for thrombin-activated platelets. J Biol Chem 259:9121–9126
76. Stenberg PE, McEver RP, Shuman MA, Jacques YV, Bainton DF (1985) A platelet alpha-granule membrane protein (GMP-140) is expressed on the platelet membrane after activation. J Cell Biol 101:880–886
77. Furman MI, Benoit SE, Barnard MR, Valeri CR, Borbone ML, Becker RC, Hechtman HB, Michelson AD (1998) Increased platelet reactivity and circulating monocyte-platelet aggregates in patients with stable coronary artery disease. J Am Coll Cardiol 31: 352–358
78. Furman MI, Kereiakes DJ, Krueger LA, Mueller MN, Pieper K, Broderick TM, Schneider JF, Howard WL, Fox ML, Barnard

MR, Frelinger AL III, Michelson AD (2001) Leukocyte-platelet aggregation, platelet surface P-selectin, and platelet surface glycoprotein IIIa after percutaneous coronary intervention: effects of dalteparin or unfractionated heparin in combination with abciximab. Am Heart J 142:790–798

79. Michelson AD, Rajasekhar D, Bednarek FJ, Barnard MR (2000) Platelet and platelet-derived microparticle surface factor V/Va binding in whole blood: differences between neonates and adults. Thromb Haemost 84:689–694

80. Gilbert GE, Sims PJ, Wiedmer T, Furie B, Furie BC, Shattil SJ (1991) Platelet-derived microparticles express high affinity receptors for factor VIII. J Biol Chem 266:17261–17268

81. Holme PA, Brosstad F, Solum NO (1995) Platelet-derived microvesicles and activated platelets express factor Xa activity. Blood Coagul Fibrinolysis 6:302–310

82. Michelson AD (1996) Flow cytometry: a clinical test of platelet function. Blood 87:4925–4936

83. Ginsberg MH, Lightsey A, Kunicki TJ, Kaufmann A, Margurie G, Plow EF (1986) Divalent cation regulation of the surface orientation of platelet membrane glycoprotein IIb. J Clin Invest 78:1103–1111

84. Frelinger AL, Furman MI, Linden MD, Li Y, Fox ML, Barnard MR, Michelson AD (2006) Residual arachidonic acid induced platelet activation via an adenosine diphosphate dependent, but cyclooxygenase-1 and cyclooxygenase-2 independent pathway: a 700 patient study of aspirin resistance. Circulation 113:2888–2896

85. Frelinger AL III, Jakubowski JA, Li Y, Barnard MR, Fox ML, Linden MD, Sugidachi A, Winters KJ, Furman MI, Michelson AD (2007) The active metabolite of prasugrel inhibits ADP-stimulated thrombo-inflammatory markers of platelet activation: influence of other blood cells, calcium, and aspirin. Thromb Haemost 98:192–200

86. Frelinger AL, Jakubowski JJ, Li Y, Barnard MR, Linden MD, Tarnow I, Fox ML, Sugidichi A, Winters KJ, Furman MI, Michelson AD (2008) The active metabolite of prasugrel inhibits adenosine diphosphate- and collagen-stimulated platelet procoagulant activities. J Thromb Haemost 6:359–365

87. Harrison P, Frelinger AL III, Furman MI, Michelson AD (2007) Measuring antiplatelet drug effects in the laboratory. Thromb Res 120:323–336

88. Michelson AD, Linden MD, Furman MI, Li Y, Barnard MR, Fox ML, Lau WC, McLaughlin TJ, Frelinger AL (2007) Evidence that pre-existent variability in platelet response to ADP accounts for 'clopidogrel resistance'. J Thromb Haemost 5:75–81

89. Frelinger AL III, Michelson AD (2005) Clopidogrel linking evaluation of platelet response variability to mechanism of action. J Am Coll Cardiol 46:646–647

90. Michelson AD (1994) Platelet activation by thrombin can be directly measured in whole blood through the use of the peptide GPRP and flow cytometry: methods and clinical studies. Blood Coagul Fibrinolysis 5:121–131

91. Michelson AD, Ellis PA, Barnard MR, Matic GB, Viles AF, Kestin AS (1991) Downregulation of the platelet surface glycoprotein Ib-IX complex in whole blood stimulated by thrombin, ADP or an in vivo wound. Blood 77:770–779

92. Grau AJ, Ruf A, Vogt A, Lichy C, Buggle F, Patscheke H, Hacke W (1998) Increased fraction of circulating activated platelets in acute and previous cerebrovascular ischemia. Thromb Haemost 80:298–301

93. Cherian P, Hankey GJ, Eikelboom JW, Thom J, Baker RI, McQuillan A, Staton J, Yi Q (2003) Endothelial and platelet activation in acute ischemic stroke and its etiological subtypes. Stroke 34:2132–2137

94. Minamino T, Kitakaze M, Sanada S, Asanuama H, Kurotobi T, Koretsune Y, Fukunami M, Kuzuya T, Hoki N, Hori M (1998) Increased expression of P-selectin on platelets is a risk factor for silent cerebral infarction in patients with atrial fibrillation: role of nitric oxide. Circulation 98:1721–1727

95. Tschoepe D, Menart-Houtermans B (2002) Diabetes mellitus. In: Michelson AD (ed) Platelets. Academic, San Diego, CA, pp 435–445

96. Tschoepe D, Roesen P, Esser J, Schwippert B, Nieuwenhuis HK, Kehrel B, Gries FA (1991) Large platelets circulate in an active state in diabetes mellitus. Semin Thromb Hemost 17:433–438

97. Kawabata K, Nakai S, Miwa M, Sugiura T, Otsuka Y, Shinzato T, Hiki Y, Tomimatsu I, Ushida Y, Hosono F, Maeda K (2002) Platelet GPIIb/IIIa is activated and platelet-leukocyte coaggregates formed in vivo during hemodialysis. Nephron 90:391–400

98. Gawaz M, Neumann FJ, Ott I, May A, Schomig A (1996) Platelet activation and coronary stent implantation. Effect of antithrombotic therapy. Circulation 94:279–285

99. Tschoepe D, Schultheiss HP, Kolarov P, Schwippert B, Dannehl K, Nieuwenhuis HK,

Kehrel B, Strauer B, Gries FA (1993) Platelet membrane activation markers are predictive for increased risk of acute ischemic events after PTCA. Circulation 88:37–42

100. Mickelson JK, Lakkis NM, Villarreal-Levy G, Hughes BJ, Smith CW (1996) Leukocyte activation with platelet adhesion after coronary angioplasty: a mechanism for recurrent disease? J Am Coll Cardiol 28:345–353
101. Ault KA, Cannon CP, Mitchell JG, McCahan J, Tracy RP, Novotny WF, Reimann JD, Braunwald E (1999) Platelet activation in patients after an acute coronary syndrome results from the TIMI-12 trial. Thrombolysis in myocardial infarction. J Am Coll Cardiol 33:634–639
102. Frelinger AL III, Jakubowski JA, Li Y, Barnard MR, Linden MD, Tarnow I, Fox ML, Sugidachi A, Winters KJ, Furman MI, Michelson AD (2008) The active metabolite of prasugrel inhibits adenosine diphosphate- and collagen-stimulated platelet procoagulant activities. J Thromb Haemost 6:359–365
103. Neumann FJ, Gawaz M, Dickfeld T, Wehinger A, Walter H, Blasini R, Schomig A (1997) Antiplatelet effect of ticlopidine after coronary stenting. J Am Coll Cardiol 29:1515–1519
104. Zeiger F, Stephan S, Hoheisel G, Pfeiffer D, Ruehlmann C, Koksch M (2000) P-selectin expression, platelet aggregates, and platelet-derived microparticle formation are increased in peripheral arterial disease. Blood Coagul Fibrinolysis 11:723–728
105. Peyton BD, Rohrer MJ, Furman MI, Barnard MR, Rodino LJ, Benoit SE, Hechtman HB, Valeri CR, Michelson AD (1998) Patients with venous stasis ulceration have increased monocyte-platelet aggregation. J Vasc Surg 27:1109–1115
106. Powell CC, Rohrer MJ, Barnard MR, Peyton BD, Furman MI, Michelson AD (1999) Chronic venous insufficiency is associated with increased platelet and monocyte activation and aggregation. J Vasc Surg 30:844–851
107. Ando M, Iwata A, Ozeki Y, Tsuchiya K, Akiba T, Nihei H (2002) Circulating platelet-derived microparticles with procoagulant activity may be a potential cause of thrombosis in uremic patients. Kidney Int 62:1757–1763
108. O'Sullivan BP, Linden MD, Frelinger AL III, Barnard MR, Spencer-Manzon M, Morris JE, Salem RO, Laposata M, Michelson AD (2005) Platelet activation in cystic fibrosis. Blood 105:4635–4641
109. Tarnow I, Michelson AD, Frelinger AL III, Linden MD, Li Y, Fox ML, Barnard MR, O'Sullivan BP (2007) Cystic fibrosis heterozygotes do not have increased platelet activation. Thromb Res 121:159–162
110. Russworm S, Vickers J, Meier-Hellmann A, Spangenberg P, Bredle D, Reinhart K, Losche W (2002) Platelet and leukocyte activation correlate with the severity of septic organ dysfunction. Shock 17:263–268
111. Joop K, Berckmans RJ, Nieuwland R, Berkhout J, Romijn FP, Hack CE, Sturk A (2001) Microparticles from patients with multiple organ dysfunction syndrome and sepsis support coagulation through multiple mechanisms. Thromb Haemost 85:810–820
112. Sevush S, Jy W, Horstman LL, Mao WW, Kolodny L, Ahn YS (1998) Platelet activation in Alzheimer disease. Arch Neurol 55:530–536
113. Fateh-Moghadam S, Bocksch W, Ruf A, Dickfeld T, Schartl M, Pogatsa-Murray G, Hetzer R, Fleck E, Gawaz M (2000) Changes in surface expression of platelet membrane glycoproteins and progression of heart transplant vasculopathy. Circulation 102:890–897
114. Janes SL, Goodall AH (1994) Flow cytometric detection of circulating activated platelets and platelet hyper-responsiveness in pre-eclampsia and pregnancy. Clin Sci 86:731–739
115. Klein B, Farildi A, Amo-Takyi BK, Heilmann L, Von Templehoff GF, Rath W (2001) Neonatal platelet activation in preeclampsia. Clin Appl Thromb Hemost 7:29–32
116. Villmow T, Kemkes-Matthes B, Matzdorff AC (2002) Markers of platelet activation and platelet-leukocyte interaction in patients with myeloproliferative syndromes. Thromb Res 108:139–145
117. Klinkhardt U, Bauersachs R, Adams J, Graff J, Lindhoff-Last E, Harder S (2003) Clopidogrel but not aspirin reduced P-selectin expression and formation of platelet-leukocyte aggregates in patients with atherosclerotic vascular disease. Clin Pharmacol Ther 73:232–241
118. Storey RF, Judge HM, Wilcox RG, Heptinstall S (2002) Inhibition of ADP-induced P-selectin expression and platelet-leukocyte conjugate formation by clopidogrel and the P2Y 12 receptor antagonist AR-C69931MX but not aspirin. Thromb Haemost 88:488–494
119. Klinkhardt U, Graff J, Graff J (2002) Clopidogrel, but not abciximab, reduces platelet leukocyte conjugates and P-selectin expression in a human ex vivo in vitro model. Clin Pharmacol Ther 71:176–185

120. Gawaz M, Ruf A, Neumann FJ, Pogatsa-Murray G, Dickfeld T, Zohlnhofer D, Schomig A (1998) Effect of glycoprotein IIb-IIIa receptor antagonism on platelet membrane glycoproteins after coronary stent placement. Thromb Haemost 80:994–1001
121. Konstantopoulos K, Kamat SG, Schafer AI, Banez EI, Jordan R, Kleiman NS, Hellums JD (1995) Shear-induced platelet aggregation is inhibited by in vivo infusion of an anti-glycoprotein IIb/IIIa antibody fragment c7E3 Fab, in patients undergoing coronary angioplasty. Circulation 91:1427–1431
122. Quinn M, Deering A, Stewart M, Cox D, Foley B, Fitzgerald D (1999) Quantifying GPIIb/IIIa receptor binding using 2 monoclonal antibodies: discriminating abciximab and small molecular weight antigens. Circulation 99:2231–2238
123. Quinn MJ, Aronow HD, Califf RM, Bhatt DL, Sapp S, Kleiman NS, Harrington RA, Kong DF, Kandzari DE, Topol EJ (2004) Aspirin dose and six-month outcome after an acute coronary syndrome. J Am Coll Cardiol 43:972–978
124. Warkentin TE, Hayward CP, Boshkov LK, Santos AV, Sheppard JA, Bode AP, Kelton JG (1994) Sera from patients with heparin-induced thrombocytopenia generate platelet-derived microparticles with procoagulant activity: an explanation for the thrombotic complications of heparin-induced thrombocytopenia. Blood 84:3691–3699
125. Aster RH, Curtis BR, Bougie DW, Dunkley S, Greinacher A, Warkentin TE, Chong BH (2006) Thrombocytopenia associated with the use of GPIIb/IIIa inhibitors: position paper of the ISTH working group on thrombocytopenia and GPIIb/IIIa inhibitors. J Thromb Haemost 4:678–679
126. Curtis BR, Swyers J, Divgi A, McFarland JG, Aster RH (2002) Thrombocytopenia after second exposure to abciximab is caused by antibodies that recognize abciximab-coated platelets. Blood 99:2054–2059
127. Frelinger AL III, Lam SCT, Plow EF, Smith MA, Loftus JC, Ginsberg MH (1988) Occupancy of an adhesive glycoprotein receptor modulates expression of an antigenic site involved in cell adhesion. J Biol Chem 263:12397–12402
128. Ginsberg MH, Frelinger AL III, Lam SCT, Forsyth J, McMillan R, Plow EF, Shattil SJ (1990) Analysis of platelet aggregation disorders based on flow cytometric analysis of membrane glycoprotein IIb-IIIa with conformation-specific monoclonal antibodies. Blood 76:2017–2023
129. Frelinger AL III, Cohen I, Plow EF, Smith MA, Roberts J, Lam SCT, Ginsberg MH (1990) Selective inhibition of integrin function by antibodies specific for ligand-occupied receptor conformers. J Biol Chem 265: 6346–6352
130. Kouns WC, Kirchhofer D, Hadvary P, Edenhofer A, Weller T, Pfenninger G, Baumgartner HR, Jennings LK, Steiner B (1992) Reversible conformational changes induced in glycoprotein IIb-IIIa by a potent and selective peptidomimetic inhibitor. Blood 80:2539–2547
131. Zamarron C, Ginsberg MH, Plow EF (1990) Monoclonal antibodies specific for a conformationally altered state of fibrinogen. Thromb Haemost 64:41–46
132. Abrams CS, Ellison N, Budzynski AZ, Shattil SJ (1990) Direct detection of activated platelets and platelet-derived microparticles in humans. Blood 75:128–138
133. Gralnick HR, Williams SB, McKeown L, Shafer B, Connaghan GD, Hansmann K, Vail M, Magruder L (1992) Endogenous platelet fibrinogen: its modulation after surface expression is related to size-selective access to and conformational changes in the bound fibrinogen. Br J Haematol 80:347–357
134. Larsen E, Celi A, Gilbert GE, Furie BC, Erban JK, Bonfanti R, Wagner DD, Furie B (1989) PADGEM protein: a receptor that mediates the interaction of activated platelets with neutrophils and monocytes. Cell 59:305–312
135. Carmody MW, Ault KA, Mitchell JG, Rote NS, Ng AK (1990) Production of monoclonal antibodies specific for platelet activation antigens and their use in evaluating platelet function. Hybridoma 9:631–641
136. Nieuwenhuis HK, van Oosterhout JJ, Rozemuller E, van Iwaarden F, Sixma JJ (1987) Studies with a monoclonal antibody against activated platelets: evidence that a secreted 53,000-molecular weight lysosome-like granule protein is exposed on the surface of activated platelets in the circulation. Blood 70:838–845
137. Febbraio M, Silverstein RL (1990) Identification and characterization of LAMP-1 as an activation-dependent platelet surface glycoprotein. J Biol Chem 265:18531–18537
138. Silverstein RL, Febbraio M (1992) Identification of lysosome-associated membrane protein-2 as an activation-dependent platelet surface glycoprotein. Blood 80:1470–1475
139. Henn V, Slupsky JR, Grafe M, Anagnostopoulos I, Forster R, Muller-Bergaus G, Kroczek RA

(1998) CD40 ligand on activated platelets triggers an inflammatory reaction of endothelial cells. Nature 391:591–594
140. Chen M, Kakutani M, Naruko T, Ueda M, Narumiya S, Masaki T, Sawamura T (2001) Activation-dependent surface expression of LOX-1 in human platelets. Biochem Biophys Res Commun 282:153–158
141. Boukerche H, McGregor JL (1988) Characterization of an anti-thrombospondin monoclonal antibody (P8) that inhibits human blood platelet functions. Normal binding of P8 to thrombin-activated Glanzmann thrombasthenic platelets. Eur J Biochem 171:383–392
142. Aiken ML, Ginsberg MH, Plow EF (1987) Mechanisms for expression of thrombospondin on the platelet cell surface. Semin Thromb Hemost 13:307–316
143. Hayward CP, Smith JW, Horsewood P, Warkentin TE, Kelton JG (1991) p-155, a multimeric platelet protein that is expressed on activated platelets. J Biol Chem 266:7114–7120
144. Hayward CP, Bainton DF, Smith JW, Horsewood P, Stead RH, Podor TJ, Warkentin TE, Kelton JG (1993) Multimerin is found in the alpha-granules of resting platelets and is synthesized by a megakaryocytic cell line. J Clin Invest 91:2630–2639
145. Sims PJ, Faioni EM, Wiedmer T, Shattil SJ (1988) Complement proteins C5b-9 cause release of membrane vesicles from the platelet surface that are enriched in the membrane receptor for coagulation factor Va and express prothrombinase activity. J Biol Chem 263:18205–18212
146. Daniel JL, Dangelmaier C, Jin JG, Ashby B, Smith JB, Kunapuli SP (1998) Molecular basis for ADP-induced platelet activation I. Evidence for three distinct ADP receptors on human platelets. J Biol Chem 273:2024–2029
147. Jin JG, Daniel JL, Kunapuli SP (1998) Molecular basis for ADP-induced platelet activation II. The P2Y1 receptor mediates ADP-induced intracellular calcium mobilization and shape change in platelets. J Biol Chem 273:2030–2034
148. Leon C, Hechler C, Vial C, Leray C, Cazenave JP, Gachet C (1997) The $P2Y_1$ receptor is an ADP receptor antagonized by ATP and expressed in platelets and megakaryoblastic cells. FEBS Lett 403:26–30
149. Hollopeter G, Jantzen H-M, Vincent D, Li G, England L, Ramakrishnan V, Yang R-B, Nurden P, Nurden A, Julius D, Conley PB (2001) Identification of the platelet ADP receptor targeted by antithrombotic drugs. Nature 409:202–207
150. Zhang FL, Luo L, Gustafson E, Lachowicz J, Smith M, Qiao XD, Liu YH, Chen GD, Pramanik B, Laz TM, Palmer K, Bayne M, Monsma FJ Jr (2001) ADP is the cognate ligand for the orphan G protein-coupled receptor SP1999. J Biol Chem 276:8608–8615
151. Williams A, Woolkalis MJ, Poncz M, Manning DR, Gewirtz A, Brass LF (1990) Identification of the pertussis toxin-sensitive G proteins in platelets, megakaryocytes and HEL cells. Blood 76:721–730
152. Woulfe D, Yang J, Prevost N, O'Brien P, Brass LF (2002). Signal transduction during the initiation, extension and perpetuation of platelet plug formation. In: Michelson AD (ed) Platelets. Academic, San Diego, CA, p 197–213
153. Smith WL (1992) Prostanoid biosynthesis and the mechanism of action. Am J Physiol 263:F118–F191
154. Santoro SA, Walsh JJ, Staatz WD, Baranski KJ (1991) Distinct determinants on collagen support a_2b_1 integrin-mediated platelet adhesion and platelet activation. Cell Regul 2:905–913
155. Jung SM, Moroi M (2000) Signal-transducing mechanisms involved in activation of the platelet collagen receptor integrin a2b1. J Biol Chem 275:8016–8026
156. Clemetson KJ (2002) Platelet receptors. In: Michelson AD (ed) Platelets. Academic, San Diego, CA, pp 65–84
157. Lopez JA, Berndt MC (2002) The GPIb-IX-V complex. In: Michelson AD (ed) Platelets. Academic, San Diego, CA, pp 85–104
158. Hato T, Ginsberg MH, Shattil SJ (2002) Integrin alphaIIb-beta3. In: Michelson AD (ed) Platelets. Academic, San Diego, CA, pp 105–116
159. Kaywin P, McDonough M, Insel PA, Shattil SJ (1978) Platelet function in essential thrombocythemia: decreased epinephrine responsiveness associated with a deficiency in platelet alpha-adrenergic receptors. N Engl J Med 299:505–509
160. Motulsky HJ, Insel PA (1982) [^{3}H] Dihydroergocryptine binding to alpha-adrenergic receptors of human platelets. A reassessment using selective radioligands (^{3}H] prazosin, [^{3}H]yohimbine, and [^{3}H]rauwolscine. Biochem Pharmacol 31:2591–2597
161. Kobilka BK, Matsui H, Kobilka TS, Yang Feng TL, Francke U, Caron MG, Lefkowitz RJ, Regan JW (1987) Cloning, sequencing, and expression of the gene coding for the human platelet a_2-adrenergic receptor. Science 238:650–656

162. Vu TK, Hung DT, Wheaton VI, Coughlin SR (1991) Molecular cloning of a functional thrombin receptor reveals a novel proteolytic mechanism of receptor activation. Cell 64:1057–1068
163. Kahn ML, Zheng YW, Huang W, Bigornia V, Zeng D, Moff S, Farese RV Jr, Tam C, Coughlin SR (1998) A dual thrombin receptor system for platelet activation. Nature 394:690–694
164. Xu W-F, Anderson H, Whitmore TE, Presnell SR, Yee DP, Ching AC, Gilbert T, Davie EW, Foster DC (1998) Cloning and characterization of the human protease-activated receptor 4. Proc Natl Acad Sci U S A 95:6642–6646
165. Michelson AD, Benoit SE, Furman MI, Barnard MR, Nurden P, Nurden AT (1996) The platelet surface expression of glycoprotein V is regulated by two independent mechanisms: proteolysis and a reversible cytoskeletal-mediated redistribution to the surface-connected canalicular system. Blood 87:1396–1408
166. Hirata T, Ushikubi F, Kakizuka A, Okuma M, Narumiya S (1996) Two thromboxane A_2 receptor isoforms in human platelets—opposite coupling to adenylyl cyclase with different sensitivity to Arg^{60} to Leu mutation. J Clin Invest 97:949–956
167. Offermanns S, Laugwitz K-L, Spicher K, Schultz G (1994) G proteins of the G_{12} family are activated via thromboxane A_2 and thrombin receptors in human platelets. Proc Natl Acad Sci U S A 91:14325–14330

Part V

Examples of Specific Assays Related to Anticoagulant Activity

Chapter 19

Anti-factor Xa (Anti-Xa) Assay

Fiona Newall

Abstract

The anti-factor Xa (anti-Xa) assay is a functional assay that facilitates the measurement of antithrombin (AT)-catalyzed inhibition of factor Xa by unfractionated heparin (UFH) and direct inhibition of factor Xa by low-molecular-weight heparin (LMWH) (Kitchen, Br J Haematol 111:397–406, 2000; Walenga et al., Semin Thromb Hemost 11:17–25, 1985; Levine et al., Arch Intern Med 154:49–56, 1994; Barrowcliffe et al., J Pharm Biomed Anal 7:217–226, 1989; Triplett, Ther Drug Monit 1:173–197, 1979; Nelson, Clin Lab Sci 12:359–364, 1999; Laffan and Manning, Dacie and Lewis: practical haematology, Churchill Livingstone, London, pp 465–479, 2001; Olson et al., Arch Pathol Lab Med 122:782–798, 1998). Whilst automated methods for the determination of the abilities of UFH and LMWH to inhibit factor Xa have been available since the 1970s, their cost was viewed to prohibit their broad use in the clinical management of UFH and LMWH until relatively recently. The anti-Xa assay can also be used to guide the determination of therapeutic APTT ranges in the clinical management of UFH (Hirsh and Raschke, Chest 126:188S–203S, 2004). As a result, the anti-Xa assay is commonly viewed as a *heparin assay*, despite the fact that it actually provides a measure of UFH effect as opposed to a measure of UFH concentration.

Key words Anti-Xa assay, Chromogenic test, Heparin monitoring, LMWH monitoring

1 Introduction

The anti-factor Xa (anti-Xa) assay is performed by chromogenic assay. Whilst the anti-Xa assay is easy to perform and automated and experiences minimal interference from biological variables, it remains more expensive than the commonly used APTT and may not be available in smaller laboratories (1). Prior to performing an anti-Xa assay, each laboratory must create a standard curve for UFH and/or LMWH using a pool of normal plasma spiked with varying amounts of unfractionated heparin (UFH) and/or low-molecular-weight heparin (LMWH). To this plasma pool, known quantities of Xa are added, and after a period of incubation, the amount of residual Xa is measured (2).

Paul Monagle (ed.), *Haemostasis: Methods and Protocols*, Methods in Molecular Biology, vol. 992,
DOI 10.1007/978-1-62703-339-8_19,

UFH molecules are chemically or enzymatically altered to produce smaller fractions of lower molecular weight. The resultant LMWHs have greater specificity, producing increased anti-Xa activity relative to anti-IIa activity (4). Therefore, APTT measurement of LMWH activity is insensitive; activity must be measured using a direct anti-Xa assay.

1.1 Principle

The reagent contains an excess of activated factor X (Xa), which is inhibited by the presence of UFH or LMWH. The amount of heparinoid in the test plasma is inversely proportional to the amount of factor Xa, with any residual Xa available to cleave a chromogenic substrate, resulting in a color change which can be detected optically.

1.2 Standardization

Standardization of anti-Xa measurement is impacted by three factors:

1. The heparinoid.
2. The laboratory analyzer.
3. The anti-Xa reagent.

1.2.1 Heparinoid

Standard curves must be created for each brand of UFH and LMWH in clinical use at each center. Multiple concentrations of UFH or LMWH should be used to create institution-specific and brand-specific standard curves. These standard curves are used to calculate UFH or LMWH concentration in the patient plasma, with results reported as anti-Xa units/mL.

1.2.2 Laboratory Analyzer

Calibration curves generated for heparinoids should be produced using the automated coagulation analyzer employed for the clinical management of patients. There is significant literature available supporting the need to standardize coagulation testing based on the local laboratory analyzer and reagents (1, 5).

1.2.3 Anti-Xa Reagent

A lack of agreement between anti-Xa levels determined by different commercially available reagent has been reported in adult populations (6, 7). This finding was confirmed by in vitro and in vivo experiments conducted in pediatric populations (8, 9) (see Note 1). The preparation of reagents designed to measure anti-Xa activity can vary significantly, with some test kits having exogenous antithrombin and/or dermatan sulfate. The impact of these exogenous agents upon the clinical utility of anti-Xa levels generated is discussed further in Subheading 4. The variability in anti-Xa levels determined using different reagents further supports the need to standardize coagulation testing based on the local laboratory analyzer and reagents in use.

1.3 Clinical Applications

1.3.1 UFH

The anti-Xa assay is a measure of UFH's AT-catalyzed inhibition of Xa (1–3, 10–14). The clinical utility of the anti-Xa assay in monitoring UFH was largely realized due to the observation that a proportion of patients exposed to therapeutic doses of UFH failed to achieve expected prolongation of the APTT. Levine et al. report the outcomes of a study comparing the use of the anti-Xa assay compared to the APTT in a cohort of patients requiring large doses of UFH (3). They demonstrated that ongoing escalations of UFH doses could be avoided by the use of anti-Xa assays, when APTT results may indicate subtherapeutic levels of anticoagulation. Outcome measures such as incidence of major bleeding and recurrent thrombosis did not differ between patients managed by the APTT and those managed by the anti-Xa assay, although the study was likely underpowered to make recommendations regarding such risk-reduction associated with choice of monitoring assay.

For the monitoring of UFH, most advisory bodies recommend therapeutic APTTs be determined by correlating APTT results with therapeutic UFH levels as measured by anti-Xa assay (0.35–0.7 U/mL) or protamine titration (0.2–0.4 U/mL) (4).

1.3.2 LMWH

Recommendations for the management of LMWH therapy in adults state that routine laboratory monitoring is generally unnecessary (4). The predictability of weight-adjusted dosing of LMWH in infants and children appears to be reduced compared to adults, making laboratory monitoring of therapy in infants and children necessary (15).

1.4 Interpretation of Results

1.4.1 UFH

The anti-Xa level can be used as a primary measure of UFH effect, as well as a tool to validate APTT measurement of UFH therapy (see Note 1).

Therapeutic UFH therapy reflects an anti-Xa assay of between 0.35 and 0.7 U/mL. Dosage of UFH therapy should be titrated to achieve this target anti-Xa assay range. If routine anti-Xa assay measurement is not available, the APTT range that corresponds to an anti-Xa level of between 0.35 and 0.7 U/mL should be determined by the laboratory within every center responsible for the management of UFH therapy in children.

Ignjatovic et al. report in vitro and ex vivo data suggesting that UFH monitoring using the APTT titrated to an anti-Xa assay of 0.35–0.7 U/mL is associated with significant age-related variation (9, 16). This effect was especially apparent in younger children, suggesting that therapeutic APTT ranges of 78–200 s were associated with an anti-Xa assay of 0.35–0.7 U/mL from in vitro samples in children aged 1–5 years, and were often un-recordable in ex vivo samples. Chan et al. and Kuhle et al. both reported poor correlation between the APTT and anti-Xa assay in ex vivo pediatric samples (17, 18). Across a population of infants and children ranging from neonates to 18-year-old adolescents, agreement between the

APTT and anti-Xa assay was 0.09 and 0.22, respectively (17, 18). Chan reported that the level of agreement was further reduced when only infants less than 2 years of age were analyzed (17). The mechanism for the discrepancies between anti-Xa and APTT are yet to be determined, but may reflect the variable anti-IIa to anti-Xa effect of UFH reported by Newall et al. (19).

1.4.2 LMWH

Current guidelines for the management of LMWH therapy in infants and children recommend an anti-Xa level be measured 4–6 h following subcutaneous injection of the LMWH (15). Ongoing dosing of LMWH should be titrated to achieve an anti-Xa level of 0.5–1.0 U/mL.

2 Materials

2.1 Specimen

Whole blood.

2.1.1 Collection

NCCLS guidelines recommend collection into plastic or siliconized glass tubes containing 3.2 % trisodium citrate (e.g., 9 volumes of whole blood to 1 volume of 0.109 M trisodium citrate) (20). One of the most important aspects of sample collection for an anti-Xa assay involves filling the collection tubes to the correct point (indicated on the tube), as to achieve the adequate ratio of blood sample to anticoagulant (21).

In cases where the anti-Xa assay is used to monitor heparinoid therapy, tubes containing citric acid theophylline adenosine dipyridamole (CTAD) anticoagulant mixture can be used. This prevents heparin inactivation by the platelet factor 4 released from activated platelets present in whole blood (22).

Once the sample is collected, the tube must be mixed immediately by gentle inversion, to allow for the anticoagulant (usually at the bottom of the tube) to mix appropriately with the sample.

Routine venipuncture is the optimal collection procedure for the anti-Xa assay, as it minimizes sample activation.

An initial discard is recommended in those situations where blood is collected from a heparinized line. However, to date, there has been no agreement on standardization of the amount of discard for specific clinical situations. The risk of heparin contamination of the sample cannot be completely removed and it is preferable that this situation is avoided whenever possible, by using the peripheral vein.

2.1.2 Stability

Once collected, the whole blood sample is prone to activation and this can in turn lead to results that are not representative of the true status of the sample. This is particularly because of the presence of platelets which are easily activated and can then lead to activation of soluble coagulation factors.

The NCCLS guidelines for stability of whole blood samples prior to testing recommend storage at room temperature for 2 h and at 4 °C for 4 h (20).

Heparinized plasma samples remain stable for up to 2 h at room temperature; following 2 h of storage at room temperature, heparin can be neutralized by plasma proteins, such as platelet factor 4 (22).

2.1.3 Processing

Recommended centrifugation protocol for obtaining a platelet-free plasma sample adequate for coagulation testing includes minimum centrifugation at 2,500 × *g* for 15 min (20).

2.1.4 Storage

Once prepared, the plasma samples can be stored for up to 2 weeks at −20 °C and for up to 6 months at −70 °C (20). It is important that the plasma sample is separated into smaller aliquots prior to storage. This will allow the sample to freeze quickly and allows for adequate thawing prior to use.

Frozen plasma must be adequately thawed prior to testing (10–15 min in a 37 °C water bath) and it is recommended that the testing is performed immediately after thawing. However, in situations where this is not possible, the plasma sample can be stored for 2 h at 4 °C prior to use (20).

2.2 Reagents

For commercially available assays, instructions provided by the manufacturer for preparation of reagents and/or instrument should be followed, in order to ensure the validity of the results.

Most reagents used to carry out the anti-Xa assay are not toxic; however working with plasma samples of unknown origin carries a certain level of risk that should be minimized by the use of gloves and eye protection.

2.2.1 Substrate

The majority of chromogenic substrates provided within commercial anti-Xa kits are lyophilized, requiring reconstitution with distilled H_2O. Following reconstitution, the substrate solution should be allowed to rest, according to manufacturer's specifications. Stability of reconstituted substrate varies, ranging from 8 days to 4 months, depending upon storage conditions and manufacturer's recommendations.

2.2.2 Activated Factor X

Activated factor X reagents within commercially available kits are generally of bovine origin and can be either lyophilized or freeze-dried. Some kits provide a specific solvent to be used for reconstitution, and others recommend reconstitution with distilled H_2O. Stability of reconstituted activated factor X varies, ranging from 7 days to 4 months, depending upon storage conditions and manufacturer's recommendations.

2.2.3 Antithrombin

Some commercial anti-Xa kits contain exogenous antithrombin. Reconstitution of the lyophilized AT with distilled H_2O produces a reagent stable for between 14 days and 4 months, depending upon storage conditions and manufacturer's recommendations.

2.2.4 Calibration Curve

Prepare calibrators according to manufacturer's specification, using the specific heparin preparation requiring measurement. Stability of calibration reagents will vary between manufacturers.

2.2.5 Quality Control

It is essential to perform quality controls to ensure the accuracy and reproducibility of the results. Prepare control solutions appropriate to the heparinoid requiring measurement. Generally two levels of controls should be performed on freshly reconstituted reagents according to laboratory guidelines. If quality control results are not within the correct range, the test procedure should be repeated using freshly reconstituted reagents.

2.3 Chromogenic Measurement

Residual activated factor X in the test plasma will cleave the chromogenic substrate, releasing a colored compound detected optically at 405 nm. The sensitivity of commercial anti-Xa kits ranges from 0 to 1.5 IU/mL for UFH and 0 to 2.0 IU/mL for LMWH preparations.

3 Methods

3.1 Assay Procedure

The plasma sample collected from patients exposed to UFH or LMWH is incubated with the substrate. Following the incubation period, the activated factor X is added (± exogenous AT) causing hydrolysis of the substrate and inhibition of activated factor X by the heparin:antithrombin complex. Once these reactions are complete, the amount of residual activated factor X activity determined by colorimetric change is inversely proportional to the heparin/LMWH concentration.

3.1.1 Automated Assay

1. 200 μL of antithrombin is added to 25–100 μL test plasma.
2. Plasma is mixed with 100–200 μL of substrate and incubated for between 1 and 4 min, according to manufacturer's specification.
3. 100–200 μL of activated factor X is added to the sample/reagent mixture.
4. Chromogenic measurement of residual activated factor X activity is measured at 405 nm.

4 Results

Anti-Xa activity measurement should be specific to the heparinoid administered to the patient. Clinical laboratories will therefore need to establish calibration curves and quality control procedures for each heparin-based therapy used within their institution.

Quality control values should be determined for each reagent lot prior to commencing experiments with patient samples. If the control values are not within the manufacturer's specifications, all components of reagent reconstitution, quality control reconstitution, and assay conditions should be examined.

Reference ranges for the clinical management of LMWH (0.5–1.0 IU/mL) and UFH (0.35–0.7 IU/mL) differ. Ensure that comments made regarding target therapeutic range achievement based upon anti-Xa levels reflect the appropriate heparinoid therapy.

5 Note

1. In vivo studies of UFH therapy in pediatric patients conducted by Ignjatovic et al. (9) demonstrated a lack of correlation between two anti-Xa assays: one assay did not have exogenous antithrombin, but did have added dextran sulfate (COAMATIC® Anti-Xa) whilst the other assay contained exogenous antithrombin (COATEST® Anti-Xa) (8, 9, 23). The added dextran sulfate in the COAMATIC® Anti-Xa kit causes any heparin in the test plasma that is bound to proteins to be released. Some of this protein-bound heparin may not have been free to catalyze AT without the influence of dextran sulfate. As a result, this assay may overestimate the heparin activity in test plasma. Exogenous AT was added to the COATEST® Anti-Xa kit in order to ensure that the heparin present in test plasma has sufficient AT to catalyze. However, for a patient deficient in AT (i.e., most pediatric patients) this exogenous AT may contribute to the non-physiological measurement of anti-Xa activity. Further investigation is required before recommendations can be made regarding which kit is likely to be most appropriate for pediatric use.

In vivo analysis of UFH therapy in pediatric patient plasma samples also suggests that the ratio between UFH inhibition of thrombin (IIa) and Xa varies with age, with infants and younger children having significantly greater anti-Xa activity than older children and adults for a given dose of UFH (19). This finding raises significant implications regarding the choice of an optimal method for monitoring UFH therapy in the pediatric population.

References

1. Olson J, Arkin C, Brandt J, Cunningham M, Giles A, Koepke J, Witte D (1998) College of American Pathologists conference XXXI on laboratory monitoring of anticoagulant therapy: laboratory monitoring of unfractionated heparin therapy. Arch Pathol Lab Med 122:782–798
2. Laffan M, Manning R (2001) Laboratory control of anticoagulant, thrombolytic and antiplatelet therapy (Chapter 18). In: Lewis S, Bain B, Bates I (eds) Dacie and Lewis: practical haematology, 9th edn. Churchill Livingstone, London, pp 465–479
3. Levine M, Hirsh J, Gent M, Turpie A, Cruisckshank M, Weitz J, Anderson D, Johnson M (1994) A randomized trial comparing activated thromboplastin time with heparin assay in patients with acute venous thromboembolism requiring large daily doses of heparin. Arch Intern Med 154:49–56
4. Hirsh J, Raschke R (2004) Heparin and low-molecular-weight heparin. Chest 126: 188S–203S
5. Monagle P, Barnes C, Ignjatovic V, Furmedge J, Newall F, Chan A, DeRosa L, Hamilton S, Ragg P, Robinson S, Auldist A, Crock C, Rowlands S (2006) Developmental haemostasis: Impact for clinical haemostasis laboratories. Thromb Haemost 95:362–372
6. Kovacs M, Keeney M, MacKinnon K, Boyle E (1999) Three different chromogenic methods do not give equivalent anti-Xa levels for patients on therapeutic low molecular weight heparin (dalteparin) or unfractionated heparin. Clin Lab Haematol 21:55–60
7. Kitchen S, Theaker J, Preston F (2000) Monitoring unfractionated heparin therapy: relationship between eight anti-Xa assays and a protamine titration assay. Blood Coagul Fibrinolysis 11:137–144
8. Ignjatovic V, Summerhayes R, Gan A, Than J, Chan A, Cochrane A, Bennet M, Shann F, Lane G, Ross-Smith M, Monagle P (2007) Monitoring unfractionated heparin (UFH) therapy: which anti factor Xa assay is appropriate? Thromb Res 120:347–351
9. Ignjatovic V, Summerhayes R, Than J, Gan A, Monagle P (2006) Therapeutic range for unfractionated heparin therapy: age-related differences in response in children. J Thromb Haemost 4:2280–2282
10. Kitchen S (2000) Problems in laboratory monitoring of heparin dosage. Br J Haematol 111:397–406
11. Walenga J, Fareed J, Hoppensteadt D (1985) In vitro coagulant and amidolytic methods for evaluating the activity of heparin and a low molecular weight heparin. Semin Thromb Hemost 11:17–25
12. Barrowcliffe T, Mulloy B, Johnson E, Thomas D (1989) The anticoagulant activity of heparin: measurement and relationship to chemical structure. J Pharm Biomed Anal 7:217–226
13. Triplett D (1979) Heparin: biochemistry, therapy, and laboratory monitoring. Ther Drug Monit 1:173–197
14. Nelson D (1999) Current considerations in the use of the APTT in monitoring unfractionated heparin. Clin Lab Sci 12:359–364
15. Monagle P, Chan A, Massicotte P, Chalmers E, Michelson A (2004) Antithrombotic therapy in children. Chest 126:645S–687S
16. Ignjatovic V, Furmedge J, Newall F, Chan A, Berry L, Fong C, Cheng K, Monagle P (2006) Age-related differences in heparin response. Thromb Res 118:741–745
17. Chan A, Black L, Ing C, Brandao L, Williams S (2007) Utility of aPTT in monitoring unfractionated heparin in children. Thromb Res 122:135–136
18. Kuhle S, Eulmesekian P, Kavanagh B, Massicotte P, Vegh P, Lau A, Mitchell L (2007) Lack of correlation between heparin dose and standard clinical monitoring tests in treatment with unfractionated heparin in critically ill children. Haematologica 92:554–557
19. Newall F, Ignjatovic V, Johnston L, Summerhayes R, Lane G, Cranswick N, Monagle P (2010) Age is a determinant factor for measures of concentration and effect in children requiring unfractionated heparin. Thromb Haemost 103:1085–1090
20. Standards N (ed) (1998) Collection, transport and processing of blood specimens for coagulation testing and general performance of coagulation assays. NCCLS, Wayne, PA
21. Reneke J, Etzell J, Leslie S (1998) Prolonged prothrombin time and activated partial thromboplastin time due to underfilled specimen tubes with 109 mmol/L (3.2 %) citrate anticoagulant. Am J Clin Pathol 109:754–757
22. Rose VL, Dermott SC, Murray BF, McIver MM, High KA (1993) Decentralized testing for PT and activated PTT using a dry chemistry portable analyzer. Arch Pathol Lab Med 117:611–617
23. Ignjatovic V, Summerhayes R, Gan A, Than J, Chan A, Cochrane A, Bennet M, Shann F, Lane G, Ross-Smith M, Monagle P (2006) Monitoring unfractionated heparin (UFH) therapy: which anti factor Xa assay is appropriate? J Thromb Haemost 120:347–351

Chapter 20

Reptilase Time (RT)

Hratsch Karapetian

Abstract

The reptilase time is a functional plasma clotting assay, which is based on the enzymatic activity of batroxobin. By specifically cleaving fibrinogen A from fibrinogen, batroxobin leads to the formation of a stable fibrin clot. The time, starting from the addition of batroxobin to the plasma sample, until clot formation is the reptilase time and is given in seconds. Clot formation can be detected manually or on automated coagulation systems. Reference values for healthy adults are 18–22 s. Healthy newborns may have a slightly prolonged reptilase time of up to 24 s.

In addition to other coagulation assays, the reptilase time is usually performed to confirm or to exclude the suspicion of dysfibrinogenemias. The reptilase time is independent of thrombin generation disturbances or disturbances in the action of thrombin on fibrinogen. Therefore, it can be used to confirm heparin contamination or to obtain similar information as with the thrombin clotting time in heparinized and hemophiliac patients.

Key words Batroxobin, Coagulation assay, Dysfibrinogenemia, Fibrin, Fibrinogen, Reptilase, Snake venom, Thrombin

1 Introduction

The reptilase time is a venom-based, plasma clotting assay using batroxobin, the thrombin-like proteolytic enzyme isolated from the venom of the South American pit viper *Bothrops atrox*. Unlike thrombin, which cleaves fibrinopeptides A and B from fibrinogen, batroxobin splits specifically fibrinopeptide A, converting fibrinogen into fibrin monomers (1). The resulting fibrin monomers polymerize spontaneously and lead to the formation of a stable fibrin clot.

The reptilase time (RT) is primarily affected by any abnormality in the fibrinogen–fibrin conversion as is the case with quantitative and qualitative fibrinogen abnormalities, the presence of fibrin/ogen degradation products (FDP) or other proteins disturbing fibrin aggregation (2–4). The clotting time obtained by RT is independent of thrombin generation disturbances and disturbances of thrombin–fibrinogen interaction and is not affected

Paul Monagle (ed.), *Haemostasis: Methods and Protocols*, Methods in Molecular Biology, vol. 992,
DOI 10.1007/978-1-62703-339-8_20, © Springer Science+Business Media New York 2013

by anticoagulants such as heparin and hirudin (2). Therefore, the RT can be used in heparinized patients and hemophiliacs to obtain similar information as with the thrombin clotting time (TCT).

1.1 Principle of the Test

The RT is based on the same principle as is the TCT and can be performed both manually and on semi/fully automated coagulation systems. A standardized amount of batroxobin leads to the formation of a stable fibrin clot. The time, starting from the addition of batroxobin to the plasma sample, until clot formation is the reptilase time and is given in seconds. Basically, clot formation can be detected manually or by electromechanical or spectrophotometrical systems. However there are differences in results obtained from different clot detection systems (see Note 1).

1.2 Clinical Applications

The reptilase time is usually performed in conjunction with, or in addition to, other coagulation assays. The main clinical application of the RT is the evaluation of patients with abnormal routine coagulation results of unknown origin. Depending on the results obtained from the RT it can be used to confirm or to exclude the suspicion of dysfibrinogenemias.

Due to its insensitivity to thrombin inhibitors the RT can be used to exclude heparin contamination, or to assess fibrin polymerization in the presence of heparin.

2 Materials

2.1 Specimen

Blood samples can be collected into plastic or siliconized glass tubes (5) containing 0.109 mol/l buffered sodium citrate solution (3.2 %) as anticoagulant in the proportion of 9 volumes of blood to 1 volume of anticoagulant solution. It is essential to maintain the adequate proportion of blood to sodium citrate as samples from both underfilled tubes and overfilled tubes lead to incorrect results. Immediately ensure that blood samples are properly mixed with the anticoagulant, by gentle inversion of each tube three to four times. Platelet-poor plasma is separated from the blood cells by centrifuging the specimen at a minimum of 2,500 × *g* for 15 min. In the case testing of plasma samples cannot be performed immediately after sample collection, plasma samples may be stored in small aliquots at 2–4 °C for up to 4 h, at −20 °C for up to 2 weeks, and for samples rapidly frozen at −70 °C for up to 6 months after blood collection (5).

2.2 Reptilase Reagent

The reptilase reagent is usually provided in a lyophilized condition and has to be dissolved, prior to its application, with deionized water. Depending on different manufacturers the lyophilisate is to dissolve to a different volume, but to a concentration of 2 batroxobin units (BU) in a 0.1 ml solution. The enzymatic activity of 1 batroxobin unit corresponds to the activity of approximately 0.17 NIH thrombin, with 2 BU achieving coagulation in 19 s in a 0.3 ml standard human plasma (see Note 2).

Unopened, lyophilized reagents are stable and may be used up to the expiry date provided by the manufacturer. Lyophilized reagents are recommended to be stored at +2 to +8 °C. After reconstitution the stability of the reagent remains for at least 8 h at 37 °C, for 5 days at 2–8 °C, or for 8 weeks at −20 °C.

3 Methods

3.1 Manual Procedure

1. Siliconized glass or plastic test tubes and reconstituted reptilase reagent have to be prewarmed to 37 °C for at least 5 min before use.
2. Incubate 0.3 ml of undiluted plasma sample into a test tube at 37 °C for 2 min.
3. Pipette 0.1 ml reconstituted reptilase reagent into the plasma sample and start immediately the stopwatch.
4. The time until formation of a stable fibrin clot is the reptilase time and is detected with a platinum hook.

3.2 Interpretation of the Results

As mentioned before, the reptilase time is affected by fibrinogen–fibrin conversion disturbances of any origin and does not indicate a specific state or a specific disorder. Therefore a careful evaluation of clinical symptoms in combination with other laboratory results is necessary for the interpretation of the RT.

3.2.1 Reference Range

Samples from healthy adults produce clotting times of 18–22 s. Healthy newborns (1–5 days) have a slightly prolonged RT of up to 24 s compared to adults (8). RT performed on automated coagulometers usually produces marginally shorter results than manually performed RT results. A prolongation of more than 3 s above the upper limit of the reference range is considered to be significantly increased and needs further evaluation. In contrast a shortening of the reptilase time is rare and, when encountered, indicates methodological errors in the accomplishment of the reptilase time (see Note 3).

3.2.2 Normal Values

Values within reference range do not exclude hyperfibrinolytic states with FDP concentration <5 μg/ml.

- In combination with increased TCT a normal RT indicates the presence of or a contamination with heparin or other thrombin inhibitors.

3.2.3 Prolongation

- A prolongation of the RT indicates the presence of structural abnormalities of fibrinogen as is the case in acquired and inherited dysfibrinogenemias.
- A reptilase time higher than 25 s in association with increased thrombin clotting time is suggestive of increased concentrations of FDP or the presence of any other proteins interfering in the fibrinogen–fibrin conversion (6).
- Both decreased and increased fibrinogen concentrations can prolong the RT (7).

4 Notes

Common sources of error in the accomplishment of RT are the following:

1. *Clot detection*. Depending on the clot detection system used there are differences between results reported from RT measured by the hook manual method, the spectrophotometrical method, or the electromechanical method. There is discordance between RT values measured by the hook manual method and the optical method in patients with high fibrinogen levels (8). Similarly, there are discrepancies between optical and electromechanical clot detection systems (9).
2. *Reagent activity*. The application of RT is based on specific enzymatic properties by the proteinase batroxobin. Previously it has been reported of inadequately purified batroxobin preparations which are offered for the application of the RT. However, inadequately purified batroxobin reagents contain various components interfering with the haemostatic system other than properly purified batroxobin reagents. Thus, using of inadequately purified reagents leads to incorrect results (7).

   Other sources disturbing reagent activity are incorrect storage, incomplete reconstitution of lyophilized reagents, or contamination with other substances.
3. Ratio of reagent to plasma. Values for RT are highly dependent on the ratio of batroxobin to plasma. Therefore, keeping the same, recommended concentration of reagent to plasma is absolutely essential.

References

1. Aronson DL (1976) Comparison of the actions of thrombin and the thrombin-like venom enzymes ancrod and batroxobin. Thromb Haemost 36(1):9–13
2. Funk C, Gmur J, Herold R, Straub PW (1971) Reptilase-R—a new reagent in blood coagulation. Br J Haematol 21(1):43–52
3. Barr RD, Ouna N, Simpson JG, Bagshawe AF (1976) Dysfibrinogenaemia and primary hepatocellular carcinoma. Q J Med 45(180):647–659
4. Wenzel E, Holzhuter H, Muschietti F, Angelkort B, Ochs HG, Pusztai-Markos S, Nowak H, Sturner H (1974) (Reliability of tests for fibrinogen (fibrin) degradation prod-

ucts in plasma with thrombin coagulase, reptilase and thrombin clotting time (author's transl)). Dtsch Med Wochenschr 99(15): 746–756
5. NCCLS (1982) Tentative guidelines for the standardized, collection, transport, and preparation of blood specimens for coagulation testing and performance of coagulation assays, vol 2, no 4. NCCLS Publication, Villanova, PA, p 103–128
6. Van Cott EM, Smith EY, Galanakis DK (2002) Elevated fibrinogen in an acute phase reaction prolongs the reptilase time but typically not the thrombin time. Am J Clin Pathol 118(2):263–268
7. Stocker K (1983) Reptilase-test. Thromb Res 31(5):765–766
8. Capel P, Roose A, Vanderpas JB (1989) Discordance between reptilase time measured by the hook manual method and the optical method in patients with high fibrinogen level. Thromb Haemost 62(4):1143
9. Lefkowitz JB, DeBoom T, Weller A, Clarke S, Lavrinets D (2000) Fibrinogen longmont: a dysfibrinogenemia that causes prolonged clot-based test results only when using an optical detection method. Am J Hematol 63(3): 149–155

Chapter 21

Protamine Titration

Fiona Newall

Abstract

Protamine titration is the gold standard method for the measurement of unfractionated heparin (UFH) concentration in plasma. Protamine titration produces reliable and reproducible results; however it is generally not considered a convenient assay for current clinical management of UFH as it is not readily automated (Olson et al. Arch Pathol Lab Med 122(9):782–798, 1998). Early clinical trials of UFH therapy determined that a heparin concentration of 0.2–0.4 U/ml by protamine titration correlated to an APTT of 1.5–2.5 times higher compared to baseline values produced desirable UFH safety and efficacy outcomes (Hull et al. N Engl J Med 315(18):1109–1114, 1986; Hull et al. N Engl J Med 322:1260–1264, 1990; Turpie et al. N Engl J Med 320:352–357, 1989; Brill-Edwards et al. Ann Intern Med 119(2):104–109, 1993; Hull Int Angiol 14(1):32–34, 1995). Such studies paved the way to the current view that it is no longer ideal to manage UFH based solely upon a 1.5–2.5 times prolongation of the "normal" APTT. Most advisory bodies recommend therapeutic APTTs be determined by correlating APTT results with therapeutic UFH levels as measured by anti-Xa assay (0.35–0.7 U/ml) or protamine titration (0.2–0.4 U/ml) (Hirsh and Raschke. Chest 126(3):188S-203S, 2004) (see Note 1).

The concentration of UFH in a sample is measured by determining the amount of protamine required to return the thrombin clotting time (TCT) test (prolonged by UFH) to a pre-UFH level (Laffan and Manning. Dacie and Lewis: practical haematology. Churchill Livingstone: London, 2001).

Key words Protamine titration, Heparin concentration, Thrombin clotting time

1 Introduction

In 1937, Chargaff and Olson discovered that protamine effectively reversed the anticoagulant properties of UFH. This discovery led to the use of protamine to titrate UFH concentrations in vitro and to neutralize UFH activity in vivo (9). The mechanism of UFH reversal by protamine is based on the electrostatic binding between the highly positively charged protamine molecule and the negatively charged UFH (10). In 1954, Refn and Vestergaard reported a method for protamine titration to determine UFH concentration, which is still used today (11).

Paul Monagle (ed.), *Haemostasis: Methods and Protocols*, Methods in Molecular Biology, vol. 992,
DOI 10.1007/978-1-62703-339-8_21,

1.1 Principle

The Thrombin Clotting Time (TCT) measures the time to clot formation following the addition of thrombin to plasma. The presence of UFH in plasma produces a dose-dependent prolongation of the TCT (8, 12). Protamine competitively binds to UFH and the protamine titration assay result represents the amount of protamine required to return the TCT to baseline.

1.2 Standardization

Protamine titration method is not expensive or technically difficult; however as it is a manual method, it is labor intensive. Efforts to standardize performance of protamine titration are limited by two key factors:

(a) Operator-dependent variability.

(b) Variability in the source/origin of thrombin.

1.2.1 Operator-Dependent Variability

Protamine titration measurement is dependent upon the operator's identification of clot formation in a test tube. As such, efforts to standardize the assay endpoint are limited. Nonetheless, reproducibility of results can be achieved by limiting the number of operators performing this assay in the laboratory and developing a clear understanding between operators of what constitutes clot formation, and therefore the test endpoint.

1.2.2 Variability in Thrombin Origin

Early published methods of protamine titration specified the use of a predetermined concentration of bovine or rabbit thrombin. This concentration was determined by identifying the amount of thrombin that produced TCT between 18 and 20 s (13). The current availability of human thrombin allows for protamine titration to be performed with improved reliability. This reflects the greater specificity between human thrombin and test plasma; human thrombin is likely to interact differently with human test plasma compared to bovine or rabbit thrombin. The use of human thrombin requires determination of the concentration of thrombin required to achieve a baseline TCT of 18–20 s. Each laboratory should determine a laboratory-specific thrombin concentration using human thrombin available to their center.

1.3 Clinical Applications

Optimal UFH therapy is achieved within a concentration of 0.2–0.4 IU/ml of UFH according to protamine titration (2–6, 8, 14). The current recommendations for UFH therapy from the American College of Chest Physicians (ACCP) suggest target APTT ranges for UFH therapy reflect heparin concentrations of 0.2–0.4 IU/ml by protamine titration or 0.35–0.7 IU/ml by an anti-Xa assay (7).

The original method for protamine titration of Refn and Vestergaard (1954) required the use of large volumes of whole blood, making this method infeasible in the pediatric setting. One method for performing protamine titration in a small volume of plasma has been previously reported (Johnston M, cited in (13)).

This micro-manual method is technically challenging due to the very small volume of protamine solution used in the method (1 μl) and specified the use of bovine thrombin.

Recently, a refined method of protamine titration using human thrombin and a small volume of plasma was established and validated (15). This method demonstrates that protamine titration can be reliably and reproducibly performed using 100 μl of plasma compared with the 500 μl volume originally described by Refn and Vestergaard (11). Given recent studies which have reported difficulties in standardizing anti-Xa assays and shown poor correlation between the anti-Xa and the APTT in children (16–19), this may be of significant clinical importance to pediatric clinical laboratories enabling them to validate their therapeutic ranges for UFH therapy against the gold standard method of protamine titration. This would necessitate determining APTT and anti-factor Xa assay results that correlate with a UFH concentration of 0.2–0.4 IU/ml. This process should be undertaken by each clinical laboratory due to the variability in reagent and analyzer systems available for use by laboratories.

1.4 Interpretation of Results

Results of protamine titration assays reflect the concentration of UFH in a plasma sample. The measurement of concentration is potentially influenced by the origin of thrombin used and inter-operator variability in human detection of the clot-based endpoint for this method (see Subheading 1.2). Limiting the number of operators performing the validation process correlating protamine titration to APTT and anti-factor Xa assays will minimize the influence of this potential variability.

Once the correlation data for protamine titration and APTT and protamine titration and anti-factor Xa assays is available, the latter measures of UFH effect can be used more reliably for monitoring UFH therapy in children.

2 Materials

2.1 Specimen

Whole blood.

2.1.1 Collection

Whole blood is collected by clean venipuncture into plastic or siliconized glass tubes containing 3.2% trisodium citrate (e.g., 9 volumes of blood to 1 volume of 0.109 M trisodium citrate).

Once the sample is collected, the tube must be mixed immediately by gentle inversion, to allow for the anticoagulant (usually at the bottom of the tube) to mix appropriately with the sample.

It is not recommended to collect whole blood for performing protamine titration from heparinized lines, even if a discard is taken beforehand. The risk of heparin contamination of the sample cannot be completely discounted and it is therefore preferable to use a peripheral vein.

2.1.2 Stability

The NCCLS guidelines for stability of whole blood samples prior to testing recommend storage at room temperature for 2 h and at 4°C for 4 h.

Non-heparinized plasma samples remain stable for up to 4 h at room temperature, while heparinized samples are stable at the same conditions for up to 2 h. This is due to the fact that heparin can be neutralized by plasma proteins, such as platelet factor 4 (20).

2.1.3 Processing

Recommended centrifugation protocol for obtaining a platelet-free plasma sample adequate for coagulation testing includes minimum centrifugation at 2,500 × *g* for 15 min.

2.1.4 Storage

Once prepared, the plasma samples can be stored for up to 2 weeks at −20°C and for up to 6 months at −70°C. It is important that the plasma sample is separated into smaller aliquots prior to storage. This will allow the sample to freeze quickly and will facilitate adequate thawing prior to use.

Thaw frozen plasma for 15 min at room temperature. It is recommended that the testing is performed immediately after thawing. However, in situations where this is not possible, the plasma sample can be stored for 2 h at 4°C prior to use.

2.2 Reagents and Reagent Preparation

2.2.1 Imidazole Buffer (Glyoxaline)

3.4 g	Imidazole
5.85 g	Sodium chloride (NaCl)
186 ml	0.1 M Hydrochloric acid (HCl)

Make up to 1,000 ml in water.
Titrate pH to 7.3.
Store at 3°C.
Check pH prior to use in the preparation of Seegers titration mixture.

2.2.2 Seegers Titration Mixture

67.0 ml	0.85% sodium chloride (NaCl)
13.2 ml	1% calcium chloride ($CaCl_2$)
26.6 ml	Acacia (1.5% solution in 0.85% NaCl) (gum arabic from acacia tree)
133.2 ml	Imidazole (glyoxaline) buffer pH 7.3

Filter by means of filter paper or a syringe filter.
Store at 3°C.
Titrate pH to 7.3 prior to performing protamine titration.

Remove stored plasma aliquots of approximately 2 ml of Seegers titration mixture from 3°C and keep at room temperature during experiments.

2.2.3 Veronal Buffer

0.0071 M	Na acetate (CH_3COOH)
0.0071 M	Sodium diethylbarbiturate ($C_8H_{11}N_2O_3Na$)
0.131 M	Sodium chloride (NaCl)

Titrate to pH 7.4.
Dilute up to 50 ml with dH_2O.

Method: Measure sodium diethylbarbiturate and NaCl and place into medium-sized glass jar. Add 45 ml dH_2O. Add Na acetate. Determine pH and titrate to a pH of 7.4. When pH is correct, make buffer solution up to a total of 50 ml. Filter solution through a 0.2 μm filter (see Note 2).

2.2.4 Thrombin

1,000 U Enzyme Research Human Alpha Thrombin HT 2490A3L.

Reconstitute in 1 ml of distilled H_2O (1,000 U/ml).

1,000 U/ml	Thrombin solution is diluted to 100 U/ml
9 ml	Distilled H_2O
1 ml	1,000 U/ml thrombin

Mix well and divide into 500 μl aliquots.

Store aliquots at −82°C.

For use, the 100 U/ml thrombin solution is diluted to approximately 6 U/ml in distilled H_2O (i.e., 1 in 17 dilution). This solution results in a baseline clotting time of 18–20 s. 50 μl of 100 U/ml thrombin is diluted in 800 μl distilled H_2O to give a working solution of 6 U/ml.

Store thrombin at 3°C until ready to use.

Keep thrombin on ice during experiments.

2.2.5 Protamine Sulfate

(Stock 10 mg/ml = 1,000 U/ml.)

Dissolve 10 mg protamine sulfate (PSO_4) in 1 ml of veronal buffer.

Prepare 1/50 working solution in veronal buffer (=0.2 mg/ml or 20 U/ml).

5 μl of 1/50 dilution + 100 μl of plasma = 1 U/ml of protamine (see Table 1).

High concentrations of UFH (i.e., >1.0 IU/ml) may require a protamine concentration greater than 0.9 U/ml. The above method may therefore require to be supplemented by the following.

Table 1
Protamine dilutions prepared using a 1/50 working solution

Protamine concentration (U/ml)	1/50 Protamine (1 U/ml)	Veronal buffer (ml)
0.9	0.9 ml	0.1
0.8	0.8 ml	0.2
0.7	0.7 ml	0.3
0.65	0.65 ml	0.35
0.6	0.6 ml	0.4
0.55	0.55 ml	0.45
0.5	0.5 ml	0.5
0.45	0.45 ml	0.55
0.4	0.4 ml	0.6
0.35	0.35 ml	0.65
0.3	0.3 ml	0.7
0.25	0.25 ml	0.75
0.2	0.2 ml	0.8
0.15	0.15 ml	0.85
0.1	0.1 ml	0.9
0.05	0.05 ml	0.95

2.2.6 Protamine Titration for High UFH Doses

Prepare a 1/25 working solution in veronal buffer (=0.4 mg/ml or 40 U/ml).

5 μl or 1/25 dilution + 100 μl of plasma = 2 U/ml of protamine (see Table 2).

Both working solutions of protamine should be prepared at the start of each experiment and should then be kept on ice for the duration of the experiment.

2.3 Clot Detection

Time to clot detection is recorded from the addition of thrombin to the test plasma. Test endpoint is the detection of a predetermined strength of clot formation by naked eye.

3 Methods

3.1 Assay Procedure

The baseline thrombin clotting time is measured by adding Seegers titration mixture followed by thrombin to a non-heparinized plasma sample. Time to clot formation following the addition of thrombin represents the baseline TCT.

Table 2
Protamine dilutions prepared using a 1/25 protamine working solution

Protamine concentration (U/ml)	1/25 Protamine (2 U/ml)	Veronal buffer (ml)
1.8	0.9 ml	0.1
1.6	0.8 ml	0.2
1.4	0.7 ml	0.3
1.2	0.6 ml	0.4
1.0	0.5 ml	0.5

To heparinized plasma, protamine and Seegers titration mixture are added. Following the addition of thrombin, time to clot formation is measured. This process is repeated until the TCT returns to baseline level. The concentration of protamine required to achieve this represents the concentration of UFH in the test plasma.

3.2 Manual Assay

All experiments are conducted at room temperature; plasma samples, protamine solution preparations, and thrombin are kept on ice until aliquoted into the test tube. Ensure that you have access to a stopwatch (timer) prior to starting the test:

1. Prepare glass test tubes for titration.
2. Pipette 100 μl un-heparinized plasma into glass tube and allow to reach room temperature for 30 s.
3. Add 100 μl Seegers titration mixture.
4. Add 100 μl thrombin and immediately start recording the clotting time.
5. This clotting time represents the baseline clotting time for non-heparinized plasma.

*It is not necessary to add NaCl to baseline titration to account for the absent volume of protamine (11).

3.3 Determination of UFH Concentration in Heparinized Plasma

Repeat assay using different concentrations of protamine (5 μl), added after plasma has reached room temperature and before Seegers titration mixture, i.e., in the following order:

(a) 100 μl plasma.
(b) 5 μl PSO4.
(c) 100 μl Seegers buffer.
(d) 100 μl thrombin.

Using varying concentrations of protamine, the smallest amount of protamine that produces the baseline clotting time is considered the point of equivalence.

3.4 Reproducibility

In the recently published micro-method for protamine titration, the mean CV% for replicated assays was 8.2% as determined by an independent observer. It is recommended that replicated testing be performed by each laboratory when establishing this method. The results of the individual (duplicate) test results should be within 10% of each other.

4 Notes

1. The ACCP recommendations suggesting target APTT ranges for UFH therapy should reflect heparin concentrations of 0.2–0.4 IU/ml by protamine titration or 0.35–0.7 IU/ml by an anti-Xa assay that assumes a level of agreement between protamine titration and anti-factor Xa assay results. A study by Kitchen et al. (14) found that protamine titration and eight commercially available anti-factor Xa assays did not necessarily correlate and that an UFH concentration of 0.2–0.4 IU/ml equated to an anti-factor Xa range of 0.25–0.5 IU/ml (21). This difference in equivalence may reflect a number of factors including concomitant vitamin K antagonists, different UFH preparations, and variability in anti-factor Xa kits and that the anti-factor Xa assay is not a measure of UFH concentration, but rather a measure of UFH effect. All these factors reinforce the need for each pediatric clinical laboratory to develop their own results for the correlation between UFH concentration using protamine titration and measures of UFH effect, such as the APTT and anti-factor Xa assay.
2. The buffers used in performing protamine titration have labile pH. Prior to performing each experiment (on a given day), the pH of all buffers should be checked and titrated to the appropriate level.

References

1. Olson J et al (1998) College of American Pathologists Conference XXXI on laboratory monitoring of anticoagulant therapy: laboratory monitoring of unfractionated heparin therapy. Arch Pathol Lab Med 122(9):782–798
2. Hull R et al (1986) Continuous intravenous heparin compared with intermittent subcutaneous heparin in the initial treatment of proximal-vein thrombosis. N Engl J Med 315(18):1109–1114
3. Hull R et al (1990) Heparin for 5 days as compared to 10 days in the initial treatment of proximal venous thrombosis. N Engl J Med 322:1260–1264
4. Turpie A et al (1989) Comparison of high-dose with low-dose subcutaneous heparin to prevent left ventricular mural thrombosis in patients with acute transmural anterior myocardial infarction. N Engl J Med 320:352–357

5. Brill-Edwards P et al (1993) Establishing a therapeutic range for heparin therapy. Ann Intern Med 119(2):104–109
6. Hull R (1995) Anticoagulant treatment. Int Angiol 14(1):32–44
7. Hirsh J, Raschke R (2004) Heparin and low-molecular-weight heparin. Chest 126(3):188S–203S
8. Laffan M, Manning R (2001) Laboratory control of anticoagulant, thrombolytic and antiplatelet therapy (Chapter 18). In: Lewis S, Bain B, Bates I (eds) Dacie and Lewis: practical haematology. Churchill Livingstone, London
9. Teng C, Yang V (1989) A facile colorimetric protamine titration method. J Lab Clin Med 113:498–504
10. Carr J, Silverman N (1999) The heparin-protamine interaction: a review. J Cardiovasc Surg 40(5):659–666
11. Refn I, Vestergaard L (1954) The titration of heparin with protamine. Scand J Clin Lab Investig 6:284–287
12. O'Shea M, Flute P, Pannell G (1971) Laboratory control of heparin therapy. J Clin Pathol 24:542–546
13. Andrew M, Monagle P, Brooker L (2000) Thromboembolic complications during infancy and childhood. Decker, Hamilton, BC
14. Kitchen S (2000) Problems in laboratory monitoring of heparin dosage. Br J Haematol 111:397–406
15. Newall F et al (2008) Refinement and feasibility testing of a manual micro-method for protamine titration. Int J Lab Hematol 31(4):457–461
16. Ignjatovic V et al (2006) Age-related differences in heparin response. Thromb Res 118(6):741–745
17. Ignjatovic V et al (2007) Monitoring unfractionated heparin (UFH) therapy: which anti factor Xa assay is appropriate? Thromb Res 120(3):347–351
18. Ignjatovic V et al (2006) Therapeutic range for unfractionated heparin therapy: age-related differences in response in children. J Thromb Haemost 4(10):2280–2282
19. Monagle P et al (2006) Developmental haemostasis: impact for clinical haemostasis laboratories. Thromb Haemost 95:362–372
20. Rose VL et al (1993) Decentralized testing for PT and activated PTT using a dry chemistry portable analyzer. Arch Pathol Lab Med 117:611–617
21. Kitchen S, Theaker J, Preston F (2000) Monitoring unfractionated heparin therapy: relationship between eight anti-Xa assays and a protamine titration assay. Blood Coagul Fibrinolysis 11(2):137–144

Chapter 22

Laboratory Methods for the Assay of Tissue Factor Pathway Inhibitor in Human Plasma

Robyn Summerhayes

Abstract

Tissue factor pathway inhibitor (TFPI) is being assayed with increasing frequency by researchers attempting to further understand the complexities of the coagulation system. There are a number of methods available for measurement of TFPI; however immunological measurement by ELIZA is the most common assay used. There are a number of commercial kits available for this assay and close attention to detail is critical for accurate results.

Key words Tissue factor pathway inhibitor, Tissue factor, Functional assay, Chromogenic substrate assay, Assay methods

1 Introduction

Tissue factor pathway inhibitor (TFPI) formerly termed lipoprotein-associated coagulation inhibitor (LACI) (1) and extrinsic pathway inhibitor (EPI) (2) is a serine protease inhibitor of coagulation.

The TFPI molecule comprises three multivalent Kunitz-type domains with an acidic amino-terminal region and a basic carboxy-terminal end. The first domain binds to FVIIa, the second binds to and inhibits FXa whilst the function of the third domain remains to be determined (3, 4).

TFPI in human plasma circulates as both a full-length molecule, exhibiting optimal aFXa inhibitory activity (5, 6), as well as variably carboxy-terminal truncated forms (7) with a molecular weight between 34 and 41 kDa (4, 8).

TFPI is synthesized primarily by microvascular endothelial cells (8, 9), with the major pool of TFPI bound to endothelial vessel walls in vivo (10). The circulating TFPI plasma pool is complexed with lipoproteins—HDL, LDL, and VLDL (>80%) (2); carrier free (10–20%); and a smaller pool (~10%) being sequestered within platelets (4, 11).

Paul Monagle (ed.), *Haemostasis: Methods and Protocols*, Methods in Molecular Biology, vol. 992, DOI 10.1007/978-1-62703-339-8_22, © Springer Science+Business Media New York 2013

TFPI inhibits the activity of factor Xa and tissue factor by formation of a TFPI–Xa complex that associates with factor VII(a)-TF (an activator of factor X and factor IX) to form a quaternary complex (1). This quaternary complex is a feedback inhibitor of tissue factor-initiated coagulation (2).

In vivo, TFPI anticoagulant activity is primarily a function of full-length, carrier-free TFPI (12, 13).

1.1 Clinical Significance of TFPI

In general, thrombotic disorders associated with a deficiency of TFPI have not been reported (14).

Patients with low levels of plasma TFPI do not suffer from thrombosis (15); however low levels of TFPI antigen are a risk factor for thrombosis (16, 17).

Elevated levels of free TFPI antigen are associated with disseminated intravascular coagulation (DIC) initiated by various conditions (18). Atherosclerotic vessels and tissues contain more TFPI antigen and consequently have higher TFPI activity than healthy tissues (9).

Administration of intravenous heparin induces the release of full-length carrier-free TFPI from vascular endothelium (10, 19–22). The anticoagulant effect of TFPI increases with the administration of heparin in vivo, and this effect is independent of heparin concentration (10). Heparin interactions with the TFPI molecule are dependent upon the presence of the carboxy-terminal region of the TFPI molecule (4). Low levels of heparin-releasable TFPI have been shown in patients with venous thrombosis when compared to healthy controls (23).

Endogenous female hormones, oral contraceptives, and hormone replacement therapy contribute to the lower mean plasma TFPI levels observed in women compared to men (16, 24) whilst plasma TFPI levels have been shown to be elevated in the third trimester of pregnancy (25).

2 Considerations for Choice of Assay Methodology

The assay of TFPI is complex in that in vivo the molecule is present in different intravascular pools and the heterogeneous nature of the TFPI molecule with regard to the degree of lipidation and truncation may influence both levels of antigen detection and the anticoagulant effect exerted.

The choice of methodology should be relevant to the patient group or research interest as the ratio between the levels of TFPI antigen and anticoagulant function varies widely between patient groups (26, 27). This may be emphasized by the subtle differences in the mechanism of the methodology employed for TFPI detection (27).

Overall TFPI activity or antigen concentration may not necessarily reflect its anticoagulant potency in vivo (12).

The types of assays commonly employed for measurement of TFPI in plasma can be broadly divided into two groups:

1. Functional assays that describe the activity of the TFPI molecule towards its substrates and its role in the coagulation processes.
2. Immunoassays that measure the overall levels of TFPI antigen in plasma.

2.1 TFPI Functional Assays: Measurement of TFPI Activity in Plasma

Activity of the TFPI molecule can be measured employing either fluid-phase or solid-phase methods utilizing chromogenic substrates sensitive to the activity of factor Xa or by a qualitative coagulation assay.

2.1.1 Amidolytic: Fluid-Phase Assay for TFPI Activity

Both fluid- and solid-phase activity assays are based on the ability of TFPI to inhibit the catalytic activity of the factor VIIa/TF complex in a reaction mixture that contains TFPI (2, 10, 13, 16, 22–24, 27–32).

Assays are relatively standardized and sensitive by the use of excess rFVIIa which negates variation of FVII(a) in assayed samples (28).

The base principle for these reactions in the assay is:

1. *The inhibition of FXa by the [TF–FVIIa] complex*

   TF + FVII (excess) + TFPI (plasma) + FXa → [TF–FVIIa–TFPI–FXa] + [TF–FVIIa residual].

2. *Reaction of FXa with the substrate resulting in the release of a chromophore*

[TF–FVIIa] + FX (excess) + chromogenic FXa substrateγ [TF–FVIIa] + FXa (residual) + peptide + chromophore.

TFPI activity in the samples is inversely proportional to the amount of FXa generated.

Note. Heat treatment of plasma pre-assay as prepared in some functional assays to reduce the interference in the assay by coagulant factors and fibrinogen has been seen to result in a loss of functional TFPI activity (26).

The addition of polybrene (hexadimethrine bromide 2 μg/ml) to the assay buffer or plasma samples will neutralize potential heparin activity in samples.

2.1.2 Binding Assay

A solid-phase assay, whereby thromboplastin is immobilized upon the wells of a microtiter plate by an overnight incubation. A prothrombin complex concentrate (source of FVII and FX) and test plasma (source of TFPI) are added, incubated at room temperature for an hour and the wells, and then rinsed with TBS. The addition of S-2222, a FXa-specific chromogenic substrate, then allows detection of the residual aFXa activity which is inversely proportional to the level of TFPI, bound as quaternary complexes, present in the test plasma sample (27, 33).

2.1.3 Commercial Functional Assays for TFPI Activity

ActichromeR TFPI Activity Assay (American Diagnostica)

A three-stage chromogenic assay which measures active TFPI activity in plasma whereby TFPI exerts an inhibitory effect upon the TF/FVIIa complex. Following incubation of test samples with TF/FVIIa and FX, the residual activity of the TF/FVIIa complex is measured using SpectrozymeR, a chromogenic substrate highly specific for FXa. The TFPI activity in the test sample is compared to a standard curve of known TFPI activity levels. This assay may be conducted as an end point or kinetic analysis (34).

The major problem limiting current functional methodologies using chromogenic substrates is that there is no way to adequately discriminate between lipid-bound TFPI and the active anticoagulant carrier-free TFPI which represents a minor component of the total TFPI profile.

Studies have shown TFPI chromogenic activity assays to correlate positively to immunoassays for TFPI total antigen in normal plasma (5, 31).

2.1.4 Clotting Assays

Coagulation assays use the addition of a low dilution of tissue factor to a plasma sample to initiate extrinsic coagulation.

Comparison of the clotting times of samples that have had the TFPI activity blocked by the addition of anti-TFPI antibody to the clotting times of uninhibited samples permits the anticoagulant effect exerted by the TFPI present in the test sample to be qualified (5, 22, 35, 36).

These assay methods have the advantage of observation of a global "in vivo" anticoagulant effect which may be interpreted as having a greater biological relevance (5, 14). Clotting assays have been used successfully in vitro to assess the positive dose-dependant relationship of carrier-free, full-length TFPI to anticoagulant activity in human plasma (13).

A recent study by Dahm et al. (2005) has shown a strong correlation between the diluted prothrombin time assay with chromogenic substrate activity and antigen assays for TFPI. It has also been determined that the anticoagulant activity assay of TFPI measures primarily the functional effect of full-length TFPI whilst remaining relatively insensitive to truncated TFPI (5).

This observation is balanced by the recognition that clotting assays examining TFPI activity are relatively qualitative as converting clotting times to a uniform measure of TFPI activity has yet to be standardized (14).

2.2 TFPI Immunoassays: Measurement of TFPI Antigen Levels in Plasma

Immunoassays are useful for quantifying free and total TFPI antigen levels and full-length and truncated TFPI antigen levels in a range of biological samples. Assays are standardized with a selection of commercially available kits. Using commercial immunoassays gives the additional advantage of providing access to technical resources and specific troubleshooting advice from the companies supplying these assays in kit form (see Note 1).

2.2.1 Imubind[R] Truncated TFPI ELISA Kit and Total TFPI ELISA Kit (American Diagnostica)

The IMUBIND[R] Truncated TFPI and Total TFPI Elisa kits are enzyme-linked sandwich immunoassays. The IMUBIND[R] Truncated TFPI combines two separate assays to measure total and full-length forms of both lipid-associated and carrier-free TFPI. The difference measured between the two assays contained in the kit is the value for truncated TFPI. The assays contain polyclonal antibody specific for Kunitz domain 1 or the C-terminus of TFPI, respectively.

The IMUBIND[R] Total TFPI Elisa kit recognizes all TFPI molecules present in a test sample including full-length, truncated, lipid-associated, and carrier-free forms.

A rabbit anti-human TFPI polyclonal antibody is used as the capture antibody which is specific for native, complexed, and free TFPI forms.

Both assays use a detection antibody conjugated to horseradish peroxidase which is reacted with a TMB substrate to detect bound TFPI antigen, the measured absorbance at 450 nm proportional to concentration of TFPI antigen present in the test sample (37, 38).

2.2.2 Asserachrom™ Total TFPI ELISA and Free TFPI ELISA (Diagnostica Stago)

The TFPI Total antigen assay detects (via the monoclonal antibody 2C6, the first 160 amino acid residues) full-length and truncated TFPI as well as lipid-bound TFPI. The detecting antibodies are conjugated to peroxidase (16).

The TFPI free antigen assay is specific for the measurement of free, circulating, full-length TFPI and does not detect lipid-bound TFPI.

The free TFPI assay uses a capture antibody (T4E2) directed against the Kunitz-2 domain and a detection antibody (HG5—directed to the lipoprotein-binding domain, specific between residues 161 and 240) of the TFPI molecule (39, 40).

The principle of the protocol as described below for the Asserachrom Total TFPI ELISA assay is applicable for general ELISA methods of antigen detection and is one that our laboratory used successfully as a standard method in the development of reference range values for TFPI antigen in both pediatric and adult plasma samples.

3 Protocol

3.1 Asserachrom™ Total TFPI ELISA Kit (Diagnostica Stago)

Principle. The internal wall of a plastic microwell is precoated with the first monoclonal antibody to TFPI (reagent 1). The second anti-total TFPI monoclonal antibody that is coupled with peroxidise (reagent 2) is added to the precoated well at the same time as the plasma whose total TFPI is to be determined.

The total TFPI of the plasma being tested is simultaneously captured on the one hand by the first monoclonal antibody that is precoated on the microwell wall and on the other by the second monoclonal antibody–peroxidase conjugate, i.e., the "sandwich" is formed in a one-step reaction.

Next, the bound peroxidise is revealed by its activity in a predetermined time on the substrate *ortho*-phenylenediamine (reagent 3a) in the presence of urea peroxide (reagent 3b). After stopping the reaction with a strong acid, the intensity of color produced bears a direct relationship with the total TFPI antigen concentration initially present in the plasma sample.

3.1.1 Specimen

Blood (9 Vol) is collected in 0.109 M (3.2%) trisodium citrate anticoagulant (1 Vol). Citrated whole blood is centrifuged at 2,500 × *g* for 10 min to obtain platelet-poor plasma.

Plasma storage: Citrated plasma—4 h at 20 ± 5°C or stored for future testing within 4 h of collection at −80°C.

Thaw stored frozen plasmas at 37°C for 10 min before testing.

Fasting before venepuncture and freeze-thawing of stored plasma samples have not been shown to affect the levels of TFPI activity (25).

Cholesterol-lowering medications do not affect the size or anticoagulant potential of the endothelial TFPI pool (21).

3.1.2 Materials

Asserachrom™ Total TFPI ELISA Kit (Diagnostica Stago)

Containing:

Reagent 1	16-well strip coated with F(ab')2 fragments from mouse anti-TFPI monoclonal antibody.
Reagent 2	Mouse anti-total TFPI monoclonal antibody–peroxidase conjugate.
Reagent 3a	Tablet containing 2 mg *ortho*-phenylenediamine (OPD, 2HCl).
Reagent 3b	Tablet containing 5 mg urea peroxide.
Reagent 4	Dilution buffer, 50 ml bottle.
Reagent 5	Washing solution, 50 ml bottle of 20× concentrate.
Reagent 6	TFPI calibrator. Freeze-dried human plasma containing ~200 ng/ml [TFPI] after reconstitution—see assay insert value.
Reagent 7	TFPI quality control. Freeze-dried human plasma containing ~120 ng/ml [TFPI] after reconstitution—see assay insert value.

Additional Materials Required

Distilled water.

3 M Sulfuric scid.

Timer.

Multichannel pipettes (see Notes 2 and 3).

Tip tubs (separate for ELISA assays only).

Plate-washing equipment.

Microplate reader set to 492 nm.

3.2 Method

3.2.1 Reagent Preparation

Reagent 1	Stand at room temperature (18–25°C) for ~0 min before step 5 (see Note 4).
Reagent 2	Reconstitute vial with 2 ml dilution buffer (reagent 4) and swirl (stable for 4 h at 20+ 5°C, 24 h at 2–8°C).
Reagents 3a and 3b	For ten strips, add four tablets of reagent 3a and four tablets of reagent 3b to 16.0 ml distilled water. Dissolve completely (stable for 1 h at room temp.).
Reagent 4	Stand at room temperature (18–25°C) for 30 min before use (stable for 1 month at 2–8°C after opening).
Reagent 5	For ten strips, dilute 50 ml with 950 ml of distilled water (presence of crystals will not affect quality, stable for 15 days after dilution at 2–8°C).
Reagent 6	Reconstitute with 0.5 ml distilled water, stand at room temperature for ~30 min (stable for 4 h at 20+ 5°C, 24 h at 2–8°C).
Reagent 7	Reconstitute with 0.5 ml distilled water, stand at room temperature for ~30 min (stable for 4 h at 20+ 5°C, 24 h at 2–8°C).

3.2.2 Dilution of Reagent 6 for Standards

1. Using reagent 4 as a diluent, prepare a 1:20 dilution of reagent 6

   50 μl reagent 6 + 950 μl reagent 4 = 1.0 ml × 1:20 dilution of reagent 6.

2. Table for Dilution of Standards.

Dilution of working solution of total TFPI calibrator	S1 (T)	S2 (T/2)	S3 (T/4)	S4 (T/8)	S5 (T/16)
Concentration of total TFPI (ng/ml) *see assay insert for exact value	200*	100*	50*	25*	12.5*
1:20 dilution of reagent 6 (μl)	500	250	125	62.5	31.25
Reagent 4 (μl)	0	250	375	437.5	468.75
Total volume for TFPI testing (200 μl)	500	500	500	500	500

3.2.3 Dilution of Reagent 7 for Quality Controls

1. Using reagent 4 as a diluent, prepare 2 dilutions (1:20 and 1:40) of reagent 7.

Dilution of reagent 7	1:20 (C1)	1:40 (C2)
Concentration of total TFPI (ng/ml) *see assay insert for exact value	High range*	Low range*
Reagent 7 (μl)	25	12.5
Reagent 4 (μl)	475	487.5
Total volume for TFPI assay (200 μl)	500	500

3.2.4 Dilution of Plasma to be Assayed for TFPI Level

1. Dilute Test Sample Plasmas with Reagent 4 as below.

   Dilution of plasma is 1:20 for expected total TFPI levels <200 ng/ml.

   Dilution of plasma is 1:40 for expected total TFPI levels up to 400 ng/ml.

Test plasma (μl)	*1:20* 12.5	*1:40* 25
Reagent 4 (μl)	237.5	225
Total volume for testing (200 μl)	250	250

To achieve greater consistency in results it is recommended, if test sample size permits, to double the volumes in table to test samples for assay in duplicate.

3.3 Assay Steps

1. Add 50 μl of reagent 2 into all precoated wells—Two strips are required for a minimum of 16 wells for blanks, standards, and controls plus additional strips for test sample wells.
2. Add the blanks, standards, and controls to the wells, in duplicate, as follows:

2 × 200 μl of reagent 4	BLANK = 2 wells
2 × 200 μl of S1, S2, S3, S4, and S5	STANDARDS = 10 wells
2 × 200 μl of C1 and C2	QUALITY CONTROL = 4 wells
200 μl Test plasma sample to be assayed per well	

3. Cover the strips with the lid provided and incubate for exactly 2 h at room temperature (18–25°C).
4. Empty wells following incubation, wash all wells exactly five times with 300 μl of reagent 5, and then immediately proceed to step 5 (see Note 5).
5. Add 200 μl of (reagents 3a and 3b) OPD/urea peroxidase substrate into every well.
6. Let each well incubate at room temperature for exactly 8 min and then add acid to stop reaction (see Note 6).
7. Add 50 μl of 3 M sulfuric acid into each well to stop reaction.
8. Wait for 30 min to 2 h at room temperature and then measure absorbance at 490 nm.

3.4 Calculation

Use log–log graph paper to plot total TFPI concentrations from the assay calibration on the *x*-axis and the corresponding A492 nm values on the *y*-axis. Draw the calibration curve (it is nonlinear).

Interpolate the absorbance values for the assayed test plasmas and controls on this calibration curve to derive their respective total TFPI values.

4 Notes

1. The enzyme-linked immunosorbent assay (ELISA) is a very sensitive assay when properly performed. Often the difference between a good assay and a poor assay result is the attention to detail in multiple steps. Often problems develop as cumulative errors. Attention to accurate pipetting, careful and thorough washing, and proper incubation will result in precise ELISA assays. Each step if not controlled may contribute only a small amount of variation. When pipetting is poor, washing is not adequate, and incubation temperatures are not controlled, the results will be inconsistent and the cause will not be evident. By understanding how each step must be controlled, the investigator can achieve acceptable results from the very beginning.
2. It is important to ensure that the pipettes used for the ELISA assay are clean and are designed to reliably deliver the volume desired. The operator instructions that accompany the pipette usually include instruction for calibration and it is good laboratory practise to ensure that routine maintenance includes calibration and adjustment as needed of regularly used equipment. Never set the volume below the minimum volume or above the maximum volume printed on the pipette.
3. Multichannel pipettes are of special concern. Be sure that the tips are appropriate for the pipette and are properly fitted and firmly attached when in use.

   Take particular care when diluting down the plate and watch to make sure that the pipette tips are all picking up and releasing the correct volume of reagent. This will greatly affect consistency of results between duplicate samples.

   In general, reagents should be dispensed into the test wells with the pipette tips touching the side of the well at a point about midsection.
4. Allow the foil packet containing the anti-TFPI AB-coated test strips to warm to room temperature for 30 min before opening (Subheading 3.2.1, Reagent 1). This step avoids condensation forming on the inner surface of the packet, which may contribute to a deterioration of the coated strips intended for future use.
5. The volume of wash should be adequate to rinse down the sides of the wells and remove any unbound reactants that might have adhered during the addition step. It is necessary during the wash steps to ensure the filling nearly to the top of all the assay test wells. The wash solution contains a detergent to help loosen proteins from the wells.

The number of washes following incubation (5 in this particular Asserachrom total TFPI assay) is to be scrupulously adhered to ensure accurate results.

Grip the middle of the microplate frame firmly, to avoid accidentally dislodging the removable test strips while emptying the wells. The microplates should be completely emptied between washes and the plate firmly rapped on a blotting paper towel after the last wash.

It is important to prevent the plates drying out between steps. While not recommended, if interruptions are unavoidable, keep all wells filled with wash solution until ready to proceed with the next step or if delay is unavoidable after removal of the last wash, leave plates upside down on a moist wipe.

After the last wash, rap the plate carefully on a dry wipe or a paper towel until no more fluid can be seen in the wells. If wetness is observed, move the plate to a new spot and rap it again on the dry towel. If the towel is dry, turn the plate upright and promptly proceed to the next step. Do not overdry the plate by knocking after all wash solution has been removed.

6. Improper incubation can lead to uneven results. Incubation should take place at room temperature with the microplate covered and placed in a darkened cupboard. The most obvious sign of improper incubation is called the "edge effect." The wells on the outside of the plate, especially the four corners, can have higher or lower than expected values. The edge effect is caused by uneven temperature, loss of enzyme activity due to drying, and exposure to light.

References

1. Broze GJ Jr, Warren LA, Novotny WF, Higuchi DA, Girard JJ, Miletech JP (1988) The lipoprotein-associated coagulation inhibitor that inhibits the factorVII-tissue factor complex also inhibits factor Xa: insight into its possible mechanism of action. Blood 71:335–343
2. Sandset PM, Abildgaard U, Pettersen M (1987) A sensitive assay of extrinsic coagulation pathway inhibitor (EPI) in plasma and plasma fractions. Thromb Res 47:389–400
3. Girard TJ, Warren LA, Novotny WF, Likert KM, Brown SG, Miletech JP, Broze GJ Jr (1989) Functional significance of the Kunitz-type inhibitory domains of lipoprotein-associated coagulation inhibitor. Nature 338:518–520
4. Novotny WF, Girard TJ, Miletech JP, Broze GJ Jr (1989) Purification and characterization of the lipoprotein-associated coagulation inhibitor from human plasma. J Biol Chem 264:18832–18837
5. Dahm AEA, Andersen TO, Rosendaal F, Sandset PM (2005) A novel anticoagulant activity assay of tissue factor pathway inhibitor 1 (TFPI). J Thromb Haemost 3:651–658
6. Wesselschmidt R, Likert KM, Girard T, Wun TC, Broze GJ Jr (1992) Tissue factor pathway inhibitor: the carboxy-terminus is required for optimal inhibition of factor Xa. Blood 79:2004–2010
7. Warshawsky I, Bu G, Mast A, Saffitz JE, Broze GJ Jr, Schwartz AL (1995) The carboxy terminus of tissue factor pathway inhibitor is required for interacting with hepatoma cells in vitro and in vivo. J Clin Invest 95:1773–1781
8. Bajaj MS, Kuppuswamy MN, Saito H, Spitzer SG, Bajaj SP (1990) Cultured normal human hepatocytes do not synthesize lipoprotein-associated coagulation inhibitor: evidence that endothelium is the principal site of its synthesis. Proc Natl Acad Sci 87:8869–8873

9. Crawley J, Lupu F, Westmuckett AD, Severs NJ, Kakkar VV, Lupu C (2000) Expression localization, and activity of tissue factor pathway inhibitor in normal and atherosclerotic human vessels. Arterioscler Thromb Vasc Biol 20:1362–1373
10. Sandset PM, Abildgaard U, Larsen ML (1988) Heparin induces release of extrinsic coagulation pathway inhibitor (EPI). Thromb Res 50:803–813
11. Novotny WF, Girard JJ, Miletech JP, Broze GJ (1988) Platelets secrete a coagulation inhibitor functionally and antigenically similar to the lipoprotein associated coagulation inhibitor. Blood 72:2020–2025
12. Lindahl AK, Jacobsen PB, Sandset PM, Abildgaard U (1991) Tissue factor pathway inhibitor with high anticoagulant activity is increased in postheparin plasma and in plasma from cancer patients. Thromb Res 2:713–721
13. Hansen JB, Huseby KR, Huseby NE, Ezban M, Nordoy A (1997) Tissue factor pathway inhibitor in complex with low density lipoprotein isolated from human plasma does not possess anticoagulant function in tissue factor induced coagulation in vitro. Thromb Res 85:413–425
14. Sandset PM, Bendz B (1997) Tissue factor pathway inhibitor: clinical deficiency states. Thromb Haemost 78:467–470
15. Novotny WF, Brown SG, Miletech JP, Rader DJ, Broze GJ Jr (1991) Plasma antigen levels of the lipoprotein-associated coagulation inhibitor in patient samples. Blood 78:387–393
16. Dahm AEA, van Hylckama Vlieg A, Bendz B, Rosendaal F, Bertina RM, Sandset PM (2003) Low levels of tissue factor pathway inhibitor (TFPI) increase the risk of venous thrombosis. Blood 101:4387–4392
17. Amini-Nekoo A, Futers TS, Moia M, Mannucci PM, Grant PJ, Ariens RAS (2001) Analysis of the tissue factor pathway inhibitor gene and antigen levels in relation to venous thrombosis. Br J Haematol 113:537–543
18. Asakura H, Ontachi Y, Mizutani T, Kato M, Saito M, Morishita E, Yamazaki M, Suga Y, Takami A, Miyamoto K, Nakao S (2001) Elevated levels of free tissue factor pathway inhibitor antigen in cases of disseminated intravascular coagulation caused by various underlying diseases. Blood Coagul Fibrinolysis 12:1–8
19. Adams MJ, Cardigan RA, Marchant WA, Grocott MPW, Mythen MG, Mutch M, Purdy G, Mackie IJ, Machin SJ (2002) Tissue factor pathway inhibitor antigen and activity in 96 patients receiving heparin for cardiopulmonary bypass. J Cardiothorac Vasc Anesth 16:59–63
20. Donahue BS, Gailani D, Mast AE (2006) Disposition of tissue factor pathway inhibitor during cardiopulmonary bypass. J Thromb Haemost 4:1011–1016
21. Hansen JB, Huseby KR, Huseby NE, Sandset PM, Hanssen TA, Nordoy A (1995) Effect of cholesterol lowering on intravascular pools of TFPI and its antigoagulant potential in type II hyperlipoproteinemia. Arterioscler Thromb Vasc Biol 15:879–885
22. Hansen JB, Sandset PM, Huseby KR, Huseby NE, Nordoy A (1996) Depletion of intravascular pools of tissue factor pathway inhibitor (TFPI) during repeated or continuous intravenous infusion of heparin in man. Thromb Haemost 76:703–709
23. Ariens RAS, Alberio G, Moia M, Mannucci PM (1999) Low levels of Heparin-releasable tissue factor pathway inhibitor in young patients with thrombosis. Thromb Haemost 81:203–207
24. Harris GM, Stendt CL, Vollenhoven BJ, Gan TE, Tipping PG (1999) Decreased plasma tissue factor pathway inhibitor in women taking combined oral contraceptives. Am J Haematol 60:175–180
25. Warr TA, Warn-Cramer BJ, Rao LV, Rapaport SI (1989) Human plasma extrinsic inhibitor activity: I. Standardization of assay and evaluation of physiologic variables. Blood 74:201–206
26. Jeske W, Hoppensteadt D, Fareed J, Bermes E (1995) Measurement of functional and immunologic levels of tissue factor pathway inhibitor. Some methodologic considerations. Blood Coagul Fibrinolysis 6:S73–S80
27. Adams MJ, Oostryck R (2000) A comparative study of functional assays for tissue factor pathway inhibitor using normal plasma and clinical samples. Blood Coagul Fibrinolysis 11:327–333
28. Bendz B, Andersen TO, Sandset PM (2000) A new sensitive chromogenic substrate assay of tissue factor pathway inhibitor type 1. Thromb Res 97:463–472
29. Ma Q, Tobu M, Schultz C, Jeske W, Hoppensteadt D, Walenga J, Cornelli U, Lee J, Linhardt R, Hanin I, Fareed J (2007) Molecular weight dependent tissue factor pathway inhibitor release by heparin and heparin oligosaccharides. Thromb Res 119:653–661
30. Kokawa T, Abumiya T, Kimura T, Harada-Shiba M, Koh H, Tsushima M, Yamamoto A, Kato H (1995) Tissue factor pathway inhibitor activity in human plasma. Arterioscler Thromb Vasc Biol 15:504–510
31. Hubbard AR, Weller LJ, Gray E (1994) Measurement of tissue factor pathway inhibitor

in normal and post-heparin plasma. Blood Coagul Fibrinolysis 5:819–823
32. Chromogenix R&D, IL (2002) Determination of TFPI activity in plasma with S-2222 (microplate method). Res Methods
33. Berrettini M, Malaspina M, Parise P, Lucarelli G, Kisiel W, Nenci G (1995) A simple chromogenic substrate assay of tissue factor pathway inhibitor activity in plasma and serum. Am J Clin Pathol 103:391–395
34. American-Diagnostica. ACTICHROME® TFPI Activity Assay, Product Information Assay Insert
35. Hansen JB, Huseby NE, Sandset PM, Svensson B, Lyngmo V, Nordoy A (1994) Tissue factor pathway inhibitor and lipoproteins: evidence for association with and regulation by LDL in human plasma. Arterioscler Thromb Vasc Biol 14:223–229
36. Nordfang O, Valentin S, Beck TC, Hedner U (1991) Inhibition of extrinsic pathway inhibitor shortens the coagulation time of normal plasma and of hemophilia plasma. Thromb Haemost 66:464–467
37. American-Diagnostica. IMUBIND® Total TFPI ELISA Kit Product No. 849, Product Information Assay Insert
38. American-Diagnostica. IMMUBIND® Truncated TFPI ELISA Product No. 850
39. Stago-Diagnostica. Asserachrom® Total TFPI ELISA assay, Product Information Assay Insert
40. Stago-Diagnostica. Asserachrom® Free TFPI ELISA assay, Product Information Assay Insert

Chapter 23

Heparin-Induced Thrombocytopenia

Andreas Greinacher, Birgitt Fürll, and Sixten Selleng

Abstract

Heparin-induced thrombocytopenia (HIT) is caused by platelet-activating immunoglobulin (Ig) G antibodies that recognize multimolecular complexes of platelet factor 4 (PF4) bound to heparin or other polyanions. Most laboratory assays for HIT have a high sensitivity for anti-PF4/heparin antibodies and a negative test generally excludes HIT (high negative predictive value), especially in a setting of a low pretest probability. The magnitude of a positive test result correlates with greater likelihood of HIT. Therefore, a combined diagnostic approach that considers the clinical picture and the magnitude of a positive test result is recommended for accurate diagnosis of HIT.

Key words Heparin-induced thrombocytopenia, Pathogenesis, Laboratory testing, Diagnosis

1 HIT Is a Clinicopathologic Syndrome

Heparin-induced thrombocytopenia (HIT) is a life- and limb-threatening prothrombotic, immune-mediated complication of heparin therapy. The antibodies are directed against complexes of positively charged chemokines [mostly platelet factor 4 (PF4)] and heparin. Platelet activation and consecutive thrombin generation result in a fundamental paradox of HIT: despite being induced by the anticoagulant heparin and associated with thrombocytopenia, the major clinical effect is an enhanced risk for venous and arterial thomboembolic events. However, antibodies against PF4/heparin complexes, whether or not platelet activating, are much more frequent than clinical HIT. Therefore, all the so-called HIT tests have a high negative predictive value and a rather low positive predictive value if not interpreted in the context of clinical picture. The diagnosis of HIT should be based on both the clinical picture and detection of pathogenic HIT antibodies (1–14).

Paul Monagle (ed.), *Haemostasis: Methods and Protocols*, Methods in Molecular Biology, vol. 992,
DOI 10.1007/978-1-62703-339-8_23, © Springer Science+Business Media New York 2013

2 Clinical Picture of HIT

The typical clinical picture of HIT is characterized by a platelet count fall >50% and/or new thrombosi(e)s occurring 5–14 days after starting heparin therapy (14). HIT can occur during prophylactic or therapeutic dose anticoagulation. The thromboembolic complications predominantly affect the venous system, with 40% of patients developing a pulmonary embolism. As a general rule, as less likely a new thromboembolic complication during heparin treatment can be explained by the underlying disease, as more likely HIT should be considered. HIT-associated thrombosis occurs in about 30% of patients on the same day of platelet count decrease >50%, in about 30% of patients within 3–4 days after the platelet count fall; however, in a considerable number (≈33%) of patients thrombosis manifests 1–2 days before the platelet count fall (12). In case of reexposure to heparin within 4 weeks (rarely up to 3 months) platelet count fall and/or thrombosis can already occur at day 1 of heparin treatment (rapid-onset HIT) when heparin-dependent antibodies are still present in the patient's plasma. A delayed onset of HIT has also been reported occurring up to 3 weeks after heparin exposure (14). In these patients the antibodies react independently of heparin with platelets and HIT has become an autoimmune disease.

3 Laboratory Assays (Immunologic and Functional)

Diagnosis of HIT requires both clinically evident symptoms and laboratory confirmation of pathogenic HIT antibodies. For the latter, there are two complementary types of assays available: The first detects antibodies based upon their binding to the major HIT antigen (PF4 bound to polyanion, i.e., immunologic or antigen assay). The second detects antibodies based upon their key functional property of heparin-dependent platelet activation (i.e., functional or activation assay).

A test for HIT antibodies should be performed only in patients presenting with clinical symptoms suggestive for HIT (see part a.). For help in "quantifying" the clinical suspicion and formulating a *pretest probability* of HIT, a clinical scoring system known as the "4 T's" has been developed (15). Patients with low (0–3) scores are unlikely to test positive for HIT antibodies (high negative predictive value), and should not be tested. Patients with intermediate (4, 5) or high (6–8) scores are more likely to test positive for HIT antibodies. The positive predictive value depends on the score level, and the experience of the physician applying the score and varies from 20 to 100% (15, 16). Therefore, a test for HIT antibodies is usually required in patients with an at least intermediate score.

HIT antibodies are transient and disappear a few weeks after acute HIT. Therefore, a test for HIT antibodies has to be performed in the acute phase of HIT. Three months after the acute phase tests will be negative in the large majority of patients (17).

3.1 Antigen Assays

Antigen assays detect antibodies upon their binding to PF4/polyanion complexes. Antibodies against other (rare) HIT antigens like IL-8/heparin or NAP-2/heparin are not detectable by PF4-based assays. A general problem of all immunological assays for HIT antibodies is the complex structure of the antigen. Test sensitivity depends on whether the purified PF4 maintains its tetrameric structure, and on the optimal ratio between the complex molecules within the PF/polyanion complexes.

3.1.1 Enzyme-Linked Immunoassay (ELISA)

Solid-Phase ELISA

This group of antigen assays detects antibodies based upon binding to PF4/polyanion complexes bound to a solid phase. Currently, two commercially available ELISA tests are widely used. One assay [from Stago (Asnieres, France)] utilizes heparin as the PF4-binding polyanion, whereas the other [Genetics Testing Institute (GTI, Waukesha, WI)] uses complexes of PF4 and polyvinyl sulfonate. Other differences include the source of PF4, which is recombinant PF4 in the former assay, and purified PF4 from outdated platelets in the latter assay. Both ELISAs utilize enzyme-conjugated goat antihuman-IgG/A/M or an antihuman IgG antibody (GTI) as secondary antibody. Test results are either evaluated using positive controls supplied by the manufacturer (as in the assay from Stago) or compared to a specified fixed cutoff (as in the assay from GTI).

A new assay for pathologic heparin-dependent antibodies, the Zymutest HIA (Aniara Corp., Mason, Ohio), was recently described. This assay utilizes a heparin-coated surface to which patient serum/plasma as well as platelet–leukocyte lysate are added. Non-PF4-dependent (e.g., anti-IL-8/heparin antibodies) antibodies as well as anti-PF4/heparin antibodies should be detected. The assay allows for separate detection of IgG, IgA, and IgM antibodies, and showed a high correlation with antibody detection by standard ELISA (18).

Custom-made solid-phase ELISAs, as used in our laboratory, utilize secondary antibodies that recognize the three major immunoglobulin classes, IgG, IgM, and IgA, separately. Test results are expressed as optical density at 450 nm. An $OD > 0.5$ is considered as a positive result. Inherent problems of solid-phase ELISAs are that surface-adsorbed proteins can undergo denaturation, potentially provoking nonspecific binding of antibodies, and compromising both test sensitivity and specificity.

Anti-PF4/heparin Enzyme Immunoassay (EIA)

Reagents and materials: $NaH_2PO_4 \times H_2O$, Merck, Darmstadt, Germany (cat. no. 1.06349.1000); EDTA Triplex, Merck, Darmstadt, Germany (cat. no. 1.08418.1000); NaCl, Merck, Darmstadt,

Germany (cat. no.1.06404.0500); $MgCl_2 \times 6H_2O$, Merck, Darmstadt, Germany (cat. no.1.05833.0250); sulfuric acid, Merck, Darmstadt, Germany (cat. no. 1.009981.001); sulfo-MBS, Pierce, Rockford, Ireland (cat. no. 22312); PF4, Chromatec, Greifswald, Germany; Goat Serum, SIGMA-Aldrich (cat. no. G-6363); TMB Substrate Reagent Set, Pharmingen (cat. no. 2642KK); Heparin (UFH), Braun, Melsungen, Germany; POD-conjugated Goat antihuman IgG, Dianova, Germany (cat. no. 109-035-088); POD-conjugated Goat antihuman IgA, Dianova, Germany (cat. no. 109-036-011); POD-conjugated Rabbit antihuman IgM, Dianova, Germany (cat. no. 309-036-043); Nunc CovaLink™ NH Modules, NUNC, Roskilde, Denmark (cat. no. 478042).

Buffers:

1. Coating buffer **1**	0.10 M $NaH_2PO_4 \times H_2O$	
	0.15 M NaCl p.a.	
	1 mM EDTA Triplex	Adjust to pH 7.5
2. Coating buffer **2**	0.05 M $NaH_2PO_4 \times H_2O$	
	0.1% NaN_3	
3. sulfo-MBS	0.125 mg/ml in Coating buffer **1**	
4. Washing buffer **1**	0.10 M $NaH_2PO_4 \times H_2O$	
	0.15 M NaCl p.a.	
	9.8 mM $MgCl_2 \times 6H_2O$	Adjust to pH 7.5
5. Washing buffer **2** (10×)	1.5 M NaCl p.a.	
	1% Tween 20	Adjust to pH 7.5

Prepare a working concentration of wash buffer **2** by mixing 1:10 with aqua dest.

6. Dilution buffer	0.05 M $NaH_2PO_4 \times H_2O$	
	0.15 M NaCl p.a.	Adjust to pH 7.5
	+ 7.5% Goat serum	

Step 1. Coating of microwell plate with cross-linker m-maleimidobenzoyl-N-hydroxysulfosuccinimide ester (sulfo-MBS)

The concentration of diluted sulfo-MBS should be 125 μg/ml in coating buffer **1**. 100 μl of diluted sulfo-MBS are given to each well, and the plate is covered and incubated at room temperature for 4 h.

Step 2. Generation of the PF4/heparin complex formation

The following stoichiometric mixture of PF4/heparin is added to allow PF4/heparin complex formation under optimal conditions: PF4 20 μg/ml f.c. and UFH 0.5 IU/ml f.c. (in coating buffer **2**) is incubated in sealed polystyrene tubes at room temperature for 1 h.

Step 3. Coating of microwell plate with PF4/heparin complexes
Plates are washed five times with washing buffer **1** as follows: Empty the plate by inversion over a sink. Tap the inverted plate against some layers of soft paper tissue to remove residual liquid. Wash the plate by filling the wells with buffer. Leave on the table for 2 min. Empty the plate as described above and repeat washing four more times. Add 100 μl of the PF4/heparin complex mixture to each well. Seal plate to prevent evaporation. Incubate for 16 h at 4°C to allow complete binding. Microwell plates can be stored at 4°C for up to 2–3 weeks.

Step 4. Incubation with test samples
Discard the solution and wash plate 5× with washing buffer **2**. Samples (serum/plasma) and negative and positive control are diluted 1:50 in dilution buffer. Add 100 μl per well to the microtiter plate and incubate at room temperature for 1 h. All experiments are performed in duplicate. Two wells are used as blank (only dilution buffer).

Step 5. Incubation with detecting antibody

(a) Discard the solution and wash the plate 5× with washing buffer **2** (200–300 μl wash buffer should be used for each washing step; an improper washing will lead to high background).

    The POD-labeled antibodies against human IgG, IgA, and IgM are diluted appropriately in dilution buffer. The dilution should be adjusted according to the desired measuring range to be determined in separate titration experiments. Usually, dilutions between 1:4,000 and 1:10,000 are suitable. Add 100 μl of diluted labeled antibody per well to the microtiter plate. Seal plate to prevent evaporation. Incubate at room temperature for 1 h.

Step 6. Incubation with substrate reagent (TMB substrate)
Discard the solution and wash the plate 5× with washing buffer **2**. Prepare a TMB substrate solution within 15 min prior to use. Add 100 μl of TMB substrate per well to the microtiter plate. Incubate at RT in the dark for color development. A blue color will develop in positive wells. The enzymatic reaction is stopped after 3 min by addition of 100 μl 2 mol/l sulfuric acid. The blue color will turn into yellow. Read the optical density (OD) for each well with a microplate reader set at 450 nm.

Data analysis
Subtract the average OD of the "blank well" from the OD of other wells. Cutoff value for detection of Ig-classes G, A, or M should be defined by determining the mean and standard deviation of 100 normal plasmas. Usually the cutoff is at 0.5 OD if the ELISA is in the appropriate sensitivity range.

Fluid-Phase ELISA

In the fluid-phase ELISA anti-PF4/heparin antibodies are detected by using biotinylated PF4/heparin complexes in the fluid phase. PF4/heparin complexes to which IgG has bound are subsequently captured by protein G-sepharose beads. After washing, the amount of anti-PF4/heparin antibody complexes immobilized to the beads is measured using a substrate reaction of labeled streptavidin, which binds to the biotinylated PF4.

The fluid-phase ELISA avoids nonspecific binding of antibodies that occurs on the solid phase, and also minimizes exposure of cryptic antigens on denatured PF4. Furthermore, it detects only anti-PF4/heparin antibodies of the IgG class (19).

Detection of anti-PF4/heparin antibodies by Fluid-Phase EIA

Reagents and materials: Dimethylsulfoxide (DMSO), Sigma-Aldrich; Protein G Sepharose 4 Fast Flow, GE Healthcare Life Science; Heparin Sepharose™ 6 Fast Flow, GE Healthcare Life Science; PF4, Chromatec, Greifswald, Germany; danaparoid, Orgaran®, Organon, The Netherlands; TMB Substrate Reagent Set, Pharmingen; Tween 20 (polyoxyethylene-sorbitan monolaurate), Sigma-Aldrich; Bicinchoninic Acid Kit for Protein Determination, Sigma-Aldrich; bovine serum albumin (BSA), Sigma-Aldrich; unfractionated heparin (UFH), Braun, Melsungen, Germany; low molecular weight heparin reviparin, Clivarin®, Abbott GmbH & Co. KG, Germany; Biotin-NHS-Ester (d-Biotinoyl-ε-aminocaproic acid *N*-hydroxysuccinimide ester), Sigma-Aldrich; streptavidin–horseradish peroxidase diluted 1:5,000 in dilution buffer, Dianova, Hamburg, Germany; Dulbecco phosphate-buffered saline (DPBS).

Buffers:

1. Washing buffer **1**	Phosphate-buffered saline (PBS) pH 7.4
2. Coating buffer **1**	0.15 M PBS, 20 mM Hepes, pH 7.4 (2.383 g Hepes in 500 ml PBS)
3. Washing buffer **2**	0.8 M NaCl, 20 mM Hepes, 5 mM EDTA, pH 7.4
4. Elution buffer	2 M NaCl, 20 mM HEPES pH 7.5, 5 mM EDTA
5. DPBS-tween	PBS + 0.05% tween 20
6. Dilution buffer	PBS-tween + 1% BSA

Procedural Steps (biotinylation of PF4)

Step 1. Coating of heparin sepharose beads with PF4
This step is required to protect PF4–heparin-binding sites. Equilibrate 5 ml heparin sepharose beads with washing buffer **1** (3 × 50 ml). 2 ml of the washed beads are mixed with 14 ml coating buffer **1**. Add 400 μl of purified PF4 [2.5 mg/ml] (=1 mg PF4) to the beads and stir for 15 min. Incubate overnight at 4°C.

Step 2. Biotinylation of PF4

The PF4–heparin–sepharose beads are mixed and brought back to room temperature (RT). 400 μl of biotin (made fresh at 10 mg/ml in DMSO) are added to the PF4–heparin–sepharose suspension. Stir at room temperature for 1 h. Pack a small column with the PF4–heparin–sepharose suspension. The beads are washed (4 × 14 ml) with washing buffer **2**. Elute the bound biotinylated PF4 with elution buffer **1**. Collect 500 μl fractions. The protein concentration in the fractions is determined using BCA protein assay reagents. Pool PF4–biotin-containing fractions.

Step 3. Removal of the unbound biotin

The biotinylated PF4 is purified using an S-sepharose column (GE Healthcare Life Science) to remove the unbound biotin. PF4 binds to the S-sepharose while unbound biotin is washed away. PF4–biotin preparation is diluted 1:3 in water and applied to a 7 ml column of S-sepharose. The column is washed with washing buffer **2**. Elute the bound biotinylated PF4 with elution buffer. Collect 500 μl fractions. The protein concentration in the fractions is determined using bicinchoninic acid kit. Pool PF4–biotin-containing fractions.

Procedural Steps (Fluid-Phase Enzyme Immunoassay)

Step 1. Generation of the PF4/heparin complexes

PF4 (20 μg/ml, 5–30% biotinylated) is mixed with an optimal concentration of heparin in PBS-tween. Depending on the PF4 used and the method of biotinylation, the optimal percent of biotinylated PF4 may range between 5 and 30%. Optimal final heparin(oid) concentrations are the following: UFH: 0.6 IU/ml; low-molecular-weight heparin (LMWH): 0.5 IU/ml; danaparoid 0.1 aFXaU/ml;

Step 2. Generation of PF4–heparin(oid)–IgG complexes

Samples (serum/plasma), negative and positive control, are diluted 1:10 in dilution buffer. Mix 200 μl diluted test samples and 200 μl antigen mixture (PF4/heparin complex, see step 1) in a microcentrifuge tube. One microcentrifuge tube is used as "blank tube" (only dilution buffer). Incubate at room temperature for 1 h.

Step 3. Immobilization of PF4–heparin(oid)–IgG complexes on Protein G Sepharose beads

Add 10 μl of protein G sepharose to 190 μl samples of PF4–heparin(oid)–IgG complexes in microcentrifuge tube in duplicate, and incubate for 1 h at room temperature. Wash sepharose beads to separate from unbound antigen three times with DPBS-tween as follows: add 500 μl DPBS-tween in the tube. Centrifuge (120 × *g*/min, 5 min) and discard the supernatant. Resuspend sepharose pellets carefully.

Step 4. Incubation with Detection antibody

Sepharose pellets are resuspended with 100 μl of streptavidin–horseradish peroxidase dilution. Incubate the tubes for 30 min at room temperature.

Step 5. Incubation with Substrate reagent (e.g., TMB substrate)
Wash the sepharose pellets three times. Add 400 μl substrate buffers to the tubes and resuspend the sepharose pellets carefully. Incubate for 15 min in the dark for color development. Centrifuge (120×*g*/min, 5 min) the tubes and transfer an aliquot of supernatant liquid in a microtiter plate (pre-add an equal volume of 2 mol/l sulfuric acid to each well to stop the enzyme reaction). Read the optical density for each well with a microplate reader set at 450 nm.

Data analysis
Subtract the average OD of the "blank well" from the OD of all other wells. Cutoff value for detection of anti-PF4/heparin antibodies should be defined by determining the mean and standard deviation of 20 normal plasmas.

3.1.2 Particle Gel Immunoassay

This assay is a column agglutination assay that utilizes PF4/heparin complexes bound to red polystyrene beads. After addition of patient serum or plasma, the anti-PF4/heparin antibodies bind to the antigen-coated beads and agglutinate them. Agglutination is further enhanced by antihuman IgG in the column. Upon centrifugation the agglutinated red-colored beads (indicating the presence of anti-PF4/heparin antibodies) do not migrate through a sephacryl gel, forming a red band at the top, whereas nonagglutinated beads (indicating the absence of antibodies) pass through the gel, thus forming a red band at the bottom of the column. Qualitative visualization of agglutination strength is provided comparable to other ID-micro-typing systems (20).

The test kit contains a positive control. Serial dilution of the patient serum enables semiquantitative assessment of the antibody titer. Weak agglutination strength is normally not associated with clinically relevant HIT. The particle gel immunoassay does not distinguish between IgG, IgA, and IgM antibodies.

This assay is only available from a commercial provider and test instructions of the manufacturer should be followed.

3.1.3 Particle Immunofiltration Assay

Patient serum is added to a reaction well containing blue-colored particles coated with PF4. Subsequently, nonagglutinated—but not agglutinated particles—will migrate through a membrane filter. A negative test is shown by a blue color in the result well, whereas no color indicates a positive test. The particle immunofiltration assay (PIFA), compared with the ELISA, appears to produce considerable false negative and false positive results (21), and seems to show a poor correlation with the 4Ts score (22). Because of its unsatisfying sensitivity and specificity, its use can currently not be recommended.

3.2 Functional (Activation) Assays

Functional assays detect HIT antibody-mediated activation of platelets from healthy donors. As this activation is mediated by platelet FcγIIa-receptors only IgG antibodies can be detected.

In contrast to antigen assays, functional assays detect also antibodies against other (rare) antigens like IL-8/heparin or NAP-2/heparin. Sensitive assays require washed platelets.

3.2.1 Aggregation Assay

Platelet-rich plasma (PRP) from a healthy donor, patient serum, and heparin are incubated in an aggregometer under stirring. HIT antibodies cause platelet aggregation after a time lag of about 5–10 min when heparin (0.5–1.0 IU/ml) is added. The aggregation assay is less sensitive than the washed platelet assays and reveals sometimes false positive results, especially in critically ill patients. Standardization is difficult. Therefore, aggregation assays utilizing PRP should not be conducted anymore for exclusion of HIT antibodies.

Detection of heparin-dependent antibodies by the aggregation test using an aggregometer

Reagents and materials:

Aggregometer (Born Method).
Aggregometer cuvette 200 μl.
Heparin (UFH): Braun, Melsungen, Germany; ACD-A: Baxter; collagenreagenz Horm®: NYCOMED Austria.

Step 1. Preparation of platelet
Collection of 20 ml citrated blood (1.6 vol adenine-citrate-dextrose (ACD) + 8.4 vol blood) from 4 healthy donors who did not receive any medication within the previous 10 days.

(a) Preparation of PRP
Centrifuge citrated blood at 120 × *g* for 20 min at room temperature, without brake to generate PRP. Take care that the centrifuge is well balanced and vibrations are avoided. After centrifugation transfer PRP in 10 ml polystyrole tubes (approximately 5–6 ml); use one tube per donor. Centrifuge the remaining whole blood at high speed to obtain platelet-poor plasma (PPP). Adjust final cell count of PRP to 3×10^8 platelets/ml with PPP of the same donor.

Step 2. Sample preparation and assay setup
Each serum is tested with platelets from 4 different platelet donors. Add to 200 μl aggregometer cuvettes: 120 μl of PRP (kept at 37°C); 75 μl of heat-inactivated (56°C, 30 min) test or control serum (kept at 37°C); calibrate the aggregometer with PPP; put cuvette into aggregometer at 1,000 rpm; adjust for basic light transmission; add 10 μl heparin (2.1 IU/ml = 0.2 IU/ml f.c.) or buffer (negative control), or 10 μl collagen (1 μg/ml final concentration, positive control for platelet reactivity); platelet aggregation is followed for 15 min.

Data Analysis
Platelets normally do not aggregate after addition of heparin. If the patient has HIT, platelet aggregation occurs within 15 min after

addition of heparin. Cross-reactivity of heparin-induced antibodies with the heparinoid danaparoid-sodium (Orgaran®, AKZO, Organon, The Netherlands) is assessed using 0.2 aFXa units (f.c.) of danaparoid-sodium instead of heparin.

3.2.2 Washed Platelet Assays

Washed platelets are resuspended in Tyrode's buffer with physiologic concentrations of Ca^{2+} and Mg^{2+}. Patient serum must be heat-inactivated to avoid thrombin- or complement-induced platelet activation. Both washed platelets and heat-inactivated plasma are incubated with heparin in different concentrations in a microtiter plate. HIT serum causes platelet activation at low (0.1–0.3 IU/ml), but not at high (100 IU/ml), heparin concentrations. This reaction is not blocked by hirudin, but blocked in the presence of the FcγIIa receptor-blocking monoclonal antibody IV.3. Currently, both the HIPA and the SRA have the best ratio of sensitivity (≈95%) to specificity (≈100%) and are regarded as confirmatory tests for HIT antibodies. But they are technically challenging and require experienced laboratory personell stuff (23). Several quality control maneuvers that ensure relatively high specificity for the presence of a potentially pathogenic HIT antibody include the following: (a) use of four platelet donors (since hierarchical variability in platelet donor reactivity to HIT sera exists); (b) use of "weak" and "strong" positive control HIT serum (to be sure that the platelets have acceptable reactivity); (c) demonstrating that high heparin concentrations (100 IU/ml) inhibit the reactivity of HIT serum; and (d) demonstrating that reactivity of HIT serum can be inhibited by an FcγIIa receptor-blocking monoclonal antibody.

Heparin-Induced Platelet Activation Test

The heparin-induced platelet activation (HIPA) test (24) is a washed platelet assay that uses platelet aggregation as platelet activation end point. Test serum and the platelets are incubated in a polysterene microtiter well containing two stainless spheres on a magnetic stirrer. The plates are read every 5 min against an indirect light source to evaluate visually a change in appearance of the reaction mixture from turbid (no aggregation) to transparent (aggregation). Aggregation with a time lag <30 min at therapeutic (0.2 IU/ml), which is inhibited at high (100 IU/ml) heparin concentration, of platelets of more than two of the four donors is a positive test result. The time lag correlates inversely to the antibody reactivity.

ASSAY LAB DETAILS START

Heparin-Induced Platelet Activation (*HIPA test*)
Reagents and materials: Stainless steel spheres: SKF, Schweinfurt, Germany; Microtiter plates: Greiner BIO-ONE, cat. no: 650101, Nürtingen, Germany; Apyrase: SIGMA-Aldrich, cat. no: A7646; Aqua ad iniectabilia: B. Braun Melsungen AG, Melsungen, Germany; Glucose solution for infusion (10%): B. Braun Melsungen AG, Germany; Hirudin: Pentapharm, Basel, Switzerland; Heparin

(UFH): Braun, Melsungen, Germany; ACD-A: Baxter; collagen reagent Horm: NYCOMED Austria; SKF-Lösung: NYCOMED Austria; Albumin bovine Fraction V: Serva, Heidelberg, Germany.

Buffers:

1. Modified Tyrode's buf fer	
80 ml a. dest	
+5.00 ml bicarbonate buffer	
+1.75 ml BSA 20% (without NaN_3)	
+1.00 ml glucose solution 10%	
Add aqua dest to 100 ml	
2. Washing buffer	
10 ml mod. Tyrode's buffer	
+25 µl apyrase (1,000 U/ml; Sigma, Germany)	
+10 µl hirudin (1,000 U/ml; Pentapharm, Ltd.)	
Adjust to pH 6.3 with 0.1 m HCl	
3. Suspension buffer	
50 ml mod. Tyrode's buffer	
+0.5 ml magnesium chloride solution	
+1.0 ml calcium chloride solution	
Adjust to pH 7.2 with 0.1 m HCl	
4. Bicarbonate buffer	
16.0 g NaCl	
0.4 g KCl	
2.0 g $NaHCO_3$	
0.1 g NaH_2PO_4	Add to 100 ml aqua dest
5. Magnesium chloride solution	
21.723 g $MgCl_2 \times 6H_2O$	Add to 500 ml aqua dest
6. Calcium chloride solution	
7.35 g $CaCl_2 \times 2H_2O$	Add to 500 ml aqua dest

The HIPA-Assay is a sensitive functional assay for the detection of heparin-dependent antibodies. The most important preanalytical step in the procedure is washing of platelets. The second important issue is the use of appropriate controls:
Preparation of platelets:

Collect 20 ml citrated blood (1.6 vol ACD + 8.4 vol blood) from four healthy donors who did not receive any medication within the previous 10 days. Incubate the citrated blood in sealed tubes at room temperature for 15 min in angle of 45°. Centrifuge citrated blood at 120 × *g* for 20 min at room temperature, without brake to generate PRP. Take care that the centrifuge is well balanced and vibrations are avoided. After centrifugation transfer PRP in 10 ml new polystyrole tubes (approximately 5–6 ml); use 1 tube per donor. Add 111 μl ACD-A (37°C) per ml PRP. Add 5 μl apyrase (1,000 U/ml) (grade IV SIGMA, Munich, Germany) per ml. Centrifuge PRP (650 × *g*, 7 min, without brake).

The next step is critical. Discard supernatant by turning the tube and putting the tube upside down on a pack of 4–6 paper towels or filter paper. This will remove the remaining plasma and makes washing more effective. Resuspend the platelet pellets carefully in 1 ml washing buffer (37°C, modified Tyrode's buffer containing 25 U apyrase, 10 U hirudin [Pentapharm, Basel, Swiss], adjusted to pH 6.3 with 0.1 M HCL). The buffer needs to be added to the pellet as soon as possible after centrifugation. Use a 1,000 μl Eppendorf pipette for resuspension aspirating several times about 300 μl; avoid any foam or bubbles. If done correctly the platelet pellet will resuspend nicely without any aggregates. There should be no red blood cells at the bottom of the pellet. After resuspension of the pellet the tube is filled up to 5 ml with washing buffer. Platelets are incubated in sealed tubes (15 min, 37°C) and centrifuged again (650 × *g*, 7 min, without brake). After centrifugation, the supernatant is discarded and platelet pellets again carefully resuspended in 1 ml suspension buffer (37°C, modified Tyrode`s buffer containing 0.212 M $MgCl_2$ and 0.196 M $CaCl_2$, adjusted to pH 7.2 with 0.1 M HCl). Details for washing and resuspending are the same as described above.

Adjust washed platelets 300×10^9/l in suspension buffer and incubate in a sealed tube for 45 min, 37°C.

Sample preparation and assay setup: (see Table 1)
Each serum is tested with platelets from 4 different platelet donors. All experiments are performed in duplicate. 20 μl heat-inactivated (56°C, 30 min) patient serum are dispensed per U-shaped well of a microtiter plate (Greiner, Nürtingen, Germany) containing two stainless steel spheres (2 mm diameter, SKF, Schweinfurt, Germany). Then 10 μl suspension buffer (negative control) and 10 μl collagen (1 μg/ml final concentration, positive control for platelet function) are placed in U-shaped wells of the microtiter tray. High concentrations (10 μl, 1,050 IU/ml = 100 IU/ml f.c.) of UFH are added to saturate all heparin-binding sites of PF4. After this, the platelet suspension (75 μl), hirudin (10 μl, 500 IU/ml = 50 IU/ml f.c.), and, finally, low concentrations of heparin (10 μl, 2.1 IU/ml = 0.2 IU/ml f.c.) are added to allow PF4/heparin complex formation under optimal conditions. The microtiter plate is incubated at room temperature on a magnetic stirrer (1,000 rpm) for 45 min.

Table 1
Pipette scheme for the HIPA Assay

	Suspension buffer	2.1 aFXa/ml Heparin[a] = 0.2 U/ml f.c. 500 IU/ml Hirudin = 50 U/ml f.c.	1,050 IE/ml Heparin[b] = 100 U/ml f.c	2.1 aFXaU/ml Heparinoid[c] = 0.2 U/ml f.c.	10 μg/ml Collagen = 1 μg/ml f.c.	Heat-inactivated patient serum	Platelet suspension (300×10^9/l)
Control with buffer (negative control)	10 μl					20 μl	75 μl
Low heparin concentration should become positive in case of HIT		10 μl				20 μl	75 μl
High heparin concentration should remain negative in case of HIT			10 μl			20 μl	75 μl
Cross-reactivity with other heparinoid/heparin				10 μl		20 μl	75 μl
Verification of the platelet function (positive control)	20 μl				10 μl		75 μl

[a]We use the low-molecular-weight heparin reviparin
[b]We use unfractionated heparin
[c]Heparinoid danaparoid

The transparency of the suspension is assessed using an indirect light source every 5 min.

Diagnostic criteria:
A sample is considered positive for HIT antibodies if the suspension becomes transparent due to platelet aggregation with 0.2 U/ml heparin (f.c.) but not with 100 U/ml heparin (f.c.). A sample is considered positive if positive results were obtained with test platelets of at least two of the four donors. If platelet activation occurs with all test platelets in the presence of low and high heparin concentrations, the sample is considered indeterminate due to nonspecific reaction. High heparin concentrations inhibit HIT–IgG-mediated platelet activation, but not activation caused by circulating immune complexes. It is possible to prevent nonspecific platelet activation caused by circulating immune complexes by the addition of Fc-receptor-blocking monoclonal antibody which inhibits HIT–IgG-mediated platelet activation. Cross-reactivity of HIT with the heparinoid danaparoid-sodium (Orgaran®, AKZO, Organon, The Netherlands) is assessed using 0.2 aFXa units (f.c.) of danaparoid-sodium instead of heparin.

Serotonin Release Assay

The serotonin release assay (SRA) (25) is a washed platelet assay that uses detection of serotonin release as platelet activation end point. Initially, platelets are radioactively labeled with ^{14}C-serotonin. After incubation the amount of radioactivity present in the supernatant is measured by scintillation counting, and is proportional to platelet activation. The result is expressed as percentage of serotonin released compared to the total amount of serotonin in the platelets. A serotonin release of >20% at therapeutic (0.1–0.3 IU/ml), which is inhibited at high (100 IU/ml) heparin concentration, is a positive test result. Laboratories require licenses to handle radioisotopes, thus limiting routine use of this assay.

Serotonin Release Test
Prepare PRP as described for the HIPA test. Then add 14C-serotonin (0.1 µCi/ml of PRP added from a stock solution of 50 µCi/ml of [14C]serotonin) (GE Healthcare) and incubate for 30 min at 37°C in sealed tubes.

From here onwards prepare platelets and run the assay exactly as described for the HIPA test. However, for the absolute value 3 additional wells containing 75 µl platelet suspension and 30 µl buffer are needed. Instead of stirring the samples with two steel spheres per well on a magnetic stirrer, the plate can also be placed on a plate shaker and rotated at about 300–500 rpm.

After a 45-min incubation add 100 µl ice-cold 5% EDTA solution, remove two times 75 µl from three wells for maximal radioactivity value, and centrifuge the microtiter plate at 800 × *g* for 10 min. Take two times 75 µl supernatant per well and transfer into a scintillation fluid, and measure radioactivity by a beta counter. Use the following formula for calculation:

$$\frac{\text{Counts patient sample} - \text{counts background} \times 100}{\text{Max counts} - \text{counts background}} = \%\ \text{serotonin release.}$$

Miscellaneous Washed Platelet Activation Assays

Further techniques allowing evaluation of the platelet activation end point include (a) quantitation of platelet-derived microparticle generation using flow cytometry; (b) quantitation of serotonin release by ELISA, and (c) assessment of ADP release by activated platelets using luminography. These assays do not differ substantially from the HIPA test or SRA as the actual method of detection of platelet activation is less important for test quality than the technique of platelet preparation itself.

4 Specimen

ELISAs are performed using plasma or serum depending on manufacturer's specifications. The specimen is relatively stable, and antibody detection is feasible within 72 h after blood withdrawal. The particle gel immunoassay should be performed using serum as fibrin clots might mimic false positive test results if plasma is used.

Functional assays should be performed using patient serum. EDTA-anticoagulated plasma is not suitable as EDTA inhibits platelet function. The specimen is relatively stable, and antibody detection is feasible within 72 h after blood withdrawal.

5 Test Sensitivities and Specificities for Clinical HIT

With exception of the platelet aggregation test using PRP, most of the current laboratory tests for HIT antibodies are very sensitive, but they differ considerably in their diagnostic specificity. Only a subset of anti-PF4/heparin antibodies is capable to activate platelets, and thereby to cause clinical HIT.

As anti-PF4/heparin antibodies of the IgM and IgA class are not able to engage the platelet FcγRIIa receptor it remains unclear to what extent anti-PF4/heparin antibodies of the IgM and IgA class are pathogenic. Accordingly, polyspecific ELISAs (detecting IgG/A/M) appear to have a higher sensitivity for clinically irrelevant antibodies (1, 26). Nevertheless, the sensitivity for detection of clinically relevant anti-PF4/heparin antibodies is similarly high (»99%) for the polyspecific ELISA (detecting IgG/A/M), for the IgG-specific ELISA, and for the washed platelet activation assays (HIPA and SRA) (1, 26). Therefore, in a patient strongly suspected as having clinical HIT laboratory testing is excellent for ruling out HIT antibodies (high negative predictive value).

Test specificities vary from »50–75% (polyspecific ELISA) to »55–90% (IgG-specific ELISA) and 95–99% (washed platelet activation assays) (1, 16, 26). Thus, the value of a positive test for HIT antibodies (positive predictive value) strongly depends on the assay performed and concomitant clinical variables (e.g., type of anticoagulant, patient population, pretest probability of HIT). Washed platelet activation assays have the most favorable sensitivity/specificity ratio.

In all assays the strength of the reaction correlates directly with the probability of clinically relevant HIT. Therefore, all results should not only be reported qualitatively as positive or negative but additionally (semi)quantitatively. For instance, probability of HIT is proportional to optical density of the ELISA. Thus HIT is probable if the patient presents with a strong positive ELISA (>1.0 OD units), but unlikely in patients with a weak positive result (0.5–1.0 OD) (1, 27).

Limited studies on the diagnostic value of the particle gel immunoassay (16, 20, 28) reveal sensitivity and specificity for HIT that may be intermediate between the washed platelet activation assays and the standard ELISA for selected samples. Its biggest advantage is its fast turnaround time of less than 15 min. Its biggest disadvantage is the difficulty to distinguish weak reactions from negative results. Diagnostic significance can be improved if plasma testing positive or borderline is progressively diluted, and a quantitative result (last positive titer) is reported (28). Patients judged clinically to have had probable or highly probable/definite HIT had antibody titers of 4 or more in 39 of 54 (72%) cases, compared with only 2 of 85 (2%) judged "unlikely" to have had HIT (28).

6 Recommendation for a Diagnostic Algorithm (29–33)

1. Assess pretest probability for HIT (e.g., using the "4Ts"). Patients with a low pretest probability for HIT need not undergo further testing and heparin can be maintained.
2. In patients with an intermediate pretest probability of HIT a combined approach using the "4Ts" together with an ELISA (27) or the particle gel immune assay (16) is a reliable strategy to rule out HIT in case of a negative test result and heparin can be maintained. Positive test results in either screening assay indicate the presence of anti-PF4/heparin antibodies and require further IgG classification. Until these results are available, anticoagulation can be switched to an alternative anticoagulant.
3. If the test for anti-PF4/heparin IgG is negative or weak positive IgG (OD < 1.0), the anti-PF4/heparin antibodies are most likely non-platelet-activating. A strong positive test for anti-PF4/heparin IgG (OD > 1.0), however, indicates an increased

risk for the presence of platelet-activating anti-PF4/heparin antibodies. In these patients, anticoagulation should be switched to an alternative anticoagulant.

4. At least sera showing a positive result in the screening test samples should be assessed by a washed platelet activation assay. A positive test demonstrates platelet-activating properties of anti-PF4/heparin antibodies and makes HIT very likely. A negative functional assay makes clinically relevant HIT unlikely.
5. Clinical reassessment and (sometimes) repeated testing (of the same sample) are required for final confirmation or exclusion of the diagnosis of HIT. However, it is a misconception to retest patients over several days. About 35% of patients after cardiac surgery will then become positive in the antigen assays without having HIT (lower part of the iceberg).

References

1. Greinacher A, Juhl D, Strobel U et al (2007) Heparin-induced thrombocytopenia: a prospective study on the incidence, platelet-activating capacity and clinical significance of antiplatelet factor 4/heparin antibodies of the IgG, IgM, and IgA classes. J Thromb Haemost 5:1666–1673
2. Lo GK, Sigouin CS, Warkentin TE (2007) What is the potential for overdiagnosis of heparin-induced thrombocytopenia? Am J Hematol 82:1037–1043
3. Warkentin TE (1999) Heparin-induced thrombocytopenia: a clinicopathologic syndrome. Thromb Haemost 82:439–447
4. Amiral J, Bridey F, Dreyfus M et al (1992) Platelet factor 4 complexed to heparin is the target for antibodies generated in heparin-induced thrombocytopenia. Thromb Haemost 68:95–96
5. Greinacher A, Potzsch B, Amiral J et al (1994) Heparin-associated thrombocytopenia: isolation of the antibody and characterization of a multimolecular PF4-heparin complex as the major antigen. Thromb Haemost 71:247–251
6. Rauova L, Poncz M, McKenzie SE et al (2005) Ultralarge complexes of PF4 and heparin are central to the pathogenesis of heparin-induced thrombocytopenia. Blood 105:131–138
7. Rauova L, Zhai L, Kowalska MA et al (2006) Role of platelet surface PF4 antigenic complexes in heparin-induced thrombocytopenia pathogenesis: diagnostic and therapeutic implications. Blood 107:2346–2353
8. Greinacher A, Gopinadhan M, Gunther JU et al (2006) Close approximation of two platelet factor 4 tetramers by charge neutralization forms the antigens recognized by HIT antibodies. Arterioscler Thromb Vasc Biol 26:2386–2393
9. Warkentin TE, Cook RJ, Marder VJ et al (2005) Anti-platelet factor 4/heparin antibodies in orthopedic surgery patients receiving antithrombotic prophylaxis with fondaparinux or enoxaparin. Blood 106:3791–3796
10. Denomme GA (2007) Platelet and leukocyte Fcγ receptors in heparin-induced thrombocytopenia. In: Warkentin TE, Greinacher A (eds) Heparin-induced thrombocytopenia, 4th edn. Informa Healthcare, New York, pp 187–208
11. Warkentin TE (1996) Heparin-induced thrombocytopenia: IgG-mediated platelet activation, platelet microparticle generation, and altered procoagulant/anticoagulant balance in the pathogenesis of thrombosis and venous limb gangrene complicating heparin-induced thrombocytopenia. Transfus Med Rev 10:249–258
12. Greinacher A, Farner B, Kroll H et al (2005) Clinical features of heparin-induced thrombocytopenia including risk factors for thrombosis. a retrospective analysis of 408 patients. Thromb Haemost 94:132–135
13. Arepally GM, Poncz M, Cines DB (2007) Immune vascular injury in heparin-induced thrombocytopenia. In: Warkentin TE, Greinacher A (eds) Heparin-induced thrombocytopenia, 4th edn. Informa Healthcare, New York, pp 209–225
14. Warkentin TE (2007) Clinical picture of heparin-induced thrombocytopenia. In: Warkentin TE, Greinacher A (eds) Heparin-induced thrombocytopenia, 4th edn. Informa Healthcare, New York, pp 21–66

15. Lo GK, Juhl D, Warkentin TE et al (2006) Evaluation of pretest clinical score (4 T's) for the diagnosis of heparin-induced thrombocytopenia in two clinical settings. J Thromb Haemost 4:759–765
16. Pouplard C, Gueret P, Fouassier M et al (2007) Prospective evaluation of the "4Ts" score and particle gel immunoassay specific to heparin/PF4 for the diagnosis of heparin-induced thrombocytopenia. J Thromb Haemost 5:1373–1379
17. Warkentin TE, Kelton JG (2001) Temporal aspects of heparin-induced thrombocytopenia. N Engl J Med 344:1286–1292
18. Vissac AM, Catala M, Amiral JJ (2007) Incidence of the various heparin dependent antibody isotypes in a group of patients with heparin induced thrombocytopenia. J Thromb Haemost 5(Suppl):P-T-318
19. Newman PM, Swanson RL, Chong BH (1998) Heparin-induced thrombocytopenia: IgG binding to PF4-heparin complexes in the fluid phase and cross-reactivity with low molecular weight heparin and heparinoid. Thromb Haemost 80:292–297
20. Eichler P, Raschke R, Lubenow N et al (2002) The new ID-heparin/PF4 antibody test for rapid detection of heparin-induced antibodies in comparison with functional and antigenic assays. Br J Haematol 116:887–891
21. Warkentin TE, Sheppard JI, Raschke R et al (2007) Performance characteristics of a rapid assay for anti-PF4/heparin antibodies: the particle immunofiltration assay. J Thromb Haemost 5:2308–2310
22. Francis JL, Drexler A, Duncan MK et al (2006) Prospective evaluation of laboratory tests for the diagnosis of heparin-induced thrombocytopenia. Blood 108:312a
23. Eichler P, Budde U, Haas S et al (1999) First workshop for detection of heparin-induced antibodies: validation of the heparin-induced platelet-activation test (HIPA) in comparison with a PF4/heparin ELISA. Thromb Haemost 81:625–629
24. Greinacher A, Michels I, Kiefel V et al (1991) A rapid and sensitive test for diagnosing heparin-associated thrombocytopenia. Thromb Haemost 66:734–736
25. Sheridan D, Carter C, Kelton JG (1986) A diagnostic test for heparin-induced thrombocytopenia. Blood 67:27–30
26. Warkentin TE, Sheppard JA, Moore JC et al (2005) Laboratory testing for the antibodies that cause heparin-induced thrombocytopenia: how much class do we need? J Lab Clin Med 146:341–346
27. Janatpour KA, Gosselin RC, Dager WE et al (2007) Usefulness of optical density values from heparin-platelet factor 4 antibody testing and probability scoring models to diagnose heparin-induced thrombocytopenia. Am J Clin Pathol 127:429–433
28. Alberio L, Kimmerle S, Baumann A et al (2003) Rapid determination of anti-heparin/platelet factor 4 antibody titers in the diagnosis of heparin-induced thrombocytopenia. Am J Med 114:528–536
29. Selleng S, Selleng K, Wollert HG et al (2008) Heparin-induced thrombocytopenia in patients requiring prolonged intensive care unit treatment after cardiopulmonary bypass. J Thromb Haemost 6:428–435
30. Crowther MA, Cook DJ, Meade MO et al (2005) Thrombocytopenia in medical-surgical critically ill patients: prevalence, incidence, and risk factors. J Crit Care 20:348–353
31. Lee DH, Warkentin TE (2007) Frequency of heparin-induced thrombocytopenia. In: Warkentin TE, Greinacher A (eds) Heparin-induced thrombocytopenia, 4th edn. Informa Healthcare, New York, pp 67–116
32. Warkentin TE, Greinacher A (2004) Heparin-induced thrombocytopenia: recognition, treatment, and prevention: the seventh accp conference on antithrombotic and thrombolytic therapy. Chest 126:311S–337S
33. Pouplard C, May MA, Regina S et al (2005) Changes in platelet count after cardiac surgery can effectively predict the development of pathogenic heparin-dependent antibodies. Br J Haematol 128:837–841

Part VI

Examples of Tests for Inhibitors of Coagulation

Chapter 24

Nijmegen-Bethesda Assay to Measure Factor VIII Inhibitors

Elizabeth Duncan, Margaret Collecutt, and Alison Street

Abstract

Hemophilia A is an inherited bleeding disorder caused by a deficiency of factor VIII coagulant activity (FVIII:C). Patients are treated with infusions of either plasma-derived or recombinant factor VIII. However, some patients develop inhibitory antibodies (inhibitors) to infused factor VIII which render it ineffective. The original Bethesda method was developed to standardize measurement of inhibitors in a factor VIII neutralization assay. One Bethesda unit is defined as that amount of inhibitor that results in 50% residual FVIII:C activity of a defined test mixture. In the Nijmegen modification of the original Bethesda method, the pH and the protein concentration of the test mixture is further standardized. As a result, the FVIII:C in the test mixture is less prone to artifactual deterioration and the test has improved specificity. Even with a standardized procedure a number of factors can affect the performance of the test and it is important for laboratory staff to be aware of their impact on the result outcome.

Key words Factor VIII, Hemophilia, Coagulation, Inhibitor

1 Introduction

Hemophilia A is a sex-linked hereditary bleeding disorder characterized by a reduced level of factor VIII (FVIII) in blood. Bleeding episodes may occur spontaneously in the severe form of hemophilia or after trauma in the milder forms. Treatment for children and adults is available with various recombinant FVIII products and plasma-derived FVIII concentrate. However, treatment may cause inhibitory antibodies (inhibitors) to form against FVIII and the reported incidence ranges from 0 to 33% of patients (1–3). The inhibitors may be transient or persistent and in the latter case they become a lifelong problem. This complication most often develops in childhood and then it usually occurs after the first 10–20 days of treatment with FVIII. However inhibitors may develop later in life, for example in mild hemophilia patients who have had little or no previous exposure to FVIII treatment (4, 5), or in rare cases following a change in product formulation (6). Infused FVIII is relatively ineffective when given to hemophilia A patients with an inhibitor. This group of patients is very difficult to treat and they

Paul Monagle (ed.), *Haemostasis: Methods and Protocols*, Methods in Molecular Biology, vol. 992,
DOI 10.1007/978-1-62703-339-8_24, © Springer Science+Business Media New York 2013

have a high rate of morbidity and mortality. Immune tolerance regimens have been developed to abolish factor VIII and IX inhibitors in up to 80% of selected patients, with best success rates if the program is started early and when the inhibitor titre is <10 Bethesda units/mL (BU/mL) (7). For those patients with persistent inhibitors >5 BU/mL, treatment with activated clotting factors (e.g., recombinant factor VIIa, activated prothrombin complex concentrates) has become the mainstay of therapy (7).

Acquired hemophilia is a serious bleeding disorder in which autoantibodies to FVIII develop in previously normal individuals and neutralize most of their available FVIII. The frequency of this condition is 1–2 per million per year. Treatment for bleeding is as for a patient with inherited hemophilia and an inhibitor. In addition, immunosuppressive treatment is used to suppress production of the antibody (7).

The detection and measurement of FVIII inhibitors are thus an important role of the haemostasis laboratory. It is necessary to diagnose inhibitors when they first arise and to measure the inhibitor concentration. Then it may be necessary to monitor the level and determine whether the inhibitor is persistent or transient (7, 8). For those patients receiving immune modulation therapy it is necessary to monitor inhibitor levels during and after treatment.

In this chapter we describe the original Bethesda method (9), with the Nijmegen modification proposed by Verbruggen et al. (10). The Scientific Standardization Committee of the International Society on Thrombosis and Haemostasis recommend the Bethesda assay with the Nijmegen modification for inhibitor measurement (10, 11). We will mainly focus on measurement of FVIII inhibitors. However, the procedure may be modified to quantitate inhibitors to factor IX or any other clotting factor measured using a functional assay, and this application will be briefly described (12–15).

In the original Bethesda method (9), test plasma is mixed with an equal volume of a normal plasma pool (NPP) and incubated for 2 h at 37°C. A control mixture is prepared by incubating an equal volume of the NPP with imidazole buffer. After 2 h the factor VIII coagulant activity (FVIII:C) of each mixture is measured using the one-stage assay. The FVIII:C of the test mixture is compared with that of the control and the percentage of residual FVIII:C is calculated. One Bethesda unit (BU) is defined as that amount of inhibitor that results in 50% residual FVIII:C activity. The BU/mL in the sample is determined from the theoretical inhibitor graph by interpolating the percentage residual activity against Bethesda units. Only percentage residual FVIII:C between 25 and 75% can be used to determine the inhibitor level. For an inhibitor >2 BU/mL, dilutions of patient plasma are also tested and the result corrected for the dilution factor.

The Nijmegen modification of the original Bethesda method (referred to here as the Nijmegen-Bethesda method) was developed to address two shortfalls of the assay and improve specificity (10). Firstly, the NPP used in the test and control mixtures is buffered to pH 7.4 using 0.1 M imidazole (final concentration). This is to maintain the test and control mixtures at pH 7.4 over the 2 h incubation period. Secondly, a source of immuno-depleted FVIII-deficient plasma is used in place of imidazole buffer to dilute NPP in the control mixture and to dilute patient samples. This maintains a similar protein concentration in control and test incubations. Together these modifications improve the stability of FVIII in the incubation mixtures and prevent artifactual deterioration of FVIII:C that may be falsely interpreted as being due to an inhibitor (10, 11). As in the original Bethesda method, in the Nijmegen modified method one Bethesda unit (BU) is defined as that amount of inhibitor that results in 50% residual FVIII:C activity (see Note 7) (10).

2 Materials

2.1 Nijmegen-Bethesda Assay

1. Buffered normal plasma pool (B-NPP).

   Commercial sources of buffered citrated plasma prepared from a pool of normal donors are available. It is essential to check the product information sheet to ensure that the lyophilized product is buffered and maintains a pH 7.4. Reconstitute according to the manufacturer's directions.

   To prepare the B-NPP in-house, collect blood from at least 20 normal donors and prepare plasma as described in Subheading 3.1. Screen individual plasma samples to ensure normal activated partial thromboplastin time, prothrombin time, and dilute Russell's viper venom time. Using polypropylene plastic containers throughout, pool the plasma, mix well, and measure the volume obtained. While stirring, add solid imidazole to achieve a final concentration of 0.1 M and then adjust the pH to 7.4 by slow addition of 1N HCl (10, 11). Dispense into aliquots of appropriate volume and freeze at −70°C until required. For safety reasons it is recommended that the B-NPP is checked for viral status and only used if negative for blood borne viruses, e.g., hepatitis B and C and HIV.

   An alternative method can be used when smaller volumes of B-NPP are processed. Prepare a 5.0 M imidazole solution and add 20 μL/mL of plasma while mixing well. Follow by immediately adjusting pH to 7.4 with 1N HCl (approximately 28 μL 1N HCl/mL plasma). This method is suitable to use with NPP that have been previously prepared and frozen for other purposes, and then required for use in an inhibitor assay.

2. Factor VIII-deficient plasma.
   Select a commercial source of FVIII-deficient plasma that is either immune-depleted or prepared from patients with severe hemophilia A. Reconstitute according to the manufacturer's directions. For many products it is possible to freeze any left-over plasma at −70°C for use in later inhibitor assays. When using an immuno-depleted FVIII-deficient plasma it is preferable to use one that contains relatively normal levels of von Willebrand factor (see Notes 16 and 17).

   Alternatively, the laboratory may prepare citrated plasma from a patient with severe hemophilia A, without an inhibitor, to use as the FVIII-deficient plasma. However the FVIII level must be <1 IU/dL which precludes donor patients who have received recent FVIII treatment. Also the viral status of the donor patient should be known to the user.
3. Quality control.
   In the absence of a commercially available inhibitor plasma, an in-house source from a patient with a FVIII inhibitor (inherited hemophilia or acquired) may be prepared and stored as described in Subheading 3.1.

   Another quality issue is the need for a program in the laboratory to ensure correct calibration of equipment. This includes regular maintenance of analyzers, pipette volume calibration, water bath temperature set at 37°C, and a timer available to ensure adherence to the 2 h incubation period.

2.2 Factor VIII 1-Stage Assay

Materials required are those that are used by the laboratory for the routine FVIII:C assay. They include FVIII-deficient plasma (see Note 16), APTT reagent, assay buffer, calibrator, and QC material (see Note 9). In the original Bethesda method the one-stage FVIII:C assay was recommended but a chromogenic assay can also be used and in some cases is preferred (see Note 19).

3 Methods

3.1 Preparation of Samples

1. The test requires a minimum of approximately 3 mL citrated whole blood to yield a 1.5 mL plasma sample. Collect blood into citrate anticoagulant concentration 0.105 or 0.129 M with a blood:citrate ratio of 9:1. In some circumstances, e.g., for children, a smaller sample can be used only if blood has been collected in the correct blood:citrate ratio and the extent of testing may be limited.
2. If the patient is also to be given an infusion of FVIII collect the sample before the infusion (see Note 14).
3. On receipt of sample in the laboratory, centrifuge specimen for at least 15 min at minimum of 2,000 × *g*, at 15–20°C. Remove plasma, taking care not to contaminate with platelet pellet, and

aliquot into approximately 0.5–1.0 mL volumes. Label adequately and store plasma at −70°C until required.

4. Samples may be used fresh or frozen. If frozen, thaw samples at 37°C for approximately 5–10 min, then mix by gentle inversion.
5. The calculations used in this assay are based on the assumption that there is no FVIII:C in the patient sample. In samples thought to contain low residual levels of FVIII this can be inactivated by heating approximately 1 mL of plasma in a small tube at 56°C for 10 min (16, 17). This inactivates FVIII present in the sample, but leaves the antibody and its inhibitory activity intact. Recent data shows complete inactivation of all other coagulation factors, even when the starting activity is 1.00 I.U./mL (or 100%) with a 90 min incubation at 58°C (18).
6. After heating, spin the sample for 1–2 min in a micro-centrifuge at full speed (approximately 20,000 × *g*) to remove any precipitated protein. Alternatively, spin for 15 min at 2,000 × *g* as above. Transfer supernatant to a fresh labelled tube, clearly stating "heat inactivated." Store at −70°C to await testing if required. This process does not apply to inhibitor detection for other factors as it does not adequately inactivate factors apart from FVIII. Other approaches are required for those factors (see Subheading 3.6).

3.2 Nijmegen-Bethesda Assay

1. For most automated analyzers a mix of equal volumes of 300 μL to yield a 600 μL final volume for all incubations will provide a sufficient final volume for analysis. This can be adjusted as required.
2. To prepare the control tube, mix an equal volume of VIII-deficient plasma (VIII-def) with B-NPP (see Note 1).
3. A full-strength test and a 1/2 dilution is recommended as a starting point for all patients previously negative for an inhibitor or those with an unknown history.
4. To test a patient sample at full strength, mix an equal volume of test plasma with B-NPP.
5. To test at 1/2, dilute test plasma 1/2 in VIII-def plasma. Then mix an equal volume of this with B-PN.
6. If a high titre of inhibitor is present, 1/5, 1/10, or higher dilutions may be required. These are also prepared by dilution of the test plasma in VIII-def plasma. Then mix with an equal volume of B-PN.
7. For very high levels of inhibitors prepare 1/10 dilution of patient plasma in FVIII-def plasma and then dilute this further to give 1/20, 1/50, and 1/100. Patient plasma can be diluted further as required.

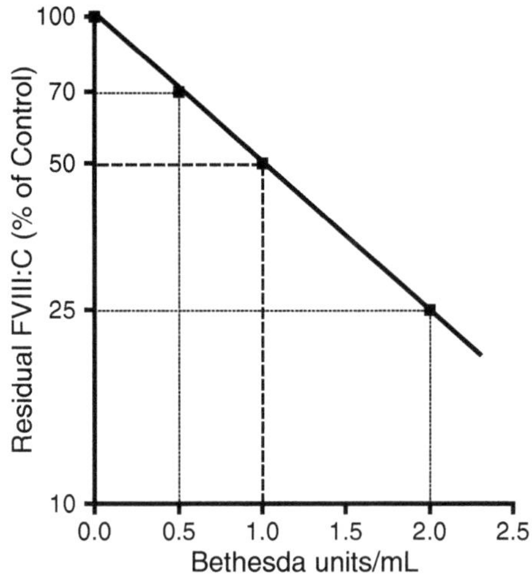

Fig. 1 Inhibitor graph to relate the percent Residual FVIII:C to the Bethesda Units/mL in test plasma

8. Prepare the mixtures in small tubes, cap and incubate at 37°C for 2 h.
9. After 2 h, measure the residual FVIII:C in the test and control mixtures using the routine method in use in your laboratory.
10. Calculate the ratio of residual factor VIII:

$$\text{Residual\_FVIII\_ratio} = \left(\frac{\text{FVIII : C\_patient\_mixture}}{\text{FVIII : C\_control\_mixture}} \right)$$

11. Convert the ratio to a percentage by multiplying by 100.
12. If the result falls between 25 and 75% residual FVIII:C, the BU/mL in the sample is determined from the theoretical inhibitor graph by interpolating the percentage residual activity against Bethesda units (Fig. 1).
13. Incubation mixtures with >75% residual FVIII:C have no detectable inhibitor, i.e., <0.5 BU/mL (see Note 2).
14. Incubation mixtures with high levels of inhibitor and <25% residual FVIII:C should have the test repeated using appropriate dilutions to lie in the 25–75% range. Multiply the answer by the dilution factor used in that mixture and average the results obtained for each valid dilution (see Notes 3–6).
15. If the inhibitor has type II kinetics it may not be possible to average a range of dilutions due to high variation of results. In this case take the lowest dilution of patient plasma to inactivate close to 50% of the FVIII in the incubation mixture, and calculate the BU/mL from this mixture (10, 19, 20).

16. One Bethesda unit/mL (BU/mL) is defined as the amount of inhibitor that causes a 50% reduction in the FVIII supplied in the control mixture (see Note 7) (9, 10).

3.3 Factor VIII Assay

Follow the usual protocol for FVIII:C assay in use in your laboratory. Generally this will be the one-stage FVIII:C assay although a chromogenic method can be used.

3.4 Internal Quality Control

1. Follow the usual quality control procedures for your laboratory for the factor VIII:C assay (see Note 9).
2. The buffered normal plasma, mixed with an equal volume of FVIII-def, should assay at approximately half of its pre-dilution value, within limits of ±10% (see Note 1).
3. If a source of sufficient patient plasma with an inhibitor is available, an internal inhibitor quality control material can be established (see Note 9). This is advisable to establish the imprecision of the assay and also to alert the laboratory of potential assay problems.

3.5 Measurement of Other Factor Inhibitors

The original Bethesda assay and the modified Nijmegen-Bethesda assay are not only applicable to measurement to FVIII inhibitors but can be used to measure inhibitors to other coagulation factors (12–15). Essentially, the test is the same as described above except that the sample is diluted in plasma deficient in the factor of interest. Also, the one-stage assay for the factor of interest is used to measure the percentage of residual factor.

3.6 Samples with Intrinsic Residual Activity of Factor of Interest

If the patient sample has only a mild or moderate reduction in factor level, it cannot be taken that the factor-deficient plasma mixed with an equal volume of B-NPP is the appropriate control for the mixture comprising patient plasma mixed with an equal volume of B-NPP. The factor activity in the test mixture must be corrected for the intrinsic residual activity (10).

1. In the case of FVIII inhibitors and low levels of FVIII:C in the patient sample, FVIII:C can be inactivated by heating the sample at 56°C for 10 min (16, 17) (see step 5 in Subheading 3.1).
2. In the case of specific inhibitors to other coagulation factors and where there are measurable levels of the factor of interest, full inactivation of all coagulation factors is achieved with a 90 min incubation at 58°C even when the starting activity is 1.00 I.U./mL (or 100%) (18).
3. A mathematical approach can be taken to the calculate percentage residual factor. Measure the factor level in the B-NPP and the patient sample before the incubation mixtures are set up. From this information calculate the theoretical factor level in the various mixtures of patient sample in the absence of an inhibitor.

This theoretical value is compared to the factor level after 2 h incubation to determine the percentage residual factor, instead of the value in the control mixture. For example, when testing a full-strength plasma containing 20 U/dL factor IX mixed in equal volume with B-NPP containing 100 U/dL factor IX, the final expected factor IX concentration is 60 U/dL. If, after 2 h incubation, the factor IX level in the mixture is 40 U/dL, this corresponds to 67% residual and approximately 0.55 BU/mL.

4 Notes

1. When testing samples from a number of patients in one batch assay a separate control mixture with every set of patient dilutions and use in the calculation for that patient. Each normal control, when mixed with an equal volume of FVIII-def, should contain approximately half of its starting FVIII:C value.
2. There is a lack of consensus between laboratories on the assay lower limit cutoff for the Nijmegen-Bethesda assay (8), with lower limits between 0.2 and 0.6 BU/mL reported in the literature. A widely used cutoff for a negative result is 0.5 BU/mL (11) which corresponds to 70% residual FVIII:C for full-strength plasma (0.4 BU/mL corresponds to 75% residual FVIII:C). The cutoff value will be influenced by the precision of the procedure (including preparation of incubation mixtures and FVIII:C assay) and should be assessed by each laboratory.
3. Where an inhibitor is detected, the final result is only valid if calculated from a percentage residual FVIII:C between 25 and 75%. If the residual FVIII:C is less than 25% the sample should be further diluted as required and retested. The inhibitor units read from the theoretical inhibitor graph should be multiplied by the dilution factor to obtain the final BU/mL (9, 10).
4. In the majority of patients with inherited hemophilia A and a FVIII inhibitor, the inhibitor shows type I kinetics, i.e., complete and irreversible binding of the antibody to FVIII. In these samples there is a linear correlation between the concentration of inhibitor and the logarithm of the percent residual FVIII:C (10, 21). Also, full-strength plasma or low dilutions of plasma will completely neutralize the added FVIII:C (21).
5. For patients with acquired FVIII Inhibitors and some hemophilia patients the sample dilutions may not show a linear correlation between concentration and percent residual FVIII:C (10, 19, 21). This is due to the type II kinetics, i.e., incomplete and reversible binding of the antibody to FVIII. In this situation, the least dilution of plasma giving close to 50% residual FVIII:C is taken to be the best estimate of the inhibitor level (10, 19). Alternatively an empirical estimation of inhibitor concentration can be used (see Note 6).

6. In another approach to calculation of results, Verbruggen et al. (10) have described an empirical method to calculate the inhibitor level for samples with >2 BU/mL. It is necessary to test a number of dilutions of the sample and prepare a log-log plot of the reciprocal of the plasma dilution (*x*-axis) against percent residual FVIII (*y*-axis). Where possible use at least four mixtures covering the range 25–75% residual FVIII:C. To determine the inhibitor level in the sample, draw a line of best fit and interpolate to the dilution factor that gives 50% residual FVIII:C—this is the BU/mL (10, 22).
7. The units used to report the Nijmegen-Bethesda assay are the same as those used for the original Bethesda method, i.e., Bethesda units/mL (BU/mL) (10). However some workers identify their use of the modified assay by reporting their results as Nijmegen-Bethesda units/mL (NBU/mL) (23, 24). Assay results and the units reported for both methods are calculated in the same way.
8. A FVIII inhibitor assay standard is under development. The aim of this standard material is to improve assay agreement between laboratories (8).
9. Internal quality control for the Nijmegen-Bethesda assay relies heavily on the quality control for the FVIII:C assay used in the measurement phase. A laboratory with access to a sufficient quantity of plasma from a patient with a FVIII inhibitor may be able to prepare in-house quality control material.
10. External quality assurance programs (QAP) for FVIII inhibitors are an ongoing challenge for organizing groups due to the need to source sufficient amounts of appropriate material. However such surveys are very instructive and help to identify assay variables which influence the result (25, 26). All laboratories performing the Nijmegen-Bethesda assay or original Bethesda assay are encouraged to enrol in a survey offering external quality control for this test, e.g., the ECAT Foundation External Quality Assessment Programme in Haemostasis and Thrombosis.
11. There is a high degree of variability between laboratories for results assayed by the Nijmegen-Bethesda method and also the original Bethesda method. In one report the Nijmegen-Bethesda method showed between-laboratory variation of 10–15% compared to variation of 13–33% for the original Bethesda method (25). We have reviewed external QAP reports received in our laboratory and observed much higher variation, with CVs from 20 to 80% for the original Bethesda method and with only a small improvement in CV shown for the Nijmegen modification.
12. The Nijmegen modification of the original Bethesda method improves the specificity of the procedure, such that a lesser

number of false-positive results in the cutoff range of 0.5 BU/mL are reported (11). However, both the original Bethesda method and the Nijmegen modified method might not detect some weak, but clinically significant inhibitors in patients with hemophilia (25, 27, 28).

13. Non-neutralizing antibodies will not be detected by the Bethesda-Nijmegen assay (17, 29). The incidence and clinical importance of such antibodies is uncertain (8, 17).
14. A FVIII inhibitor bound in an immune complex with FVIII will not be detected by the Bethesda-Nijmegen assay (30). Inhibitor detection after infusion of FVIII therapy in patients known or suspected to have an inhibitor may be unsuccessful.
15. The designation of Bethesda units in an inhibitor plasma does not imply that any specific number of factor VIII units infused into the patient would neutralize the circulating inhibitor (9).
16. The type and source of FVIII-deficient plasma used in the procedure can influence inhibitor assay results. Use of a FVIII-deficient plasma that contains relatively normal levels of von Willebrand factor is recommended (23). Also, use of the same FVIII-deficient plasma for both the sample dilution and FVIII:C assay is preferred (23). FVIII-deficient plasma prepared by chemical depletion should be avoided (11, 23).
17. Speculation has been raised that FVIII-deficient plasma prepared using immuno-depletion column technology may, on occasions, be contaminated with anti-FVIII monoclonal antibodies (23). These contaminating antibodies may cause a lower than usual FVIII:C level in the normal plasma control and decrease the inhibitor level determined (23). Inhibitor assessment of the FVIII-deficient plasma used in a procedure may be helpful for quality control or troubleshooting purposes.
18. To reduce the cost of the Nijmegen-Bethesda assay, a 4% bovine-serum albumin buffer can be used to dilute patient samples, instead of factor-deficient plasma (24). This modification maintains similar specificity to the method when factor-deficient plasma is used. However, it is unclear whether this modification causes a loss of the previous gain in performance from the presence of von Willebrand factor when FVIII-deficient plasma is used as the diluent (23).
19. Lupus anticoagulants (LA) may cause a false-positive result as they inhibit the phospholipid-dependent clotting pathway and cause prolongation of assay clotting times. LA can be excluded if the patient has a normal dilute Russell's viper venom clotting time. A coexisting LA and FVIII inhibitor may be suspected if, for example, the patient is positive for LA with a bleeding phenotype and has a FVIII:C that is substantially reduced compared to other clotting factor levels. A chromogenic FVIII

method can be used for the Bethesda assay as this method is not affected by LA and has been shown to be more specific (31). Also, a commercial ELISA developed to detect FVIII inhibitors can help to discriminate between these and a lupus anticoagulant or other factor inhibitors (22).

20. Heparin may cause a false-positive result or falsely elevates the inhibitor level due to inhibition of APTT-dependent tests (26, 32). Blood collected through a port or catheter line is at risk of heparin contamination. Performing a thrombin time (TT) using routine methods can be helpful. A TT within normal limits can exclude the presence of heparin, whereas a prolonged TT is suggestive of heparin, raised D-dimers, or an impairment of fibrinogen conversion to fibrin (e.g., low or dysfunctional fibrinogen, antibody interference at this step). A heparin assay using routine anti-Xa methods can both detect heparin and measure the concentration. If it is necessary to test a sample containing heparin, the sample can be pre-treated with heparinase (32).

21. Recombinant VIIa does not interfere with the determination of inhibitor level for factors VIII, IX, or XI in patients receiving treatment with this product. However, the measurement of inhibitors to factors II, V, VII, or X is unreliable in samples containing recombinant VIIa (33).

22. Recombinant porcine FVIII, for treatment of patients with inhibitors, is undergoing clinical trial (34). In future, laboratories may be required to check the cross-reactivity of inhibitors to porcine FVIII before a patient receives this form of therapy. This requires a source of porcine FVIII in the assay incubation mixture (16, 34, 35).

References

1. Ehrenforth S, Kreuz W, Scharrer I, Linde R, Funk M, Gungor T, Krackhardt B, Kornhuber B (1992) Incidence of development of factor VIII and factor IX inhibitors in haemophiliacs. Lancet 339:594–598
2. Scharrer I, Neutzling O (1993) Incidence of inhibitors in haemophiliacs. A review of the literature. Blood Coagul Fibrinolysis 4: 753–758
3. Wright J, Paisley S (2003) The epidemiology of inhibitors in haemophilia A: a systematic review. Haemophilia 9:418–435
4. Hay CRM (1998) Factor VIII inhibitors in mild and moderate-severity haemophilia A. Haemophilia 4:558–563
5. Oldenburg J, El-Maarri O, Schwaab R (2002) Inhibitor development in correlation to factor VIII genotypes. Haemophilia 8(Suppl 2):23–29
6. Peerlink K, Hermans C (2006) Epidemiology of inhibitor formation with recombinant factor VIII replacement therapy. Haemophilia 12:579–590
7. Hay CRM, Brown S, Collins PW, Keeling DM, Liesner R (2006) The diagnosis and management of factor VIII and IX inhibitors: a guideline from the United Kingdom Haemophilia Centre Doctors Organization. Brit J Haematol 133:591–605
8. Dimichele DM (2006) Inhibitor treatment in haemophilias A and B: inhibitor diagnosis. Haemophilia 12(Suppl 6):37–42
9. Kasper CK, Aledort LM, Counts RB, Edson JR, Frantantoni J, Green D et al (1975) A more uniform measurement of factor VIII inhibitors. Thrombos Diath Haemorrh 34:869–872
10. Verbruggen B, Novakova I, Wessels H, Boezeman J, van den Berg M, Mauser-

Bunschoten E (1995) The Nijmegen modification of the Bethesda assay for factor VIII:C inhibitors: improved specificity and reliability. Thromb Haemost 73:247–251
11. Giles AR, Verbruggen B, Rivard GE, Teitel J, Walker I, and the Association of Haemophilia Centre Directors of Canada (1998) A detailed comparison of the performance of the standard versus the Nijmegen modification of the Bethesda assay in detecting factor VIII:C inhibitors in the haemophilia A population in Canada. Thromb Haemost 79:872–875
12. Gadarowski JJ, Czapek EE, Ontiveros JD, Pedraza JL (1988) Modification of the Bethesda assay for factor VIII and IX inhibitors to improve efficiency. Acta Haematol 80:134–138
13. Hay CRM, Baglin TP, Collins PW, Hill FGH, Keeling DM (2000) The diagnosis and management of factor VIII and IX inhibitors: a guideline from the UK Haemophilia Centre Doctors' Organization (UKHCDO). Brit J Haematol 111:78–90
14. Salomon O, Zivelin A, Livnat T, Dardik R, Loewenthal R, Avishai O et al (2003) Prevalence, causes, and characterization of factor XI inhibitors in patients with inherited factor XI deficiency. Blood 101:4783–4788
15. Favaloro EJ, Posen J, Ramakrishna R, Soltani S, McRae S, Just S et al (2004) Factor V inhibitors: rare or not so uncommon? A multi-laboratory investigation. Blood Coagul Fibrinolysis 15:637–647
16. Gatti L, Mannucci PM (1984) Use of porcine factor VIII in the management of seventeen patients with factor VIII antibodies. Thromb Haemost 51:379–384
17. Ling M, Duncan EM, Rodgers SE, Street AM, Lloyd JV (2003) Low detection rate of antibodies to non-functional epitopes on factor VIII in patients with haemophilia A and negative for inhibitors by Bethesda assay. J Thromb Haemost 1:2548–2553
18. Verbruggen B, Novakova I, van Heerde W (2009) Detecting and quantifying functional inhibitors in haemostasis. In: Kitchen S, Olson JD, Preston FE (eds) Quality in laboratory haemostasis and thrombosis, 1st edn. Blackwell Publishing, Oxford, Chapter 20
19. Kasper CK (1995) Laboratory diagnosis of factor VIII inhibitors. In: Kessler C, Garvey MB, Green D, Kasper C, Lusher J (eds) Acquired haemophilia, 2nd edn. Excerpta Medica, Princeton, NJ, Chapter 2
20. Goldsmith J (1993) Diagnosis of factor VIII versus nonspecific inhibitors. Semin Haematol 30(Suppl 1):3–6
21. Ling M, Duncan EM, Rodgers SE, Somogyi AA, Crabb GA, Street AM, Lloyd JV (2001) Classification of the kinetics of factor VIII inhibitors in haemophilia A: plasma dilution studies are more discriminatory than time-course studies. Brit J Haematol 114:861–867
22. Sahud MA (2000) Laboratory diagnosis of inhibitors. Semin Thromb Hemostas 26:195–203
23. Verbruggen B, Giles A, Samis J, Verbeek K, Mensink E, Novakova I (2001) The type of factor deficient plasma used influences the performance of the Nijmegen modification of the Bethesda assay for factor VIII:C inhibitors. Thromb Haemost 86:1435–1439
24. Verbruggen B, van Heerde W, Novakova I, Lillicrap D, Giles A (2002) A 4% solution of bovine serum albumin may be used in the place of factor VIII:C deficient plasma in the control sample in the Nijmegen modification of the Bethesda factor VIII:C inhibitor assay. Thromb Haemost 88:362–364
25. Reber G, Aurousseau MH, Dreyfus M, Delahousse B, Caron C, Trzeciack MC et al (1999) Inter-laboratory variability of the measurement of low titer factor VIII:C inhibitor in haemophiliacs: improvement by the Nijmegen modification of the Bethesda assay and the use of common lyophilized plasmas. Haemophilia 5:292–293
26. Favaloro EJ, Bonar R, Duncan E, Earl G, Low J, Aboud M et al (2006) Identification of factor inhibitors by diagnostic haemostasis laboratories: a large multi-centre evaluation. Thromb Haemost 96:73–78
27. Ewing NP, Kasper CK (1982) In Vitro detection of mild inhibitors to factor VIII in hemophilia. Am J Clin Pathol 77:749–752
28. Keeling D, Beavis J, Sukhu K (2005) A simple inhibitor screen is more sensitive than a Bethesda assay in monitoring for the development of inhibitors in haemophilia A and B. Brit J Haematol 128:885
29. Dazzi F, Tison T, Vianello F, Radossi P, Zerbinati P, Carraro P et al (1996) High incidence of anti-FVIII antibodies against non-coagulant epitopes in haemophilia A patients: a possible role for the half-life of transfused FVIII. Brit J Haematol 93:688–693
30. White GC (1994) Factor VIII inhibitor assay: quantitative and qualitative assay limitations and development needs. Semin Haematol 31(Suppl 4):6–10
31. Blanco AN, Peirano AA, Grosso SH, Gennari LC, Bianco RP, Lazzari MA (2002) A chromogenic substrate method for detecting and titrating anti-factor VIII antibodies in the presence of lupus anticoagulant. Haematologica 87:271–278
32. Manco-Johnson MJ, Nuss R, Jacobson LJ (2000) Heparin neutralization is essential for

accurate measurement of factor VIII activity and inhibitor assays in blood samples drawn from implanted venous access devices. J Lab Clin Med 136:74–79

33. Keeney M, Allan DS, Lohmann RC, Chin Yee IH (2005) Effect of recombinant human factor 7 (Niastase) on laboratory testing of inhibitors of factors VIII and IX. Lab Haematol 11:118–123

34. Barrow RT, Lollar P (2006) Neutralization of antifactor VIII inhibitors by recombinant porcine factor VIII. J Thromb Haemost 4:2223–2229

35. Lloyd JV, Duncan EM, Street AM, Maxwell EL, Berry E, Rowell J et al (1997) Cross-reactivity to porcine factor VIII of factor VIII inhibitors in patients with haemophilia in Australia and New Zealand. Aust N Z J Med 27:658–664

Chapter 25

Kaolin Clotting Time

Kottayam Radhakrishnan

Abstract

The kaolin clotting time (KCT) is a sensitive test used in the laboratory detection of lupus anticoagulants (LA) (Derksen and de Groot, Thromb Res 114:521–526, 2004). It is essentially an activated partial thromboplastin time (APTT) test with no added phospholipid. Kaolin acts as the activator in the KCT. In the absence of additional phospholipid reagent, the quality of the test sample is extremely important since the generation of thrombin completely depends on the presence of residual cell membranes and plasma lipids (Derksen and de Groot, Thromb Res 114:521–526, 2004). Since the test contains no exogenous phospholipid, a confirmatory test using excess phospholipid is required to confirm the presence of lupus anticoagulant in the sample (Court, Br J Biomed Sci 54:287–298, 1997).

Key words Kaolin clotting time (KCT), Lupus anticoagulant (LA), Activated partial thromboplastin time (APTT), Phospholipids, Kaolin

1 Introduction

The kaolin clotting time (KCT) is essentially an APTT test with no added phospholipid. Lupus anticoagulants, if present in the test plasma, bind to phospholipid complexes thereby prolonging the clotting time of the test plasma. The test is performed not only on the test plasma but also a mixture of 80% normal and 20% patient's plasma. This allows differentiation between the presence of LA, deficiency of one or more coagulation factors, and the lupus cofactor effect (3). Lupus anticoagulants were discussed in detail in Chapter 7.

The KCT is considered a sensitive test for the detection of circulating anticoagulants. However, it is relatively nonspecific, detecting all classes of inhibitors including factor VIII and contact activation-specific inhibitors as well as heparin. The KCT is extremely sensitive to shortening by activated platelets. Therefore, plasma specimen for testing should be as free of platelets as possible (a platelet count $<10 \times 10^9/l$ is recommended).

Paul Monagle (ed.), *Haemostasis: Methods and Protocols*, Methods in Molecular Biology, vol. 992,
DOI 10.1007/978-1-62703-339-8_25, © Springer Science+Business Media New York 2013

2 Materials

2.1 Specimen and Sample Preparation

1. Whole venous blood is collected in a 3.2% citrate anticoagulant tube (1.4 or 3 ml tubes) with a blood to citrate ratio of 9:1. The blood should be collected by a rapid draw and minimal venous stasis (see Notes 1 and 2).
2. Platelet-free plasma should be prepared from the sample within 1 h of blood collection (see Note 3).
3. Centrifuge the citrated blood tube, after checking to make sure there are no clots in the sample, at 3,000 × g-force for 10 min at 10°C.
4. Platelet poor plasma (PPP) is obtained from the above step.
5. From the PPP obtained in the previous step, platelet-free plasma (PPFP with a platelet count <10 × 109/l) is obtained by filtering the PPP through a 0.22 mm filter (see Notes 4 and 5).
6. This platelet-free plasma is used to perform the KCT.
7. Specimen stability:

   PFP—4 h at 2–8°C.

   – 6 months at −70°C.

   PPFP—4 h on STA Compact Analyzer.

   – 8 h at 2–8°C.

   – 12 months at −70°C.

2.2 Reagents

1. Kaolin: 20 mg/ml in Tris buffer, pH 7.4.
2. Normal PPP: Platelet count reduced by microfiltration or double centrifugation.
3. Patient's PPP: Platelet count <10 × 109/l.
4. CaCl2: 0.025 mol/l.

3 Methods

1. Normal plasma and patient plasma are mixed in plastic tubes with the following ratios of normal to patient's plasma:

   10:0, 9:1, 8:2, 5:5, 2:8, 1:9, and 0:10.

2. From each mixture pipette 0.2 ml into a glass tube at 37°C.
3. To the pipetted mixtures, add 0.1 ml of Kaolin as an activator.
4. Incubate the plasma kaolin mixture for 3 mins at 37°C.
5. Now add 0.2 ml of CaCl2.

6. Record the time taken for the samples to clot after the addition of $CaCl_2$.
7. Similarly the clotting time of patient and control plasma is recorded.
8. The ratio of the clotting time of the mixture containing 80% normal plasma and 20% test plasma to the clotting time of the mixture containing 100% normal plasma is calculated as given by the formula, i.e., mixture ratio:

$$\frac{\text{KCT (80\% N : 20\% Test)}}{\text{KCT (100\% N)}}.$$

9. The ratio of clotting time of the test to clotting time of control is also calculated.
10. A test-control ratio of >1.2 indicates an abnormal result and a mixture ratio of >1.2 indicates the presence of LA.
11. The KCT of a normal control sample is simultaneously determined. A control KCT of <60 s may indicate contamination of the control plasma with phospholipids and invalidates the test result.

4 Automated Assays

The method described previously is a manual method; however, in routine diagnostic laboratories, the assay is usually performed on an automated analyzer (e.g., STA—COMPACT) using specific test kits, such as KaocLot—Gradipore™. In this instance, the kit contains the relevant reagents, and the method is as per the kit insert. KaocLot requires no calibration (see Notes 6 and 7).

The results are calculated as follows:

1. $\text{KCT ratio}\frac{\text{KCT patient(s)}}{\text{KCT PPFP(s)}}.$
2. $\text{KCT mix ratio} = \frac{\text{KCT patient mix(s)}}{\text{KCT PPFP(s)}}.$

And then interpreted as described in Table 1 (see Notes 8–10).

4.1 Quality Control

The quality control material for the KCT is normal pooled platelet-free plasma which serves as a normal control. The pooled normal plasma may be prepared in-house or is commercially available. For each new batch of pooled platelet-free plasma new reference ranges for the KCT must be established. For each new batch of KaocLot reference range for pooled platelet-free plasma must be established.

Table 1
Interpretation of results for automated assays

KCT ratio	KCT mix ratio	Diagnosis
<1.2	<1.2	LA not detected
< or ≥1.2	>1.2	LA detected
>1.2	<1.1	Factor deficiency/oral anticoagulation
>1.2	1.1–1.2	Equivocal results Possible heparin contamination of sample
>1.2	>1.2	LA detected LA + oral anticoagulation Heparin ± LA detected Factor inhibitor + LA detected

Quality control is performed:

1. Automatically every 4 h (where a patient test is requested).
2. Prior to testing first patient sample.
3. Following loading of freshly prepared reagents.
4. Following calibration (loading of a new lot of reagents).
5. For trouble shooting.

In diagnostic laboratories, quality control should be checked prior to the release of patient's results. If quality control is outside acceptable limits patient results are not released until the issues are resolved.

5 Notes

1. Sample collection and preparation are important variables that affect the sensitivity and specificity of the KCT.
2. An adequate volume of blood should be collected into a suitable anticoagulant. The tube should be filled appropriately.
3. Prior to preparation of platelet-free plasma, the blood tube should be visually inspected for the presence of clots. Clotted samples should be rejected and fresh samples requested.
4. The sensitivity of the KCT to LA depends to a major extent on the influence of residual red cell membrane fragments and plasma lipid on coagulation. Hence the KCT is extremely sensitive to platelet contamination of the plasma sample.

5. The platelet content of the plasma sample should be $<10 \times 10^9/l$ (5). To obtain platelet-free plasma double centrifugation is now recommended (4) as an alternative to filtration.
6. KaocLot—Gradipore™ and STA®—CaCl2 0.025 M contain sodium azide. If disposing of the products down the sink, always flush with large volume of water to avoid the possibility of an explosive residue forming in metal plumbing.
7. STA®—Desorb is hazardous and may cause irritation to eyes and skin. Wear suitable gloves and eye/face protection when handling this product.
8. A KCT ratio and KCT mix ratio of >1.2 is suggestive of the presence of LA, heparin, or specific factor inhibitors.
9. If a factor inhibitor is present, the patient will have bleeding symptoms while a patient with LA will not have bleeding symptoms (with very rare exceptions).
10. If the patient is receiving heparin, testing should be delayed until heparin treatment has ceased for a reasonable period of time.

References

1. Derksen RHWM, de Groot PG (2004) Tests for lupus anticoagulant revisited. Thromb Res 114:521–526
2. Court EL (1997) Lupus anticoagulants: pathogenesis and laboratory diagnosis. Br J Biomed Sci 54:287–298
3. Laffan M, Manning R (2006) Investigation of a thrombotic tendency. In: Lewis SM, Bain BJ, Bates I (eds) Dacie and Lewis practical haematology. Churchill Livingstone, Philadelphia, PA, pp 443–445
4. Pengo V, Tripodi A, Reber G, Rand JH, Ortel L, Galli M, De Groot PG (2009) Update of the guidelines for lupus anticoagulant detection. J Thromb Haemost 7:1737–1740
5. Tripodi A (2007) Laboratory testing for lupus anticoagulants: a review of issues affecting results. Clin Chem 53:1629–1635

Chapter 26

The Dilute Russell's Viper Venom Time

Kottayam Radhakrishnan

Abstract

The dilute Russell's viper venom time is a clot-based test used in the detection of the lupus anticoagulant in the laboratory. Lupus anticoagulants and the overall approach for their detection are described in Chapter 7.

Key words Lupus anticoagulant, Antiphospholipid antibody, Dilute Russell's viper venom time, Activated partial thromboplastin time, Mixing studies, Pooled normal plasma, Diagnosis, Anticoagulants

1 Introduction

Lupus anticoagulants can be detected by a variety of phospholipid-dependent coagulation tests, the most robust of which is the dilute Russell's viper venom time (DRVVT) (1–6). This test is completed in two stages, namely, the DRVVT screen and the DRVVT confirm (where the test is repeated after the addition of excess phospholipid).

The Russell's viper venom (RVV) contains an enzyme that directly activates factor X, in the coagulation pathway and in the presence of phospholipid, calcium ions, factor V, and prothrombin leads to the formation of a fibrin clot (2). LAs prolong the clotting time by interfering with the interaction between phospholipids and clotting factor proteins. The test is then repeated with the addition of excess phospholipids. Addition of the excess phospholipid results in shortening of the clotting time, thus demonstrating the phospholipid-dependent nature of the anticoagulant and confirming its presence in the sample. Since RVV directly activates factor X, defects of the contact system and factor VIII, IX, or XI deficiencies do not interfere with the test (2). Thus, this test is more specific for lupus anticoagulants than the APTT tests.

Paul Monagle (ed.), *Haemostasis: Methods and Protocols*, Methods in Molecular Biology, vol. 992,
DOI 10.1007/978-1-62703-339-8_26, © Springer Science+Business Media New York 2013

In most laboratories today, the DRVVT test is performed in an automated system. This test is commonly performed on the STAGO STA-COMPACT® analyzer as the DRVVT screen and DRVVT confirm procedure. The method for the test is as described below.

2 Materials

2.1 Equipment

1. STA-R evolution® analyzer.
2. Pipettes variable to 1 and 5 mL.
3. Disposable tips to fit the 1 and 5 mL pipettes.
4. STA®-mini reducers.
5. STA®-micro cups.
6. STA®-micro cup holders.
7. Eppendorf tube.
8. Water bath at 37°C.

2.2 Reagents

1. Water for injection BP.
2. STA®-STACLOT® DRVV screen.

   Contains RVV, anti-heparin agent, and calcium in buffered medium (see Notes 9 and 10).
3. STA®-STACLOT® DRVV confirm.

   Contains, in addition to the above, phospholipids.
4. STA®-$CaCl_2$ 0.025 M.
5. STA®-Desorb (see Note 12).
6. STA®-control LA 1 + 2 (see Note 11).

2.3 Stability of Reagents/Samples

1. STA®-STACLOT® DRVV screen is stable for 1 month at −80°C and stable for 72 h on STA-R Evolution® (15–19°C).
2. STA®-STACLOT® DRVV confirm is stable for 1 month at −80°C and stable for 72 h on STA-R Evolution® (15–19°C).
3. Platelet-free plasma (PFP) patient is stable for 4 h at 20°C and stable for 6 months at −80°C.
4. Quality control material (QC material).

STA®-control 1 + 2 is stable for 8 h on STA-R Evolution (15–19°C) and stable for 1 month at −80°C. Pooled platelet-free plasma (PPFP) is stable for 4 h on STA-R Evolution (15–19°C); stable for 8 h at 2–8°C; and stable for at least 12 months at −80°C.

3 Methods

3.1 Blood Collection

1. Fresh venous whole blood should be collected into 3.2% citrate anticoagulated tubes (1.4 or 3 mL) ensuring a blood:citrate ratio of 9:1. As with all coagulation tests, minimal venous stasis, rapid draw, and immediate anticoagulation should be ensured (6) (see Note 1).
2. Ideally, blood should be collected before the start of anticoagulation or a sufficient period after its discontinuation (5) (see Notes 6–8).
3. Plasma should preferably be prepared written 1 h of blood collection (6) (see Note 2).
4. To obtain platelet-poor plasma from whole blood centrifuge the citrated blood tube (1.4 or 3 mL) at 2,500 × *g* for 10 min at 10°C.
5. To obtain PFP, fill the platelet-poor plasma obtained in the previous step through a 0.22 μm filter. A platelet count of $<10\times10^9$/L should be ensured. It is currently recommended (5) that double centrifugation rather than filtration of the sample be performed to ensure that the sample is platelet poor (see Notes 4). This can be done by transferring the product of the initial centrifugation process to a non-activating plastic centrifuge tube using a plastic pipette and then recentrifuging the plasma for 10 min and a higher speed (>3,000 RPM). Care should be taken not to include residual platelets which may have collected at the base of the centrifuge tube, when aliquoting to a secondary tube. As plasma filtration introduces variables (such as type of filter, amount of plasma filtered, etc.) and adds to the cost, it is no longer recommended (see Notes 3 and 4).
6. If testing is not performed immediately after preparation of the PFP, it should be stored at −80°C to prevent loss of coagulation factors (7) (see Note 5).

3.2 Preparation of Reagents

3.2.1 STA®-STACLOT® DRVV Screen (Reconstitution)

1. Add 5 mL distilled water.
2. Allow reconstituted reagent to stand at room temperature for 30 min.
3. Swirl gently to obtain a homogenous solution.

3.2.2 STA®-STACLOT® DRVV Confirm

1. Add 2 mL distilled water.
2. Allow reconstituted reagent to stand at room temperature for 30 min.
3. Swirl gently to obtain a homogenous solution.

Table 1
The reagent volumes required for DRVVT

Reagent	Dead vol (μL)	QC (μL)	Test (μL)	Mix (μL)	Minimum volume
DRVV screen	700*	200	100	100*	$900+(100\times n)$
DRVV confirm	700*	200*	100*	100*	$900+(100\times n)$
PPFP	50	100-DRVV screen, 100-DRVV confirm	N/A	50-DRVV screen, 50-DRVV confirm	$150+(150\times n)^*$, $100+(50\times n)^*$

*200 microliters if microcups are used (adjust minimum volume accordingly)

3.2.3 STA®-Control LA 1+2

1. Add 1 mL distilled water to each vial.
2. Allow reconstituted reagent to stand at room temperature for 30 min.
3. Swirl gently to obtain a homogenous solution.

3.3 Quality Control

Quality control with STA®-Control LA 1+2 should be performed:

1. Prior to testing the first patient sample.
2. Following loading of freshly prepared reagent.
3. Following calibration (loading a new lot of reagent).
4. Automatically every 4 h when tests are requested while reagents are still on the analyzer.
5. For troubleshooting.

If quality control data are outside acceptable limits, patient results should not be released until the issue is resolved.

3.4 Establishment of Local Reference Ranges (4)

1. Local reference ranges must be established for the DRVVT test and the type of coagulometer.
2. This should be done by performing the LA test on at least 20 individual plasma samples from healthy normal subjects. When ratios are used, the clotting time of each plasma is divided by the mean time and the mean ± 2 SD range is determined.
3. Pooled normal plasma used for the calculation of LA clotting time ratios must include donations from at least 12 healthy normal subjects.

3.5 Procedure

1. DRVVT tests are usually batched.
2. Calculate the reagent volumes required (total of 200 μL if microcups are used—adjust minimum volume accordingly) to complete the tests as per Table 1, where n = number of patient specimens.
3. The "standard operating procedures" manual for the instrument gives the full details on how to perform the testing. The various

Table 2
Interpretation of complex DRVVT results

DRVV screen		DRVV confirm		
Patient plasma	Mixing test	Patient plasma	Mixing test	Diagnosis
N	N	N	N	LA not detected
ABN	ABN	N	N	LA detected
ABN	N	ABN	N	Factor deficiency/oral anticoagulation
ABN	ABN	ABN	N	LA plus factor deficiency/ oral anticoagulation
ABN	ABN	ABN	ABN	Other inhibitor

samples are loaded onto the analyzer as per the instructions in the standard operating procedure manual. In summary, the clotting time determination of the plasmas to be tested is automatically carried out by the analyzer as soon as the samples have been loaded.

4. Calculations:

(a) $$\text{DRVV Screen ratio} = \frac{\text{DRVV Scrren patient (s)}}{\text{DRVV Screen PPFP (s)}}.$$

(b) $$\text{DRVV Screen-mix ratio} = \frac{\text{DRVV Sreen patient mix (s)}}{\text{DRVV Screen PFPP (s)}}.$$

(c) $$\text{DRVV Confirm ratio} = \frac{\text{DRVV Confirm patient (s)}}{\text{DRVV Confirm PFPP (s)}}.$$

(d) $$\text{DRVV Confirm mix ratio} = \frac{\text{DRVV Confirm patient}}{\text{DRVV Confirm PPF}}$$

(e) $$\text{DRVV normalized ratio} = \frac{\text{DRVV Screen ratio (s)}}{\text{DRVV Confirm ratio (s)}}.$$

(f) $$\text{DRVV normalized mix ratio} = \frac{\text{DRVV Screen mix r}}{\text{DRVV Confirm mix}}$$

3.6 Interpretation of Results

1. A normalized mix ratio of >1.2 is indicative of the presence of LA.
2. Table 2 helps to interpret more complex results.
3. Normal reference ranges and ratios should be established for each analyzer–reagent combination. For each lot of STA®-STACLOT®DRVV screen and STA®-STACLOT®DRVV confirm, establish reference ranges from at least 20 individual normal plasma samples.

4 Manual Method for the DRVVT (2)

The manual method for the DRVVT test is outdated and most laboratories now perform the automated assay. The procedure and other details for the manual method for the test are described here:

4.1 Reagents

1. Platelet-poor plasma—from patient and a normal control (as described earlier in the chapter).
2. Pooled normal plasma—a suggested minimum for the normal pool is 20 donors.
3. Glyoxaline buffer—0.05 mol/L, pH 7.4.
4. RVV—commercially available. Dilute approximately 1 in 200 in buffer to obtain a working solution. This solution is stable at 4°C for several hours.
5. Phospholipid—platelet substitute; also available commercially.
6. $CaCl_2$—0.025 mol/L.

4.2 Preparation of Reagent

1. The concentration of the RVV is adjusted so as to produce a clotting time of 30–35 s when 0.1 mL of the venom is added to a mixture 0.1 mL of normal plasma and 0.1 mL of undiluted phospholipid.
2. The procedure is then repeated using doubling dilutions of the phospholipid reagent. The dilution of phospholipid selected is the last dilution before the clotting time is prolonged by 2 s or more (i.e., prolongation of the clotting time to 35–37 s).

4.3 Method

1. In a glass tube at 37°C place 0.1 mL of pooled normal plasma and 0.1 mL of the dilute phospholipid reagent as determined in the step above.
2. Warm the mixture, i.e., the pooled normal plasma and dilute phospholipid reagent, for 30 s after the addition of 0.1 mL dilute RVV to the mixture.
3. Then add 0.1 mL of $CaCl_2$.
4. Record the clotting time.
5. Steps 1–4 are repeated using the test plasma instead of pooled normal plasma.
6. The ratio of the clotting times of test and control is then calculated.

5 Interpretation

1. As mentioned earlier the normal ratio should be determined separately in each laboratory.
2. In general, the normal ratio is usually between 0.9 and 1.05.

3. A ratio more than 1.05 could indicate:
   (a) Deficiency of factor II, V, X, or fibrinogen. Addition of normal plasma corrects the prolonged DRVVT due to factor deficiency but does not correct the prolonged clotting time due to an inhibitor.
   (b) Presence of an inhibitor. Lupus inhibitor or anticoagulants being phospholipid dependent, a platelet neutralization procedure should be used to confirm this phospholipid dependence, wherein addition of freeze-thawed/fractured platelets (which serves as a source of phospholipid) leads to normalization of the previously prolonged clotting time.

6 Notes

1. After blood collection the tubes should be inverted gently several times to ensure adequate mixture of blood and anticoagulant (4). Prior to testing the blood tubes should be checked for clots. If clots are present, the sample should be rejected and a fresh sample requested.
2. If not tested within 2 h the platelet-free test sample should be stored at –80°C until the time of testing, to prevent the loss of coagulation factors.
3. Plasma filtration is not recommended as this introduces variable such as filter type, amount of plasma to be filtered, added costs, and loss of von Willebrand factor (8).
4. A platelet count of $<10\times10^9$/L must be achieved in the sample to be tested. An excess of platelets in the sample will reduce the sensitivity of the test by serving as a source of phospholipids. This can result in false negative test results. The ability to obtain a platelet-free sample (platelet count $<10\times10^9$/L) is the single most important factor affecting test results.
5. Prior to actual testing, the frozen samples and reagent should be thawed strictly in a water bath at 37°C for 5 min. This will avoid formation of cryoprecipitate. The thawed sample should then be mixed thoroughly.
6. It is recommended that, wherever possible, LA testing be withheld while patients are on anticoagulation. The test may be performed after anticoagulation is stopped for a reasonable period of time. However, it should be noted that the commercial DRVVT assay reagents incorporate an unfractionated heparin neutralizer which can neutralize unfractionated heparin concentrations of up to 0.8 U/mL in the sample.
7. Oral anticoagulation can result in false positive DRVVT results with prolongation of the clotting times. Mixing studies on the

sample will help to differentiate factor deficiency and presence of LA (see Table 2 on interpretation of results).

8. If it is suspected that LA may be present in a patient on oral anticoagulation, an approximate and clear comment should be included in the test results that are released to the clinician.
9. STA®-STACLOT® DRVV screen and DRVV confirm are derived from human and/or animal origin and though tested for blood-borne diseases should be handled as potentially infectious.
10. STA®-STACLOT® DRVV screen and DRVV confirm contain sodium azide. If disposing of these products down the sink, always flush with large volumes of water to avoid the possibility of an explosive residue forming in the metal plumbing.
11. STAx-control LA 1 + 2 are derived from human and/or animal origin and though tested for blood-borne diseases should be handled as potentially infectious.
12. Desorb U is hazardous and may cause irritation to eyes and skin. Wear suitable gloves and eye/face protection when handling this product.

References

1. Kristi JS, Rodgers GM (2009) Laboratory identification of lupus anticoagulants. Am J Hematol 84: 440-442
2. Laffan M, Manning R (2006) Investigation of a thrombotic tendency. In: Lewis SM, Bain BJ, Bates I (eds) Dacie and Lewis practical haematology. Churchill Livingstone, Philadelphia, PA, pp 442–443
3. Brandt JT, Barna LK, Triplett DA (1995) Laboratory identification of lupus anticoagulants: results of the second international workshop for identification of lupus anticoagulants. On behalf of the subcommittee on lupus anticoagulants/antiphospholipid antibodies of the ISTH. J Thromb Haemost 76:1597–1603
4. Greaves M, Cohen H, MacHin SJ, Mackie I (2000) Guidelines on the investigation and management of the antiphospholipid syndrome. Br J Haematol 109:704–715
5. Pengo V, Tripodi A, Reber G, Rand JH, Ortel L, Galli M, De Groot PG (2009) Update of the guidelines for lupus anticoagulant detection. J Thromb Haemost 7:1737–1740
6. Urbanus RT, Derksen RH, de Groot PG (2008) Current insights into diagnostics and pathophysiology of the antiphospholipid syndrome. Blood Rev 2:93–105
7. Clinical and Laboratory Standards Institute (CLSI) (2008) Collection, transport, and processing of blood specimens for testing plasma based coagulation assays and molecular hemostasis assays; approved guideline-fifth edition. Clinical and Laboratory Standards Institute, Pennsylvania, USA
8. Favalaro EJ (2007) Preanalytical variables in coagulation testing. Blood Coagul Fibrinolysis 18:86–89

Chapter 27

Platelet Neutralization Test

Kottayam Radhakrishnan

Abstract

The platelet neutralization test is used in the laboratorvy diagnosis of the lupus anticoagulant (Laffan and Manning, Dacie and Lewis practical haematology. Churchill Livingstone, Philadelphia, PA, pp 445–446, 2006). The lupus anticoagulant typically causes prolongation of phospholipid-dependent coagulation tests such as APTT, DRVVT, etc.

The phospholipid-dependent nature of the LA can be demonstrated by adding washed and "fractured" platelets as a source of phospholipid and repeating the tests. If an LA is present in the sample, the addition of platelets will correct the prolonged clotting times. This appears to be due to the ability of the platelets to absorb the LA and negate its effect on the clotting time (Br J Haematol 109:704–715, 2001).

Key words Platelet neutralization, Phospholipid, Lupus anticoagulant, Clotting time, Activated partial thromboplastin time, Dilute Russell's viper venom time, Centrifuge

1 Introduction

In the platelet neutralization test, the platelets are used as a source of phospholipid to demonstrate the phospholipid dependence of the lupus anticoagulant. Before they can be used in the test, the platelets should be washed and then activated (to expose the coagulation factor-binding sites) by repeated thawing and refreezing 3–4 times. The activated platelets can then be used in the dilute RVV test as a confirmatory test or in the APTT in place of the usual phospholipid reagent (1).

2 Materials

See Chapter 26 for materials needed for DRVVT.

Paul Monagle (ed.), *Haemostasis: Methods and Protocols*, Methods in Molecular Biology, vol. 992,
DOI 10.1007/978-1-62703-339-8_27, © Springer Science+Business Media New York 2013

2.1 Reagents

1. Commercial platelet extract reagent or washed normal platelets.
2. Acid-citrate-dextrose (ACD) anticoagulant solution. Washed platelets require a pH of 5.4.
3. Na2 EDTA 0.1 mol/l in saline.
4. Calcium-free Tyrode's buffer: Disolve 8 g NaCl, 0.2 g KCl, 0.625 g Na2HPO4, 0.415 g MgCl2, and 1.0 g NaHCO2 in 1 l of water. If necessary, adjust the pH to 6.5 with 1 mol/l HCl.

3 Methods (1)

3.1 Preparation of Washed Activated Platelets

1. Whole venous blood is collected into an ACD tube maintaining a ratio of 6 parts of blood to 1 part anticoagulant (see Note 2).
2. Check sample to exclude clots.
3. Centrifuge the ACD tube at 270 × g for 10 min.
4. Platelet-rich plasma (PRP) obtained as a supernatant.
5. Pipette the supernatant PRP into a plastic container.
6. Centrifuge again to obtain more PRP.
7. Add the PRP thus obtained to the first lot of PRP in the plastic container.
8. Now, dilute the PRP with an equal volume of calcium-free Tyrode's buffer and add one-tenth volume of EDTA to give a final concentration of 0.01 mol/l.
9. Centrifuge this mixture in a conical or round-bottom tube at 2,000 × g for 10 min.
10. Discard the supernatant.
11. Very gently resuspend the platelet pellet in buffer and 0.01 mol/l EDTA.
12. Centrifuge again and discard the supernatant.
13. Resuspend the pellet in buffer alone.
14. This gives a platelet count of at least 400×10^9/l.
15. The platelets have been washed and may now be stored at below −20°C in 1–2 volumes.
16. Please note that before they can be used in the platelet neutralization procedure they must be activated by repeated thawing and refreezing 3–4 times.

3.2 Platelet Neutralization Method

The platelet neutralization is performed by adding the washed and activated platelets in the dilute RVV test (instead of the commercial confirm reagent) or in the APTT test in place of the usual phospholipid reagent. The details of the performance of the APTT tests and the DRVVT tests have been explained in earlier chapters. The clotting times of the patient and normal plasmas are recorded and a correction ratio is derived by the following formula:

$$\mathrm{CR} = \frac{\frac{P_s}{N_s} - \frac{P_c}{N_c}}{\frac{P_s}{N_s}}$$

where CR is correction ratio; *s* screening procedure; P_s clotting time of patient plasma in the screening procedure; N_s clotting time of normal plasma in the screening procedure; *C* confirmation procedure; P_c clotting time of patient plasma in the confirmation procedure (i.e., platelet neutralization test); and N_c clotting time of normal plasma in the confirmation procedure.

3.3 Interpretation of Results

1. In general, a correction of >10% is regarded as a positive test and indicative of the presence of LA (see Note 1).
2. However, it is recommended that every lab establishes its own local normal ranges.
3. False positive results may be obtained in patients on heparin anticoagulation.
4. Interpretation of results may be difficult in patients on oral anticoagulation. This problem can be overcome by performing mixing studies of normal and patient plasmas.

4 Notes

1. In the platelet neutralization procedure, the extent to which correction of a prolonged clotting time occurs is crucially dependent on the ability of different batches of platelets. Therefore, a plasma sample known to contain a lupus anticoagulant should be tested in parallel with the test sample (2).
2. Given the poor batch-to-batch variability in the efficacy of freeze/thawed platelets, the International Society of Thrombosis and Hemostasis currently does not recommend freeze/thawed platelets as a source of phospholipid for the confirmatory tests in lupus anticoagulant testing (3).

References

1. Laffan M, Manning R (2006) Investigation of a thrombotic tendency. In: Lewis SM, Bain BJ, Bates I (eds) Dacie and Lewis practical haematology. Churchill Livingstone, Philadelphia, PA, pp 445–446
2. Greaves M, Cohen H, Machin SJ, Mackie I (2000) Guidelines on the investigation and management of the antiphospholipid syndrome. Br J Haematol. 109:704–715
3. Pengo V, Tripodi A, Reber G, Rand JH, Ortel L, Galli M, De Groot PG (2009) Update of the guidelines for lupus anticoagulant detection. J Thromb Haemost 7:1737–1740

Part VII

Examples of Tests for Increased Risk of Thrombosis

Chapter 28

Antithrombin

Mirta Hepner and Vasiliki Karlaftis

Abstract

Antithrombin (AT) is a heparin cofactor and a member of the serine protease inhibitor family (serpin). The mature AT molecule is composed of 432 amino acids and it is produced mainly in the liver. Initially, several different AT activities in plasma were reported, leading to the classification of antithrombin in a range from I to IV. It was subsequently shown that these various antithrombin activities were the function of one molecule, antithrombin III, whose name was reduced to antithrombin at the meeting of the International Society in Thrombosis and Haemostasis in 1993. AT is an important protease inhibitor of thrombin and factor Xa. However, AT is also able to inhibit factors IXa, XIa, XIIab, kallikrein, and plasmin.

Given that AT is one of the major naturally occurring inhibitors of coagulation, acquired or hereditary deficiencies of this protein result in excessive thrombin generation. As a vast array of mutations are responsible for hereditary AT deficiencies, screening for their presence by DNA testing would require sequencing each entire gene involving numerous exons. Moreover, the knowledge of the gene mutation does not offer any benefit in the treatment of affected families, so the routine molecular characterization is not indicative. These defects are detected by functional or immunological assays. AT amidolytic assays are recommended for initial testing for AT deficiency. There is no need to routinely perform AT immunological assays. However, they are useful in order to distinguish type I from type II hereditary AT deficiency.

Key words Antithrombin, Thrombophilia, Functional assay, Immunological assay, Blood coagulation inhibitor, Acquired deficiency, Hereditary deficiency

1 Introduction

Antithrombin (AT) is a heparin cofactor and a member of the serine protease inhibitor family (serpin). The mature AT molecule is composed of 432 amino acids and it is produced mainly in the liver (1). Initially, several different AT activities in plasma were reported, leading to the classification of antithrombin in a range from I to IV (2). It was subsequently shown that these various antithrombin activities were the function of one molecule, antithrombin III, whose name was reduced to antithrombin at the meeting of the International Society in Thrombosis and Haemostasis in 1993. AT is an important protease inhibitor of thrombin (3) and factor Xa (4). However, AT is also able to inhibit factors IXa (5), XIa (6),

Paul Monagle (ed.), *Haemostasis: Methods and Protocols*, Methods in Molecular Biology, vol. 992,
DOI 10.1007/978-1-62703-339-8_28, © Springer Science+Business Media New York 2013

XIIa (7), kallikrein and plasmin (8). Given that AT is one of the major naturally occurring inhibitors of coagulation, acquired or hereditary deficiencies of this protein result in excessive thrombin generation. As a vast array of mutations are responsible for hereditary AT deficiencies, screening for their presence by DNA testing would require sequencing each entire gene involving numerous exons (9). Moreover, the knowledge of the gene mutation does not offer any benefit in the treatment of affected families, so the routine molecular characterization is not indicative. These defects are detected by functional or immunological assays. AT amidolytic assays are recommended for initial testing for AT deficiency. There is no need to routinely perform AT immunological assays. However, they are useful in order to distinguish type I from type II hereditary AT deficiency (9).

1.1 Functional Assays

At present, functional levels of AT protein are measured with synthetic substrates using amidolytic methods assessed photometrically (10, 11). Commercially available functional assays are made to measure AT inhibitory activity against either factor Xa or thrombin in the presence of heparin. Residual thrombin or factor Xa is measured through reaction with specific chromogenic substrates. The decrease in absorbance at 405 nm is proportional to AT concentration. The new commercial AT assays have protease inhibitors, such as aprotinin, which minimizes nonspecific substrate cleavage, and bovine thrombin, which is resistant to heparin cofactor II. The choice between factor Xa or thrombin is debatable (12). However, the United Kingdom National External Quality Assessment Scheme found varying results of certain AT deficiency variants depending on the assay conditions that were chosen (13). Overall, given that very few documented discrepancies have been reported (14), running both tests seems to be rarely needed (13). Assays can be performed in an automated way on a coagulation analyzer, or following a microplate method. Both procedures can be performed either by measuring the rate of cleavage of substrate (kinetic method) or by measuring absorbance after a fixed incubation time (end point method) (see Note 1).

1.2 Antigenic Assays

Once AT functional deficiency has been identified, the second stage of investigation should consist in completing an antigen assay to establish the nature of the defect: defective synthesis of a normal protein or normal synthesis of a defective protein.

One of the first assays developed for detection of AT deficiency quantified the antigen form of the molecule by radial immunodiffusion techniques (RID) or electroimmunoassay (15).

AT antigen also may be measured by enzyme-linked immunosorbent assay (ELISA). The RID assay may be the simplest assay to set up, but the other methods have greater precision. Dysfunctional ATs may be investigated by running double cross-immunoelectrophoresis in the presence and absence of heparin (16) (see Note 2).

In a proficiency survey carried out in 2000 by the College of American Pathologists, the antigen AT assays had a CV percentage of approximately 40–50%, while the amidolytic assays had a much lower CV percentage, between 9 and 14% (CG2-A 2000) (see Notes 3, 4–6).

In the Laurell rocket procedure, an agarose gel is impregnated with antibodies against AT. Plasma samples are added in wells and then electrophoresed. The antibody-antigen complexes precipitate during electrophoresis, and the height of the precipitin arc is proportional to the amount of AT in plasma. The results are calculated from a standard curve that should be constructed using serial dilutions of a pooled normal plasma calibrated against the corresponding WHO international standard for AT (National Institute for Biological Standards and Control). Otherwise, results can be calculated using a commercial calibrator calibrated against the corresponding international standard. Final results are reported as a percentage of the calibrator.

In the ELISA, human AT will bind to a capture antibody coated on a microtiter plate. After appropriate washing steps, peroxidase-labeled polyclonal anti-human AT primary antibody binds to the captured protein. The excess antibody is then washed away and TMB substrate is used for color development at 450 nm. A standard calibration curve is prepared using dilutions of purified AT and measured along with the test samples. The color development is proportional to the concentration of AT in the samples (see Note 1).

2 Materials

2.1 Radial Immunodiffusion Technique

2.1.1 Antithrombin Antigen Rocket Plates

1. Glass plate 80 × 100 × 2 mm.
2. Agarose type I-A: Low EEO (Sigma A -0169).
3. Tris glycine buffer: 0.05 M Tris-HCl, glycine 0.10 M, ethylenediaminetetraacetic acid (EDTA) 5 mM, natrium barbital (0.05 M), pH 8.6. Store at room temperature.
4. Antiserum: Rabbit anti-human Antithrombin (Dako, code A296).
5. Punch (2 mm diameter).

2.1.2 Electrophoresis

1. Running buffer:

   Tris glycine buffer: 0.05 M Tris-HCl, glycine 0.10 M, ethylenediaminetetraacetic acid (EDTA) 5 mM, natrium barbital (0.05 M), pH 8.6. Store at room temperature.
2. Distaining solution:

   Methanol 0.45% (v/v) (Merck), glacial acetic acid 0.1% (v/v).

3. Staining solution:

   Coomassie Brilliant Blue (Merck R 250), 0.25% (w/v) in distaining solution: Store at room temperature. Mix thoroughly, keep dark at room temperature for 48 h, and filter before use. Keep dark at room temperature.

4. Pooled normal plasma:

   Calibrated against the corresponding WHO international standard for AT (National Institute for Biological Standards and Control). Otherwise, results can be calculated using a commercial calibrator calibrated against the corresponding international standard (the current WHO international standard for AT is code number 93/768). Final results are reported as a percentage of the calibrator (see Notes 7–10).

2.2 ELISA Technique

Citrate anticoagulated whole blood (see Note 11).

2.2.1 Specimen

2.2.2 Collection

NCCLS guidelines recommend collection into plastic or siliconized glass tubes containing 3.2% trisodium citrate (e.g., 9 volumes of blood to 1 volume of 0.109 M trisodium citrate). Immediately after sample collection, the tube is gently inverted to allow for the anticoagulant to mix with the sample (see Note 12).

2.2.3 Processing

Recommended centrifugation protocol for obtaining a platelet-free plasma sample adequate for coagulation testing includes minimum centrifugation at 2,500 × *g* for 15 min.

2.2.4 Storage

Once prepared, the plasma samples can be stored for up to 6 months at −70°C (see Notes 13 and 14).

3 Methods

3.1 Preparation of Rocket Plates

1. Prepare a 1% (w/v) agarose solution: Dissolve 100 mg of agarose in 10 ml Tris glycine buffer with boiling water. The agarose solution is allowed to cool to 50–56°C.
2. Add an appropriate amount of antiserum (about 50 μl) and mix quickly and carefully.
3. Pour onto the glass plate placed on a flat surface to obtain a uniform thickness. Let the plate gel at room temperature or in refrigerator at least 30 min.
4. A row of wells (2 mm diameter) with their centers at least 6 mm apart is punched in the gel. It is advisable to leave 2 cm between the border of the frame and the first well. Make an extra well to include a dye plasma mix and visualize the migration front. Keep in wet environment inside the refrigerator.

3.2 Preparation of Standard Curve

The dilutions are carried out with a standard or calibrator in Tris glycine buffer as 1:5, 1:10, 1:20, and 1:40 to obtain AT levels for the nominal percent activity of 100%, 50%, 25%, and 12.5%, respectively.

3.3 Preparation of Sample Dilutions

Prepare two dilutions of each patient's plasma samples in Tris glycine buffer: 1:5 dilution (1 part patient sample and 4 parts buffer) and a 1:10 dilution (4 parts patient sample and 9 parts buffer) (see Note 15).

3.4 Preparation of Electrophoresis Chamber

Add the running buffer into each inner section of the chamber.

3.5 Application of Samples

1. Remove the plate from the refrigerator.
2. Position the gel so that the edges of the agar are in the buffer and the wells are toward the cathode (−) side of the chamber.
3. The anodal and cathodal ends of the gel are connected with the electrode vessel by paper contact strips (10 × 10 cm); let stand approximately 20 min to reach room temperature.
4. Apply 2 μl of each patient sample dilution to the designated wells taking care not to damage the wells. Duplicate applications of patient samples must be run on each plate.
5. The standard curve dilutions must be applied in each side of the row.
6. To secure a reasonably uniform diffusion time for all of the samples in a set, the interval between application of the first and last sample should not exceed 10 min.

3.6 Electrophoresis

1. Place cover on the chamber. Connect to a power supply and electrophorese the plate at a constant current of 12 mA per plate (80 V) for 6 h. To assure the run is performing in the right way, check the migration of the dye. Stop the electrophoresis when the colored dot reaches the cathode edge.

3.7 Drying

1. Remove the glass plate from the electrophoresis chamber and rinse with deionized water for around 1 h.
2. After that wash it in 0.85% saline solution for 1 h.
3. Rinse the plate with deionized water.
4. Place the plate on a flat surface and cover it with a wet filter paper, care being taken to avoid inclusion of any air bubbles.
5. This filter paper is covered by a 2–3 cm layer of soft blotting paper, on top of which is placed a weight exerting a pressure.
6. Within 10 min the gel layer contracts to a thin film.

7. The weight and the blotting paper are removed.
8. The gel surface, still covered by the filter paper, is placed in front of a hot air fan. The filter paper soon dries and may be removed after about 10 min.

3.8 Staining

1. Place the plate into a plastic container and cover it with the staining solution for 15 min.
2. Remove the staining solution and cover with the destaining solution, slightly shaking it up to clearly visualize the precipitation peaks (1–3 min).
3. Discontinue destaining as soon as the background sufficiently clears in order to easily distinguish rocket peaks. Excessive destaining may fade the rockets, making correct measurements difficult. If over destaining does occur, stain the rockets again.
4. Let the plate dry at room temperature.

3.9 Measurements and Calculation of Antigen Concentration

1. Place the plate on white paper for easier viewing of the rockets. Mark the apex of each rocket peak with a marker. Turn the plate upside down and place it on a millimetered paper.
2. Measure the length of each peak in millimeters from the base or the middle of the well to the rocket apex.
3. Plot the values of the standard curve versus each rocket height on three-cycle semi-logarithmic paper.
4. Draw the best fit line for the standard points.
5. Calculate the patient values from the standard curve and multiply each by the appropriate dilution factor. Patient samples with antithrombin antigen levels greater than the range of the standard curve must be re-assayed using the appropriate dilutions.

3.10 AT Antigen ELISA

Using a commercially available kit, the assay measures total human AT in the 0.01–10 ng/ml range. It is recommended that samples which give AT levels above 10 ng/ml should be diluted (1:50,000–1:100,000) in blocking buffer before use to obtain the best results.

3.10.1 Reagents and Reagent Preparation

For commercially available assays, instructions provided by the manufacturer for the preparation of reagents and/or instrument should be followed, in order to ensure the validity of the results. Most reagents used to carry out the ELISA are not toxic; however working with plasma samples of unknown origin carries a certain level of risk that should be minimized by the use of gloves and eye protection.

3.10.2 Antithrombin Standard

The antithrombin standard which is used in this assay comes lyophilized and is stored at 4°C. The reconstitution is performed with the addition of distilled water to give a 50 ng/ml solution. Dilutions (0–10 ng/ml) for the standard curve and the zero standard must be made and applied to the plate immediately (see Note 16).

3.10.3 Assay Procedure

1. Add 100 μL of standards in duplicate and unknowns to wells in a plate which is coated with anti-human AT capture antibody, blocked, and dried and carefully record positions.
2. Shake plate at 300 rpm for 30 min.
3. Wash wells three times with 300 μL wash buffer.
4. Remove excess wash buffer by gently tapping plate on paper towel or Kimwipe.
5. Add 100 μL of primary antibody to all wells.
6. Shake plate at 300 rpm for 30 min.
7. Wash wells three times with 300 μL wash buffer.
8. Remove excess wash buffer by gently tapping plate on paper towel or Kimwipe.
9. Add 100 TMB substrate to all wells and shake plate for 5–10 min.

   Quench reaction by adding 50 μL of 1 N H_2SO_4 stop solution.

   Mix thoroughly.

3.10.4 Measurement

1. Set the absorbance at 450 nm in a microtiter plate spectrophotometer.
2. Measure the absorbance in all wells at 450 nm.
3. Subtract zero point from all standards and unknowns to determine corrected absorbance.

3.10.5 Assay Calibration

1. Plot A_{450} against the amount of human AT in the standards.
2. Fit a straight line through the points using a linear fit procedure.
3. Amount of total human AT in the unknowns can be determined from this curve.

4 Notes

1. A reference range for AT activity to antigen ratio can be of help to differentiate method variation in type II defect. Further investigations might include AT assays with a different enzyme. For example, if the original assay was Xa-based, the next assay can be done with bovine or human thrombin.
2. Detection of AT deficiency by functional and/or immunological testing is associated with a degree of uncertainty because

the interpretation of results can be influenced by the accuracy of normal ranges and also by other genetic and environmental factors. Hence, repeat testing is often required. Family studies may be beneficial to establish hereditary AT deficiency.

3 Accuracy should be verified by using normal and abnormal quality-control plasma samples and also by taking part in national and/or international quality assurance programs. Internal quality control (IQC) and external quality assessment (EQA) are distinct complementary components of a laboratory quality assurance program. IQC is used to identify the degree of precision of the technique, precision being the degree of agreement among repeat measurements on one sample. EQA is used to identify the degree of agreement between results from one laboratory and those obtained by other centers. EQA for thrombophilia tests are available from several international EQA providers (13). In all cases, the control material must be treated exactly like test samples if possible. Since some variation will necessarily occur as a result of biological, technical, and analytical variation, each quality-control result should be recorded and assessed against the target range considered to be acceptable.

4. Detection of AT deficiency by functional and/or immunological testing is associated with a degree of uncertainty because the normal range for AT concentration is narrow. The assay with a higher degree of precision is the chromogenic assay.

5. The specificity of amidolytic assays for AT is greatly increased by bovine thrombin, which reacts minimally with heparin cofactor (HCII), or by the use of FXa, which is not a target for HCII (20). The sensitivity of amidolytic assays for AT depends on the type of enzyme-based assay used to distinguish different variants of type II AT deficiency.

6. When performing AT by end point chromogenic assay, note that this assay can be influenced by elevated bilirubin, hemolysis, or lipemia in samples. Therefore, it is essential to perform a blank, where water is added instead of enzyme. The absorbance value for the blank is subtracted from that of the test and then the AT concentration is calculated.

7. The results are calculated from a standard curve that should be constructed using serial dilutions of a pooled normal plasma calibrated against the corresponding WHO international standard for AT (National Institute for Biological Standards and Control). Otherwise, results can be calculated using a commercial calibrator calibrated against the corresponding international standard. Final results are reported as a percentage of the calibrator. The current WHO international standard for AT is code number 93/768 (STH 2007).

8. Every batch of assays should be tested with its own calibration curve using plasma calibrated against the appropriate standard. The number of dilutions of the standard curve depends on the linear relationship between the variables being measured. If test results fall outside the linear region (linear regression plot) of the standard curve, the test should be repeated at an appropriate dilution. Do not extrapolate out of the calibration curve.
9. Calculation of local laboratory reference ranges is very important, owing to variability in test methodology from site to site and variability in population parameters. It should be based on the 2.5–97.5 centile or constructed from log-transformed data given that distribution of results is not Gaussian. There is a possibility of obtaining a potential false-positive, as a normal reference range only captures ~95% of population values.
10. AT levels are age dependent. AT levels are low in neonates and infants, and on average they either increase to adult levels by approximately 1 year of age or they attain adult levels by 16 years of age (17, 18). Therefore, it is strongly recommended to employ local reference ranges according to age group (19). Gender, oral contraceptive use, and circadian rhythm may influence AT levels, but it is acceptable to use an adult reference range including similar numbers of men and women.
11. Heparin therapy can cause an acquired AT deficiency. Therefore, this point should be taken into consideration when interpreting AT results if these pharmacological agents have been used. At least 5 days should have passed after stopping heparin therapy before AT measurement can be performed (21). In patients receiving direct thrombin inhibitors, such as hirudin, do not use thrombin-based assays, as these could lead to overestimation of AT levels.
12. Adequate performance of assays should include consideration of preanalytic variables, so careful collection and processing is required. AT levels in clotted samples are decreased. The needle size should be appropriate to the blood vessel (19–21 gauges for adults and 21–23 gauges for children). Syringes should not be bigger than 10 ml. The time that blood remains without anticoagulant should be minimized.
13. If testing is not going to occur on the day of collection, the plasma samples should be frozen (ideally stored at -70°C below), but must be thawed once only for functional assays; for antigenic assays they can be reused.
14. Once complete reconstitution of reagents has been attained, frozen samples should be kept at 37°C for 3–5 min until completely thawed; mixed thoroughly, ensuring that all cryo-precipitation has been completely dissolved; and then immediately assayed.

15. Duplicate AT measurements on a sample should vary by no more than 5 IU/dL. The expected imprecision for chromogenic assays is 1–3% that of automated assays.
16. After the reconstitution of each reagent vial, the solutions should be allowed to stand at room temperature (18–25°C) for 60 min, and then should be mixed before use. When controls and calibrators are lyophilized, they must be reconstituted at the same time as reagents. When using normal pool plasma as a calibrator, it must be thawed at the same time as the samples.

References

1. Bock SC, Harris JF, Balazs I, Trent JM (1985) Assignment of the human antithrombin III structural gene to chromosome 1q23-25. Cytogenet Cell Genet 39:67–69
2. Seegers WH, Johnson JF, Fell C (1954) An antithrombin reaction to prothrombin activation. Am J Physiol 176:97–103
3. Rosenberg RD, Damus PS (1973) The purification and mechanism of action of human antithrombin-heparin cofactor. J Biol Chem 248:6490–6505
4. Buchanan MR, Boneu B, Ofosu F, Hirsh J (1985) The relative importance of thrombin inhibition and factor Xa inhibition to the antithrombotic effects of heparin. Blood 65:198–201
5. Kurachi K, Fujikawa K, Schmer G, Davie EW (1976) Inhibition of bovine factor IXa and factor Xabeta by antithrombin III. Biochemistry 15:373–377
6. Scott CF, Colman RW (1989) Factors influencing the acceleration of human factor XIa inactivation by antithrombin III. Blood 73:1873–1879
7. Stead N, Kaplan AP, Rosenberg RD (1976) Inhibition of activated factor XII by antithrombin-heparin cofactor. J Biol Chem 251:6481–6488
8. Highsmith RF, Rosenberg RD (1974) The inhibition of human plasmin by human antithrombin-heparin cofactor. J Biol Chem 249:4335–4338
9. Lane DA, Bayston T, Olds RJ et al (1997) Antithrombin mutation database: 2nd (1997) update. For the Plasma Coagulation Inhibitors Subcommittee of the Scientific and Standardization Committee of the International Society on Thrombosis and Haemostasis. Thromb Haemost 77:197–211
10. Abildgaard U, Lie M, Odegard OR (1977) Antithrombin (heparin cofactor) assay with "new" chromogenic substrates (S-2238 and Chromozym TH). Thromb Res 11:549–553
11. Odegard OR, Lie M, Abildgaard U (1975) Heparin cofactor activity measured with an amidolytic method. Thromb Res 6:287–294
12. Kristensen SR, Rasmussen B, Pedersen S, Bathum L (2007) Detecting antithrombin deficiency may be a difficult task—more than one test is necessary. J Thromb Haemost 5:617–618
13. Jennings I, Kitchen S, Woods TA, Preston FE (2005) Multilaboratory testing in thrombophilia through the United Kingdom National External Quality Assessment Scheme (Blood Coagulation) Quality Assurance Program. Semin Thromb Hemost 31:66–72
14. Ungerstedt JS, Schulman S, Egberg N, Antovic J, Blombäck N (2002) Discrepancy between antithrombin activity methods revealed in Antithrombin Stockholm: do factor Xa-based methods overestimate antithrombin activity in some patients? Blood 99:2271–2272
15. Laurell C (1977) Electroimmunoassay. Scand J Clin Lab Invest 29:21–37
16. Sas G, Pepper DS (1976) Detection of thrombin-antithrombin III complex by crossed immunoelectrophoresis. Thromb Res 9:95–97
17. Andrew M, Paes B, Milner R et al (1987) Development of the human coagulation system in the full-term infant. Blood 70: 165–172
18. Andrew M, Vegh P, Johnston M, Bowker J, Ofosu F, Mitchell L (1992) Maturation of the hemostatic system during childhood. Blood 80:1998–2005
19. Monagle P, Barnes C, Ignjatovic V et al (2006) Developmental haemostasis—impact for clinical haemostasis laboratories. Thromb Haemost 95:362–372
20. Demers C, Henderson P, Blajchman MA et al (1993) An antithrombin III assay based on factor Xa inhibition provides a more reliable test to identify congenital antithrombin III deficiency than an assay based on thrombin inhibition. Thromb Haemost 69:231–235
21. Refvem O, Fagerhol MK, Abildgaard U (1973) Changes in antithrombin III levels following cessation of anticoagulant therapy. Acta Med Scand 193:307–309

Chapter 29

Protein C

Mirta Hepner and Vasiliki Karlaftis

Abstract

Protein C (PC) is a 62-kDa vitamin K-dependent plasma zymogen which, after activation to serine protease, plays an important role in the physiologic regulation of blood coagulation.

Given that PC is one of the major naturally occurring inhibitors of coagulation, acquired or hereditary deficiencies of this protein result in excessive thrombin generation. As a vast array of mutations are responsible for hereditary PC deficiencies, screening for their presence by DNA testing would require sequencing each entire gene involving numerous exons. Moreover, the knowledge of the gene mutation does not offer any benefit in the treatment of thrombophilic families, so the routine molecular characterization is not indicative. These defects are detected by functional or immunological assays. Measurement of PC activity is essential to identify subjects with both type I and type II PC defects. There is no need to routinely perform PC immunological assays. However, they are useful in order to distinguish type I from type II PC hereditary deficiency.

Key words Protein C, Thrombophilia, Functional assay, Immunological assay, Blood coagulation inhibitor, Acquired deficiency, Hereditary deficiency

1 Introduction

Protein C (PC) is a 62-kDa vitamin K-dependent plasma zymogen which, after activation to serine protease, plays an important role in the physiologic regulation of blood coagulation (1). Human protein C, produced principally in the liver, is composed of a heavy 41 kDa chain with 250 amino acids, and a light 21 kDa chain with 155 amino acids; these chains are held together by disulfide bond (2).

Vitamin K is required for a posttranslational modification of PC, where glutamic acid residues are converted to gamma carboxyglutamic acid, required for calcium binding and interaction with phospholipid surfaces. PC binds to a membrane receptor, the endothelial cell PC receptor (EPCR). It is then activated by thrombin bound to an adjacent membrane protein, thrombomodulin (TM). Activated PC (APC), together with its cofactor, protein S (PS),

Paul Monagle (ed.), *Haemostasis: Methods and Protocols*, Methods in Molecular Biology, vol. 992,
DOI 10.1007/978-1-62703-339-8_29,

forms a complex on cell membrane surfaces and proteolytically degrades activated and VIII, thus inactivating them (3). In addition to activating PC, the TM/Thrombin complex is also able to activate the thrombin activatable fibrinolysis inhibitor (TAFI), which results in inhibition of fibrin degradation.

Given that PC is one of the major naturally occurring inhibitors of coagulation, acquired or hereditary deficiencies of this protein result in excessive thrombin generation. As a vast array of mutations are responsible for hereditary PC deficiencies, screening for their presence by DNA testing would require sequencing each entire gene involving numerous exons (4). Moreover, the knowledge of the gene mutation does not offer any benefit in the treatment of thrombophilic families, so the routine molecular characterization is not indicative. These defects are detected by functional or immunological assays. Measurement of PC activity is essential to identify subjects with both type I and type II PC defects. There is no need to routinely perform PC immunological assays. However, they would be useful in order to distinguish type I from type II PC hereditary deficiency (5).

1.1 Functional Assays

Functional assays were designed to measure the inhibitory activity of protein C against the natural substrates (activated factors VIII and V). This measurement can be achieved through the activated partial thromboplastin time (aPTT) (clotting assay), or using synthetic substrates assessed photometrically (amidolytic assay) (see Notes 1–3). There are commercial methods based on these principles. Both these assays use the PC activator from southern copperhead venom (*Agkistrodon contortrix contortrix*, Protac), which is a rapid activator that can be used without prepurification of protein C. The amidolytic assay uses a synthetic peptide substrate for the activated PC, to which a para-nitroaniline group is attached. The increase in absorbance at 405 nm is proportional to PC concentration. Assays can be performed in an automated way on a coagulation analyzer, or following a microplate method. Both procedures can be performed either by measuring the rate of cleavage of substrate (kinetic method) or by measuring absorbance after a fixed incubation time (end point method). The methods based on activation with snake venom and measurements of the activity with synthetic substrates are much simpler and devoid of artifacts, and are recommended for initial testing for PC deficiency (5). The chromogenic substrates used in the amidolytic assay bind only to the active site of activated PC. A rare case of dysfunctional PC deficiency affecting protein C ability to interact with thrombin, endothelial Protein C receptor, phospholipid, or PS has been published, but has not been detected by amidolytic assays.

1.2 Antigenic Assays

Antigenic assays for PC measure the amount of PC in plasma, but do not assess functionality. The available assays include enzyme-linked immunosorbent assays (ELISAs) (6) electroimmunoassay (7) and radioimmunoassay (8). Both ELISA and radioimmunoassay can detect PC levels below 5%, but Laurell rocket method may not be able to detect levels that low.

In the Laurell rocket procedure, an agarose gel is impregnated with antibodies against PC. Plasma samples are added in wells and then electrophoresed. The antibody-antigen complexes precipitate during electrophoresis, and the height of the precipitin arc is proportional to the amount of PC in plasma.

It is necessary to include EDTA in both gel and running buffer to ensure that both carboxylated and acarboxylated forms migrate at the same rate (9). This assay is time-consuming and has very poor sensitivity and precision.

Radioimmunoassay and ELISA are assays that quantify PC antigen using an antibody specific to PC. In ELISA, a capture antibody directed against human PC is immobilized on the surface of a microtiter plate. After patient plasma specimen is added, the amount of PC bound is detected by a secondary anti-PC antibody, which is directly coupled to an enzyme (peroxidase or alkaline phosphatase) for colorimetric detection. (6). The color generated is proportional to the concentration of PC in the sample. The radioimmunoassay is performed using a similar principle, but with a solution-based technique using a single, radiolabeled antibody (8).

1.3 Reference Ranges

Calculation of local laboratory reference ranges is very important, owing to variability in test methodology from site to site and variability in population parameters. It should be based on the 2.5–97.5 centile or constructed from log-transformed data given that distribution of results is not Gaussian. There is a possibility of obtaining a potential false-positive, as a normal reference range only captures ~95% of population values.

The wide range of antigen and functional PC values in normal adults could be caused by an overlap in values between heterozygous and normal individuals at the low end of the reference ranges.

Gender, oral contraceptive use, and circadian rhythm may influence PC levels, but it is acceptable to use an adult reference range including similar numbers of men and women. PC levels may be higher in postmenopausal women.

PC levels are age dependent. PC levels are low in neonates and infants, and on average they either increase to adult levels by approximately 1 year of age, or they attain adult levels by 16 years of age (10, 11). Therefore, it is strongly recommended to employ local reference ranges according to age group (12).

A reference range for PC activity to antigen ratio can be of help to differentiate method variation in type II defect.

Accuracy should be verified by using normal and abnormal quality control plasma samples and also by taking part in national and/or international quality assurance programs. Internal quality control (IQC) and external quality assessment (EQA) are distinct complementary components of a laboratory quality assurance program. IQC is used to identify the degree of precision of the technique, precision being the degree of agreement among repeat measurements on one sample. EQA is used to identify the degree of agreement between the results from one laboratory and those obtained by other centers. EQA for thrombophilia tests are available from several international EQA providers (13). In all cases, the control material must be treated exactly like test samples if possible. Since some variation will necessarily occur as a result of biological, technical, and analytical variation, each quality control result should be recorded and assessed against the target range considered to be acceptable.

1.4 Clinical Applications

The PC immunological assays would be useful in order to distinguish type I from type II PC hereditary deficiency (5). The antigen assay can also be useful in confirming a low PC level in the investigation of patients stabilized on oral anticoagulation, by means of rate comparison with other protein vitamin K antigen (for example FII or FX antigen). Use of this rate was also suggested to identify some carriers of type I deficiency whose PC levels are within the normal range (14).

Detection of PC deficiency by functional and/or immunological testing is associated with a degree of uncertainty because the interpretation of results can be influenced by the accuracy of normal ranges and also by other genetic and environmental factors. Hence, repeat testing is often required.

Oral vitamin K inhibitors, such as warfarin or acenocoumarol should be taken into consideration when interpreting PC results. It is best to perform assays 30 days after discontinuation of vitamin K antagonists. Phenprocoumon, which has a 132-h half life, requires a longer delay before testing (15). Given that PC is a vitamin K-dependent factor, prothrombin time should be performed along with assays of two other vitamin K-dependent factors (for example FVII and FX) in order to demonstrate a specific deficiency.

In the clotting method, falsely low levels have been reported in plasma with high levels of factor VIII (16), and plasmas from carriers of factor V Arg506Gln (FV Leiden), particularly homozygous FV Leiden (17). Some of the clot-based PC functional assays are sensitive to coagulation inhibitors, such as heparin, direct thrombin inhibitors (e.g., hirudin or argatroban), and lupus anticoagulants (LA), which may lead to an overestimation of PC levels. The influence of LA on a particular test will depend largely on the concentration and composition of phospholipids in the test system.

Assays for PC are not recommended while on oral contraceptive or hormone replacement therapy (15).

Family studies may be beneficial to establish hereditary PC deficiency. Around 75% of patients with PC hereditary deficiency are type I (low function and antigen levels). Approximately 98% of the remaining patients have type II deficiency with low levels of PC in both clotting and chromogenic assays (18). A few cases of type II PC deficiency have been reported where amidolytic and antigen assay results have been normal, but clotting assay results have been abnormal (19). The advantages of chromogenic assays over clotting-based assays are related to specificity and precision, but the disadvantage is a lack of sensitivity to the rare defects. The consequences of failing to detect these rare defects must be evaluated at each medical center (see Notes 4 and 5).

2 Materials

2.1 Specimen

Citrate anticoagulated whole blood.

2.2 Collection

The needle size should be appropriate to the blood vessel (19–21 gauges for adults and 21–23 gauges for children). Syringes should not be bigger than 10 ml. The time for blood remains without anticoagulant should be minimized. NCCLS guidelines recommend collection into plastic or siliconized glass tubes containing 3.2% trisodium citrate (e.g., 9 volumes of blood to 1 volume of 0.109 M trisodium citrate) (see Note 6).

Immediately after sample collection, the tube is gently inverted to allow for the anticoagulant to mix with the sample.

2.3 Processing

Recommended centrifugation protocol for obtaining a platelet-free plasma sample adequate for coagulation testing includes minimum centrifugation at 2,500 × *g* for 15 min.

2.4 Storage

If testing is not going to occur on the day of collection, the plasma samples can be stored for up to 6 months at −70°C but must be thawed once only for functional assays; for antigenic assays they can be reused.

Once complete reconstitution of reagents has been attained, frozen samples should be kept at 37°C for 3–5 min until completely thawed, mixed thoroughly, ensuring that all cryoprecipitation has been completely dissolved, and then immediately assayed.

After the reconstitution of each reagent vial, the solutions should be allowed to stand at room temperature (18–25°C) for 60 min, and then should be mixed before use.

3 Methods

3.1 PC Antigen ELISA

3.1.1 Assay Procedure

1. Add 100 μl purified monoclonal anti-PC antibody which has been diluted in coating buffer (50 mM) to every well on a microplate.
2. Incubate overnight at 2–8°C or for 2 h at 22°C.
3. Empty contents of wells.

4. Add 150 μl blocking buffer (PBS-BSA (1%, w/v)) to every well and incubate for 90 min at 22°C.
5. Wash plate three times with wash buffer [PBS-Tween (0.1%, v/v)].
6. Dilute reference plasma 1/100 and then serial 1/2's down to 1/3,200 (3.13%) in HBS-BSA-T20 sample diluents (see Notes 5 and 6).
7. Dilute sample plasma 1/200, 1/400, and 1/800 in HBS-BSA-T20 sample diluents (see Notes 7 and 8).
8. Apply 100 μl to appropriate wells.
9. Incubate plate at 22°C for 90 min.
10. Wash plate three times with wash buffer.
11. Dilute the peroxidase conjugated polyclonal anti-PC antibody 1/100 using HBS-BSA-T20 sample diluent.
12. Apply 100 μl to each well.
13. Incubate the plate at 22°C for 90 min.
14. Wash plate three times with wash buffer.
15. Apply 100 μl of freshly prepared OPD substrate to every well.
16. Allow the color to develop for 10–15 min then stop color reaction with the addition of 50 μl/well of 2.5 M H_2SO_4.

3.1.2 Measurement

1. Set the absorbance at 490 nm in a microtiter plate spectrophotometer.
2. Measure the absorbance in all wells at 490 nm (see Note 9).

3.1.3 Assay Calibration

1. Plot A_{490} against the amount of PC in the standards (see Note 10).
2. Amount of PC in the unknowns can be determined from this curve (see Note 11).

4 Notes

1. In the case of clotting assays, although the manual procedure method is included in the "paper inside the kit" (insert), measuring the clotting time with a stopwatch is almost impossible.
2. For clotting assays, the procedure can be made in either an automated or a semi-automated way. When using a semi-automated method, reagents must be kept at 4–8°C (cryo-racks/on melting ice) during the test run.
3. For clotting assays, keeping a consistent pace throughout the procedure is essential to reproduce values and save reagents. The automated method provides the possibility of working master, as dilutions are not performed by the technician,

thereby allowing for higher performance rates. Duplicate clotting times may be required at each dilution.

4. PC clotting assay results are significantly lower than PC chromogenic results in samples from individuals who are heterozygous or homozygous for factor V Arg506Gln, but the predilution of test samples in PC-deficient plasma removes the effect (13). Moreover, the predilution of the patient's plasma in PC-deficient plasma allows for the correction of other abnormalities such as PS deficiency.
5. When performing PC measurement by end point chromogenic assay, note that this assay can be influenced by elevated bilirubin, hemolysis, or lipemia in samples. Therefore, it is essential to perform a blank, where water is added instead of viper activator. The absorbance value for the blank is subtracted from that of the test and then the PC concentration is calculated.
6. Adequate performance of assays should include consideration of preanalytic variables, so extremely careful collection and processing is required. PC levels in clotted samples are low.
7. When controls and calibrators are lyophilized, they must be reconstituted at the same time as reagents. It is advisable that plasma sample, calibrator, and control dilutions be carried out using vortex mixer. When using normal pool plasma as a calibrator, it must be thawed at the same time as the samples.
8. The results are calculated from a standard curve that should be constructed using serial dilutions of a pooled normal plasma calibrated against the corresponding WHO international standard for PC (National Institute for Biological Standards and Control). Otherwise, results can be calculated using a commercial calibrator calibrated against the corresponding international standard. Final results are reported as a percentage of the calibrator. The current WHO international standard for PC is code number 02/342 STH 2007.
9. Duplicate measurements of PC levels on a sample should vary by no more than 5 IU/dl. The expected imprecision for chromogenic assays is 1–3% that of automated assays. The assay with a higher degree of precision is the chromogenic assay.
10. Every batch of assays should be tested with its own calibration curve using plasma calibrated against the appropriate standard.
11. The number of dilutions of the standard curve depends on the linear relationship between the variables being measured. If test results fall outside the linear region (linear regression plot) of the standard curve, the test should be repeated at an appropriate dilution. Do not extrapolate out of the calibration curve. PC activity of the samples should be determined immediately after calibration.

References

1. Kisiel W (1979) Human plasma protein C: isolation, characterization, and mechanism of activation by alpha-thrombin. J Clin Invest 64:761–769
2. Stenflo J, Fernlund P (1982) Amino acid sequence of the heavy chain of bovine protein C. J Biol Chem 257:12180–12190
3. Sadler JE (1993) Structure-function-relationships of the thrombin-thrombomodulin interaction. Haemostasis 23:183
4. Reitsma PH, Bernardi F, Doig RG et al (1995) Protein C deficiency: a database of mutations, 1995 update. On behalf of the Subcommittee on Plasma Coagulation Inhibitors of the Scientific and Standardization Committee of the ISTH. Thromb Haemost 73:876–889
5. Richards SM, Olson T, Keyes LD (1990) Quantitative and functional assays compared for determination of zymogen and activated human protein C. Clin Chem 36:1892–1896
6. Amiral J, Adalbert B, Adam M (1984) Application of enzyme immunoassays to coagulation testing. Clin Chem 30:1512–1516
7. Laurell C (1977) Electroimmunoassay. Scand J Clin Lab Invest 29:21–37
8. Ikeda K, Stenflo J (1985) A radioimmunoassay for protein C. Thromb Res 39:297–306
9. Mikami S, Tuddenham EG (1986) Studies on immunological assay of vitamin K dependent factors. II. Comparison of four immunoassay methods with functional activity of protein C in human plasma. Br J Haematol 62:183–193
10. Andrew M, Paes B, Milner R et al (1987) Development of the human coagulation system in the full-term infant. Blood 70:165–172
11. Andrew M, Vegh P, Johnston M, Bowker J, Ofosu F, Mitchell L (1992) Maturation of the hemostatic system during childhood. Blood 80:1998–2005
12. Monagle P, Barnes C, Ignjatovic V et al (2006) Developmental haemostasis—impact for clinical haemostasis laboratories. Thromb Haemost 95:362–372
13. Jennings I, Kitchen S, Woods TA, Preston FE (2005) Multilaboratory testing in thrombophilia through the United Kingdom National External Quality Assessment Scheme (Blood Coagulation) Quality Assurance Program. Semin Thromb Hemost 31:66–72
14. Pabinger I, Allaart CF, Hermans J, Briet E, Bertina RM (1992) Hereditary protein C-deficiency: laboratory values in transmitters and guidelines for the diagnostic procedure. Report on a study of the SSC Subcommittee on Protein C and Protein S. Protein C Transmitter Study Group. Thromb Haemost 68: 470–474
15. Kottke-Marchant K, Comp P (2002) Laboratory issues in diagnosing abnormalities of protein C, thrombomodulin, and endothelial cell protein C receptor. Arch Pathol Lab Med 126:1337–1348
16. de Moerloose P, Reber G, Bouvier CA (1988) Spuriously low levels of protein C with a Protac activation clotting assay. Thromb Haemost 59:543
17. Faioni EM, Franchi F, Asti D, Mannucci PM (1996) Resistance to activated protein C mimicking dysfunctional protein C: diagnostic approach. Blood Coagul Fibrinolysis 7:349–352
18. Faioni EM, Hermida J, Rovida E et al (2000) Type II protein C deficiency: identification and molecular modelling of two natural mutants with low anticoagulant and normal amidolytic activity. Br J Haematol 108:265–271
19. Bovill EG, Tomczak JA, Grant B et al (1992) Protein CVermont: symptomatic type II protein C deficiency associated with two GLA domain mutations. Blood 79:1456–1465

Chapter 30

Protein S

Mirta Hepner and Vasiliki Karlaftis

Abstract

Protein S (PS) is a vitamin K-dependent plasma glycoprotein. Around 60–70% of PS in plasma is noncovalently bound to C4-binding protein (C4BP). Free PS functions as a cofactor that enhances the activity of activated protein C (APC) in the proteolytic degradation of activated factors V and VIII. PS also has a more recently described APC-independent ability to directly inhibit prothrombinase and tenase by direct binding of activated factors V, VIII, and X.

Given that PS is one of the major naturally occurring inhibitors of coagulation, acquired or hereditary deficiencies of this protein result in excessive thrombin generation. As a vast array of mutations are responsible for hereditary PS deficiencies, screening for their presence by DNA testing would require sequencing each entire gene involving numerous exons. Moreover, the knowledge of the gene mutation does not offer any benefit in the treatment of thrombophilic families, so the routine molecular characterization is not indicative. These defects are detected by functional or immunological assays for free and total PS forms. Given that functional PS assays may detect some forms of PS deficiency that free PS immunoassays may miss, it is recommended to include them for initial testing along with immunoassays for free PS, although they should be used with caution. Functional PS assays are subject to multiple interference. For example in the presence of lupus anticoagulant (LA), only free PS immunoassays are recommended for initial testing. PS antigen assays are more popular with most laboratories.

Key words Protein S, Functional assay, Immunological assays, Blood coagulation inhibitor, Acquired deficiency, Hereditary deficiency

1 Introduction

Protein S (PS) is a vitamin K-dependent plasma glycoprotein. Around 60–70% of PS in plasma is noncovalently bound to C4-binding protein (C4BP) (1). Free PS functions as a cofactor that enhances the activity of activated protein C (APC) in the proteolytic degradation of activated factors V and VIII. PS also has a more recently described APC-independent ability to directly inhibit prothrombinase and tenase by direct binding of activated factors V, VIII, and X (2, 3).

Protein S is composed of 635 amino acids and is produced mainly in the liver (4). However, it has also been identified in

Paul Monagle (ed.), *Haemostasis: Methods and Protocols*, Methods in Molecular Biology, vol. 992,
DOI 10.1007/978-1-62703-339-8_30, © Springer Science+Business Media New York 2013

megakaryocytes (5), endothelial cells (4), the brain, and Leydig cells (6). This binding interaction complicates the measurement and interpretation of PS concentrations in plasma.

Given that PS is one of the major naturally occurring inhibitors of coagulation, acquired or hereditary deficiencies of this protein result in excessive thrombin generation. As a vast array of mutations are responsible for hereditary PS deficiencies, screening for their presence by DNA testing would require sequencing each entire gene involving numerous exons (7). Moreover, the knowledge of the gene mutation does not offer any benefit in the treatment of thrombophilic families, so the routine molecular characterization is not indicative. These defects are detected by functional or immunological assays for free and total PS forms. Given that functional PS assays may detect some forms of PS deficiency that free PS immunoassays may miss, it is recommended to include them for initial testing along with immunoassays for free PS, although they should be used with caution. Functional PS assays are subject to multiple interference. For example in the presence of lupus anticoagulant (LA), only free PS immunoassays are recommended for initial testing. PS antigen assays are popular with most laboratories.

1.1 Functional Assays

PS functional assays were designed to measure the inhibitory activity of this protein as an APC cofactor in the inactivation of activated factors VIII and V. There are commercial methods based on this principle that apply either the prothrombin time or the aPTT test. In the aPTT methodology, diluted patient plasma is added to PS-depleted plasma in the presence of purified APC and factor Va (see Notes 1–3). In the PT format, a similar approach can be taken or else, the native plasma PC in the depleted plasma can be activated by Protac, an enzyme from the southern copperhead venom (*Agkistrodon contortrix contortrix*). However, the specificity of these methods has proven to be rather poor, because of the influence of factor V Arg506Gln (8), APC resistance, high concentrations of prothrombin, factor VIII, and factor VII. Lupus anticoagulant may also interfere, although its effect is minimized by the dilution of patient plasma used in the assay.

The results are calculated from a standard curve that should be constructed using serial dilutions of pooled normal plasma calibrated against the corresponding WHO international standard for PS (National Institute for Biological Standards and Control). Otherwise, results can be calculated using a commercial calibrator calibrated against the corresponding international standard. Final results are reported as a percentage of the calibrator.

There is a considerable availability of commercial PS activity assay kits today. However, it should be noted that discrepancies have been reported (9) particularly when using the manufacturer's reference range. Therefore, it is strongly recommended to employ locally determined reference ranges when protein S assays are performed.

1.2 Immunologic Assays

Antigenic assays for PS measure the amount of PS in plasma, but do not assess functionality. The available assays include enzyme-linked immunosorbent assays (ELISA), electroimmunoassay (10), and latex-based ITB assays. ELISA can detect PS levels below 5%, but Laurell rocket method may not be able to detect levels that low.

Until more reliable methods for measuring PS activity are available, the laboratory should rely on the measurement of the antigen with ELISA-based methods. Because of the distribution of PS in plasma (60–70% of PS is bound to C4BP), it is possible to measure the total or the free antigen depending on assay conditions. Pretreatment of the test plasma with polyethylene glycol (PEG) precipitates the bound form of PS, leaving the free form in the supernatant. Both free and total PS can be conveniently measured by commercial methods using an ELISA system with monoclonal or polyclonal antibodies. Laboratories have a number of commercially available polyclonal ELISAs which, together with the addition of 3.75% polyethylene glycol 6000 (PEG) precipitation, measure free PS. However, PEG precipitation is not reproducible and time-consuming. At present, commercially available monoclonal ELISAs can accurately measure free and total PS. These assays do not require PEG precipitation of C4BP bound PS.

In 1996, at a meeting held by the International Society of Thrombosis and Haemostasis and the World Health Organization (WHO), it was found that measurement of free PS may be more useful than total PS for the diagnosis of PS deficiency. Indeed, recent studies investigating members of large kindreds affected with genetically proven PS deficiency revealed that the free antigen is more reliable than the total antigen for discriminating carriers from noncarriers of PS deficiency (11, 12). The only drawback of performing only PS assays is that rare cases of type II PS deficiency might be missed. The practical gold standard is clearly ELISA with or without PEG precipitations.

In the Laurell rocket procedure, an agarose gel is impregnated with antibodies to PS. Plasma samples should be treated with and without PEG precipitation, depending on whether free or total PS is being measured. The samples should be added in wells and electrophoresed. The antibody-antigen complexes precipitate during electrophoresis, and the height of the precipitin arc is proportional to the amount of PS in plasma. The results are calculated from a standard curve that should be constructed using serial dilutions of a pooled normal plasma calibrated against the corresponding WHO international standard for PS (National Institute for Biological Standards and Control), treated both with and without PEG precipitation. Otherwise, results can be calculated using a commercial calibrator calibrated against the corresponding international standard. Final results are reported as a percentage of the calibrator.

ELISA assays quantify PS antigen using an antibody specific to PS. In ELISA, a capture antibody directed against human PS is immobilized on the surface of a microtiter plate. After patient plasma specimen is added, the amount of PS bound is detected by a secondary anti-PS antibody, which is directly coupled to an enzyme (peroxidase or alkaline phosphatase) for colorimetric detection (13). ELISA is precise and very sensitive to low levels of PS.

1.3 Reference Ranges

Calculation of local laboratory reference ranges is very important, owing to variability in test methodology from site to site and variability in population parameters, considering that there is a possibility of obtaining a potential false-positive rate of ~2.5% (given that distribution of results is Gaussian, a normal reference range is defined as the mean ± 2 standard deviations, which only capture ~95% of normal values).

PS levels are gender dependent. PS levels are lower in women than in men and can be further decreased by the use of certain oral contraceptives. Therefore, specific reference ranges for women should be considered. Hormone replacement therapy may reduce levels of total PS but not of free PS. PS levels obtained during pregnancy or postpartum period are lower because they are influenced by physiologic changes.

PS levels are age dependent. PS levels are low in neonates and infants, and on average they either increase to adult levels by approximately 1 year of age or they attain adult levels by 16 years of age (14, 15). Therefore, it is strongly recommended to employ local reference ranges according to age group (16).

Accuracy should be verified by using normal and abnormal quality control plasma samples and also by taking part in national and/or international quality assurance programs. Internal quality control (IQC) and external quality assessment (EQA) are distinct complementary components of a laboratory quality assurance program. IQC is used to identify the degree of precision of the technique, precision being the degree of agreement among repeat measurements on one sample. EQA is used to identify the degree of agreement between the results from one laboratory and those obtained by other centers. EQA for thrombophilia tests are available from several international EQA providers (9). In all cases, the control material must be treated exactly like test samples. Since some variation will necessarily occur as a result of biological, technical, and analytical variation, each quality control result should be recorded and assessed against the target range considered to be acceptable.

1.4 Clinical Applications

There is no need to routinely perform total PS immunological assays. However, they are useful to distinguish subtypes of hereditary deficiencies. Hereditary PS deficiency is classified as type I, II, or III. Type I is characterized by reduced levels of total PS antigen, free PS antigen, and PS activity. Type II is defined by isolated PS activity. Type III has normal levels of total PS but reduced levels of both free and PS activity. Family studies may be beneficial to establish hereditary PS deficiency.

Detection of PS deficiency by functional and/or immunological testing is associated with a degree of uncertainty because the interpretation of results can be influenced by the accuracy of normal ranges and also by other genetic and environmental factors. Hence, repeat testing is often required. Assays for PS are not recommended while on oral contraceptive or hormone replacement therapy (17).

The antigen assay can also be useful in confirming a low PS level in the investigation of patients stabilized while on oral anticoagulation, by means of rate comparison with other protein vitamin K antigen (for example FII or FX antigen). Use of this rate was also suggested to identify some type I deficiency carriers whose PS levels are within the normal range (18).

Given that PS is a vitamin K-dependent factor, prothrombin time should be performed along with assays of two other vitamin K-dependent factors (for example FVII and FX) to demonstrate a specific deficiency. Oral vitamin K inhibitors, such as warfarin or acenocoumarol, should be taken into consideration when interpreting PS results. It is best to perform assays 30 days after discontinuation of vitamin K antagonists. Phenprocoumon, which has a 132-h half life, requires a longer delay before testing (17).

2 Materials

2.1 Specimen

Citrate anticoagulated whole blood.

2.2 Collection

The needle size should be appropriate to the blood vessel (19–21 gauges for adults and 21–23 gauges for children). Syringes should not be bigger than 10 ml. The time for blood remains without anticoagulant should be minimized. NCCLS guidelines recommend collection into plastic or siliconized glass tubes containing 3.2% trisodium citrate (e.g., 9 volumes of blood to 1 volume of 0.109 M trisodium citrate) (see Note 4).

Immediately after sample collection, the tube is gently inverted to allow for the anticoagulant to mix with the sample.

2.3 Processing

Recommended centrifugation protocol for obtaining a platelet-free plasma sample adequate for coagulation testing includes minimum centrifugation at 2,500 $\times g$ for 15 min.

2.4 Storage

If testing is not going to occur on the day of collection, the plasma samples can be stored for up to 6 months at –70°C but must be thawed once only for functional assays; for antigenic assays they can be reused.

Once complete reconstitution of reagents has been attained, frozen samples should be kept at 37°C for 3–5 min until completely thawed, mixed thoroughly, ensuring that all cryoprecipitation has been completely dissolved, and then immediately assayed.

After the reconstitution of each reagent vial, the solutions should be allowed to stand at room temperature (18–25°C) for 60 min, and then should be mixed before use.

3 Methods

3.1 Total PS

3.1.1 Assay Procedure

1. Coat microplate with the first mouse monoclonal anti-human total PS antibody.
2. Dilute plasma samples 1:21 with phosphate buffer (50 μl plasma +1 ml phosphate buffer) (see Notes 5–7).
3. Apply 50 μl of second mouse monoclonal anti-human total PS antibody coupled with peroxidase to each well.
4. Apply 200 μl of the diluted plasma samples to each well.
5. Cover all wells.
6. Incubate plate for 1 h at room temperature.
7. Wash wells five times with wash buffer.
8. Apply 200 μl TMB solution to each well.
9. Incubate plate for 5 min at room temperature.
10. Quench the reaction with 50 μl 1 M H_2SO_4.
11. Wait 15 min and then measure the absorbance at 450 nm within an hour.

3.1.2 Measurement

1. Set the absorbance at 450 nm in a microtiter plate spectrophotometer.
2. Measure the absorbance in all wells at 450 nm.

3.1.3 Assay Calibration

1. Plot *A*450 nm against the amount of total PS in the standards (see Note 8).
2. Amount of total PS in the unknowns can be determined from this curve (see Notes 9 and 10).

3.2 Free PS

3.2.1 Assay Procedure

1. Coat microplate with the first mouse monoclonal anti-human free PS antibody.
2. Dilute plasma samples 1:21 with phosphate buffer (50 μl plasma + 1 ml phosphate buffer) (see Notes 5–7).
3. Apply 50 μl of second mouse monoclonal anti-human free PS antibody coupled with peroxidase to each well.

4. Apply 200 μl of the diluted plasma samples to each well.
5. Cover all wells.
6. Incubate plate for 1 h at room temperature.
7. Wash wells five times with wash buffer.
8. Apply 200 μl TMB solution to each well.
9. Incubate plate for 5 min at room temperature.
10. Quench the reaction with 50 μl 1 M H_2SO_4.
11. Wait 15 min and then measure the absorbance at 450 nm within an hour.

3.2.2 Measurement

1. Set the absorbance at 450 nm in a microtiter plate spectrophotometer.
2. Measure the absorbance in all wells at 450 nm.

3.2.3 Assay Calibration

1. Plot *A*450 nm against the amount of total PS in the standards (see Note 8).
2. Amount of total PS in the unknowns can be determined from this curve (see Notes 9 and 10).

4 Notes

1. In the case of clotting assays, although the manual procedure method is included in the "paper inside the kit" (insert), measuring the clotting time with a stopwatch can be very difficult.
2. For clotting assays, the procedure can be made in either an automated or a semi-automated way. When using a semi-automated method, reagents must be kept at 4–8°C (cryo racks or melting ice) during the test run.
3. For clotting assays, keeping a consistent pace throughout the procedure is essential to reproduce values and save reagents. The automated method provides the possibility of working master, as dilutions are not performed by the technician, thereby allowing for higher performance rates.
4. Adequate performance of assays should include consideration of preanalytic variables, so careful collection and processing is required (Arkin, NCCLS). PS levels in clotted samples are decreased.
5. When controls and calibrators are lyophilized, they must be reconstituted at the same time as reagents. It is advisable that plasma samples, calibrator, and control dilutions be carried out using vortex mixer. When using normal pool plasma as a calibrator, it must be thawed at the same time as the samples.
6. When measuring free PS by ELISA with monoclonal antibodies, the dilutions should be tested without delay, and incubation

times and temperatures should be controlled appropriately because they can result in overestimation of free PS.

7. The results are calculated from a standard curve that should be constructed using serial dilutions of a pooled normal plasma calibrated against the corresponding WHO international standard for PS (National Institute for Biological Standards and Control). Otherwise, results can be calculated using a commercial calibrator calibrated against the corresponding international standard. Final results are reported as a percentage of the calibrator. The current WHO international standard for PS is code number 03/228.
8. Every batch of assays should be tested with its own calibration curve using plasma calibrated against the appropriate standard. PS activity of the samples should be determined immediately after calibration.
9. The number of dilutions of the standard curve depends on the linear relationship between the variables being measured. If test results fall outside the linear region (linear regression plot) of the standard curve, the test should be repeated at an appropriate dilution. Do not extrapolate in the calibration curve. Duplicate measurements of clotting times may be required at each dilution.
10. Duplicate PS levels on a sample should vary, but the data should be analyzed to ensure a good precision (<5% variation between replicate values is advised).

References

1. Dahlback B, Hildebrand B, Malm J (1990) Characterization of functionally important domains in human vitamin K-dependent protein S using monoclonal antibodies. J Biol Chem 265:8127–8135
2. van Wijnen M, van't Veer C, Stam JG et al (1996) The interaction of protein S with the phospholipid surface is essential for the activated protein C-independent activity of protein S. Thromb Haemost 76:397–403
3. Koppelman SJ, van't Veer C, Sixma JJ, Bouma BN (1995) Synergistic inhibition of the intrinsic factor X activation by protein S and C4b-binding protein. Blood 86:2653–2660
4. Fair DS, Marlar RA (1986) Biosynthesis and secretion of factor VII, protein C, protein S, and the protein C inhibitor from a human hepatoma cell line. Blood 67:64–70
5. Ogura M, Tanabe N, Nishioka J, Suzuki K, Saito H (1987) Biosynthesis and secretion of functional protein S by a human megakaryoblastic cell line (MEG-01). Blood 70:301–306
6. Malm J, He XH, Bjartell A, Shen L, Abrahamsson PA, Dahlback B (1994) Vitamin K-dependent protein S in Leydig cells of human testis. Biochem J 302(Pt 3):845–850
7. Gandrille S, Borgel D, Sala N et al (2000) Protein S deficiency: a database of mutations–summary of the first update. Thromb Haemost 84:918
8. Faioni EM, Franchi F, Asti D, Sacchi E, Bernardi F, Mannucci PM (1993) Resistance to activated protein C in nine thrombophilic families: interference in a protein S functional assay. Thromb Haemost 70:1067–1071
9. Jennings I, Kitchen S, Woods TA, Preston FE (2005) Multilaboratory testing in thrombophilia through the United Kingdom National External Quality Assessment Scheme (Blood Coagulation) Quality Assurance Program. Semin Thromb Hemost 31:66–72
10. Laurell C (1977) Electroimmunoassay. Scand J Clin Lab Invest 29:21–37
11. Simmonds RE, Ireland H, Lane DA, Zoller B, de Frutos PG, Dahlback B (1998) Clarification of the risk for venous thrombosis associated with hereditary protein S deficiency by investigation of a large kindred with a characterized gene defect. Ann Intern Med 128:8–14

12. Makris M, Leach M, Beauchamp NJ et al (2000) Genetic analysis, phenotypic diagnosis, and risk of venous thrombosis in families with inherited deficiencies of protein S. Blood 95:1935–1941
13. Amiral J, Adalbert B, Adam M (1984) Application of enzyme immunoassays to coagulation testing. Clin Chem 30:1512–1516
14. Andrew M, Paes B, Milner R et al (1987) Development of the human coagulation system in the full-term infant. Blood 70:165–172
15. Andrew M, Vegh P, Johnston M, Bowker J, Ofosu F, Mitchell L (1992) Maturation of the hemostatic system during childhood. Blood 80:1998–2005
16. Monagle P, Barnes C, Ignjatovic V et al (2006) Developmental haemostasis–impact for clinical haemostasis laboratories. Thromb Haemost 95:362–372
17. Kottke-Marchant K, Comp P (2002) Laboratory issues in diagnosing abnormalities of protein C, thrombomodulin, and endothelial cell protein C receptor. Arch Pathol Lab Med 126:1337–1348
18. Pabinger I, Allaart CF, Hermans J, Briet E, Bertina RM (1992) Hereditary protein C-deficiency: laboratory values in transmitters and guidelines for the diagnostic procedure. Report on a study of the SSC Subcommittee on Protein C and Protein S. Protein C Transmitter Study Group. Thromb Haemost 68:470–474

Chapter 31

Testing for Hyperhomocysteinemia in Subjects with a History of Thromboembolic Events Using HPLC Technique

Jonas Denecke

Abstract

An elevated homocysteine level is a well-known thrombophilic risk factor. Determination of total plasma homocysteine therefore is an integrated part of the diagnostic setting after thromboembolic events; about 5–7% of the population do have elevated homocysteine levels. Some forms of hyperhomocysteinemia are treatable; thus a standardized and reliable diagnostic setting has to be at hand. HPLC analysis is widely available in routine diagnostic laboratories. We use the fluorogenic reagent SBD-F to derivate with plasma homocysteine after release of the amino acid from homo- and heterodimers and protein bond using TBP. Separation is performed using a c18 reverse-phase column with aqua and acetonitrile as solvent. Due to continuous release of homocysteine from blood cells centrifugation and separation of plasma within 30 min after venous puncture are crucial for reproducible results.

Key words Homocysteine, Thromboembolic risk factors, HPLC

1 Introduction

The amino acid homocysteine was first described in 1950 by Du Vignoud as a product of methionine metabolism. Homocysteine is a product of the intermediary metabolism without any known ulterior function and plays a role for the methyle-donating function of methionine that is important for several metabolic pathways. Homocysteine is metabolized either by transsulfuration to cysteine using the enzyme cystathionine-β-synthase that requires vitamin B6 as a cofactor or by remethylation to methionine catalyzed by the enzyme betaine-homocysteine methyltransferase which depends on vitamin B12. Homocysteine can be increased in blood due to an impaired intracellular metabolism that can for example be a result from vitamin B12 deficiency (decreased remethylation to methionine) or due to genetic defects or variants affecting the catabolism of homocysteine (1, 2). Additionally some drugs and conditions decreasing the homocysteine excretion are able to raise

Paul Monagle (ed.), *Haemostasis: Methods and Protocols*, Methods in Molecular Biology, vol. 992,
DOI 10.1007/978-1-62703-339-8_31, © Springer Science+Business Media New York 2013

plasma homocysteine levels (3). Patients with homocysteinuria, an autosomal recessive defect in the homocysteine metabolism, have excessively increased blood homocysteine level and a high risk of thrombosis. Homocysteine levels in healthy subjects are known to be age dependent rising especially during childhood and in women after the menopause. Three categories of hyperhomocysteinemia were defined by Chen et al. classifying groups with mildly (15–25 μmol/l), moderately (25–50 μmol/l), and severely increased homocysteine levels (>50 μmol/l); normal homocysteine concentrations range between 5 and 15 μmol/l (4). However, other classifications exist. About 5–7% of the population have at least a mild elevation of homocysteine in plasma, most of them due to known genetic variants that directly or indirectly affect homocysteine metabolism (5).

Evidence suggests that elevated homocysteine increases the risk of cerebrovascular and coronary heart disease and of venous thromboembolic events. Thus determination of plasma homocysteine should be performed in every case where evaluation of thrombophilic risk factors is indicated (5).

Some authors propose that fasting homocysteine should be determined; however, Thirup et al. showed that postprandial homocysteine levels do not systematically deviate from fasting homocysteine levels (6).

Homocysteine is continuously released from blood cells independent of the plasma homocysteine levels. Thus reliable and constant homocysteine levels should be determined from EDTA-plasma after centrifugation of the blood sample within 30 min after venous puncture. In the plasma homocysteine is stable for several days.

2 Materials

1. C18 HPLC-Column (XTerra columns, USA, XTerra RP18, 5 μm).
2. SBD-F (4-Fluoro-7-sulfobenzofuranzan, ammonium salt, Dokindo Laboratories, Japan).
3. Plasma Control Homocysteine Level 1 (10.9 μmol/l) and Level 2 (22.2 μmol) (Chromosystems, Germany).
4. Acetic buffer: 11.4 ml of 100% acetic acid (HPLC grade) are mixed with 1,400 ml of aqua (HPLC grade). pH is adjusted to 3.5 using a solution of 6.8 g sodium acetate in 250 ml aqua. Finally fill up to 2 l. Have to be prepared weekly.
5. TBP-stock-solution: Add 200 μl of Tri-*n*-butylphosphine (flammable, stored under argon) to 1.8 ml DMF, store at RT (see Note 1).
6. Perchloric acid 0.5 M with 1 mM EDTA: Mix 0.5 M perchloric acid (100 ml aqua and 4.3 ml perchloric acid 70–72%) with 37.2 mg EDTA.

7. 2 M potassium borate buffer pH 10.5: 300 ml aqua is carefully added to 33.67 g KOH. Boric acid is added till pH 10.5 is adjusted.
8. 2 M potassium borate buffer pH 10.5 with 5 mM EDTA: Add 372.2 mg EDTA to 2 M potassium borate buffer pH 10.5.
9. 0.1 M potassium borate buffer pH 9.5 with 2 mM EDTA: 10 ml of 2 M potassium borate buffer pH 10.5 are restocked to 200 ml using aqua and 148.9 mg EDTA is added. Adjust to pH 9.5.
10. SBD-F solution: Prepare a solution containing 1 mg SBD-F in 1 ml 0.1 M potassium borate buffer pH 9.5 with 2 mM EDTA (ultrasonic bath may be useful to dissolving SBD-F), store in the dark, useable for 3 weeks.
11. Homocystein-standards will be prepared using pure homocysteine solved in 0.1 M potassium borate buffer pH 9.5 with 2 mM EDTA.

3 Methods

Only 1% of plasma homocysteine is free, reduced homocysteine, about 5–10% is oxidized homocysteine, 5–10% is associated with cysteine as mixed disulfide, and 80–90% is bound to plasma proteins, especially albumin (7). The entire homocysteine concentration in the plasma, free homocysteine, oxidized and protein-bound homocysteine, is termed total plasma homocysteine. Since total plasma homocysteine is to be determined, homocysteine has to be released from disulfide and protein bonds by reduction preanalytically (8). Thiol oxidation is inhibited by adding EDTA to the following reactions. Finally homocysteine is derivate with the fluorogenic reagent SBD-F and derivated homocysteine is separated from other derivates and quantified by HPLC (9).

3.1 Plasma Sample Preparation

1. 10 μl of TBP-stock-solution is added to 100 μl of plasma (or prepared standard), mixed, and incubated for 30 min at 4°C (see Notes 2–4).
2. Add 100 μl of perchloric acid 0.5 M with 1 mM EDTA for protein precipitation, mix, and incubate at RT for 10 min. Centrifuge at 14,000 × *g* for 10 min.
3. 50 μl of the supernatant of step 2 is transferred to 125 μl of 2 M potassium borate buffer pH 10.5 with 5 mM EDTA and 50 μl of SBD-F solution is added. Mix and incubate for 60 min at 60°C, put samples on ice subsequently, and store at 4°C until use.

3.2 HPLC-Run

1. Inject 20 μl of prepared sample.
2. HPLC with fluorescence monitor (385 nm excitation, 515 nm emission).

3. HPLC-gradient:

Time (min)	Acetic buffer (%)	Acetonitrile (%)
0	100	0
3.5	98	2
7.5	96	4
8.7–13	100	0

4. Clean column with 50% aqua, 50% acetonitrile.
5. Peaks are quantified by reference to a calibration curve constructed by triplicate analysis of homocysteine standards 2.5–100 μmol/l.

4 Notes

1. TBP in our hands is more stable when solved in DMF. Solve the original liquid completely in 2 ml portions.
2. Homocysteine is stable in plasma at RT for at least 2 days.
3. Homocysteine is stable in plasma at −20°C for months.
4. Homocysteine is stable in whole blood for up to 4 h when cooled in ice water.

References

1. D' Angelo A, Coppola A, Madonna P, Fermo I, Pagano A, Mazzola G, Galli L, Cerbone AM (2000) The role of vitamin B12 in fasting hyperhomocysteinemia and its interaction with the homozygous C677T mutation of the methylenetetrahydrofolate reductase (MTHFR) gene. A case-control study of patients with early-onset thrombotic events. Thromb Haemost 83:563–570
2. Gaustadnes M, Rudiger N, Rasmussen K, Ingerslev J (2000) Intermediate and severe hyperhomocysteinemia with thrombosis: a study of genetic determinants. Thromb Haemost 83:554–558
3. Desouza C, Keebler M, McNamara DB, Fonseca V (2002) Drugs affecting homocysteine metabolism: impact on cardiovascular risk. Drugs 62:605–616
4. Chen P, Poddar R, Tipa EV, Dibello PM, Moravec CD, Robinson K, Green R, Kruger WD, Garrow TA, Jacobsen DW (1999) Homocysteine metabolism in cardiovascular cells and tissues: implications for hyperhomocysteinemia and cardiovascular disease. Adv Enzyme Regul 39:93–109
5. McCully KS (1996) Homocysteine and vascular disease. Nat Med 2:386–389
6. Thirup P, Ekelund S (1999) Day-to-day, postprandial, and orthostatic variation of total plasma homocysteine. Clin Chem 45:1280–1283
7. Jacobsen DW (1998) Homocysteine and vitamins in cardiovascular disease. Clin Chem 44:1833–1843
8. Araki A, Sako Y (1987) Determination of free and total homocysteine in human plasma by high-performance liquid chromatography with fluorescence detection. J Chromatogr 422: 43–52
9. Garcia AJ, Apitz-Castro R (2002) Plasma total homocysteine quantification: an improvement of the classical high-performance liquid chromatographic method with fluorescence detection of the thiol-SBD derivatives. J Chromatogr B Analyt Technol Biomed Life Sci 779:359–363

Chapter 32

Anticardiolipin Antibody and Anti-beta 2 Glycoprotein I Antibody Assays

Anne Raby, Karen Moffat, and Mark Crowther

Abstract

Antiphospholipid syndrome (APS) is an autoimmune disease and is a risk factor for a number of clinical manifestations; the classic presentations include fetal death or thrombosis (arterial or venous thromboembolism), in the presence of persistently increased titers of antiphospholipid (aPL) antibodies . The actual cause of APS is unknown but thought to be multifactorial. The disease is characterized by the presence of a heterogenous population of autoantibodies against phospholipid-binding proteins. APS presents either in isolation with no evidence of an underlying disease or in concert with an autoimmune disease such as systemic lupus erythematosus or rheumatoid arthritis. The wide diversity in clinical presentation often causes difficulty in identifying and treating patients and therefore a concise laboratory report containing interpretative comments is required to provide needed guidance to the clinician.

For a diagnosis of APS to be made both clinical and laboratory classification criteria must be met. Laboratory testing to identify aPL antibodies includes lupus anticoagulant (liquid-based clotting assays) and immunological solid-phase assays (usually enzyme-linked immunosorbent assay formats) for IgG and/or IgM anticardiolipin (aCL) antibodies and anti-beta 2 glycoprotein I (β2-GPI) antibodies. Other autoantibodies, such as those directed against anionic phospholipids, can also be assayed; however they are not of clinical significance.

Participation in a quality assurance program and an in-depth technical and clinical understanding of testing for aPL antibodies are required, as methods are limited by poor robustness, reproducibility, specificity, and standardization. Testing is further complicated by the lack of a "gold standard" laboratory test to diagnose or classify a patient as having APS.

This chapter discusses the clinical and laboratory theoretical and technical aspects of aCL and anti-β2GPI antibody assays.

Key words Antiphospholipid syndrome, Guidelines, Lupus anticoagulant, Anticardiolipin antibody, Anti-β2 glycoprotein I antibody, External quality assurance

1 Introduction

Antiphospholipid syndrome (APS) is an autoimmune disease and a risk factor for a number of commonly encountered clinical manifestations. The classic presentations include fetal death or thrombosis (arterial or venous thromboembolism), in the presence of

Paul Monagle (ed.), *Haemostasis: Methods and Protocols*, Methods in Molecular Biology, vol. 992,
DOI 10.1007/978-1-62703-339-8_32,

persistently increased titers of antiphospholipid (aPL) antibodies (1–3). The cause of APS is unknown; it presents either in isolation with no evidence of an underlying disease or in concert with an autoimmune disease such as systemic lupus erythematosus (SLE) or rheumatoid arthritis.

The term "APS" is misleading as the autoantibodies of interest are not directed against anionic phospholipids but are a group of heterogenous autoantibodies/immunoglobulins directed against glycoproteins in concert with anionic phospholipids (4). They were originally described in 1906 in a study by Wassermann et al. among patients with positive serologic test results for syphilis. The frequency of aPL antibodies in patients with SLE and the connection of aPL antibodies with a falsely positive Venereal Disease Research Laboratory (VDRL) test remain the explanation for the inclusion of a false positive VDRL in diagnostic criteria for SLE (1).

aPL antibodies are present with APS but may also be present when stimulated by infection or drugs (5). The concept of the APS requires the patient to have both an appropriate clinical manifestation and a positive aPL antibody test. A laboratory testing panel to identify aPL antibodies includes lupus anticoagulant (liquid-based clotting assays) and immunological solid-phase assays (usually enzyme-linked immunosorbent assay [ELISA] formats) for IgG and/or IgM anticardiolipin (aCL) antibodies and anti-beta 2 glycoprotein I (β2GPI) antibodies (5–7). Other autoantibodies, such as those directed against anionic phospholipids, can also be assayed; however they are not of clinical significance.

aCL antibodies and lupus anticoagulants have clinical, laboratory, and biochemical differences and therefore solid-phase assays should not be considered as confirmatory procedures for lupus anticoagulant activity (8–10). aCL antibodies are much more prevalent than the lupus anticoagulant, the ratio being 5 or 6:1 (11). The presence of a lupus anticoagulant in APS is the strongest risk factor associated with thrombosis in adults, especially when it results from the activity of antibodies to β2GPI, in particular those specific for epitope Gly40-Arg43 directed to domain I of the beta 2 glycoprotein (2, 12–15).

Frequently, uninformed clinicians will ask laboratories for "aPL antibody testing" without specifying an assay. Laboratories should develop policies and procedures to determine which assays (including isotypes) or combinations of assays will be performed should this request be received. Often, these tests will be ordered for patients with systemic autoimmune conditions or as part of an assessment for "APS" where selected clinical problems may relate to the presence of an aPL antibody. Ordering physicians may not understand the ambiguity of antiphospholipid testing caused by the variation in test selection and laboratory practices that can influence test results.

The differences in laboratory practice relate to technical or clinical expertise, assay formulations, selection and limitations of existing methods (test kits and instruments), and subsequent interpretation (1, 6, 15). Therefore, if a physician with a patient with clinical classic features of APS requiring treatment uses these tests solely as diagnostic criteria for APS the physician may inappropriately exclude APS because of false-negative results. This finding is sometimes referred to as non-aPL APS or seronegative APS, or SNAPS. In contrast, patients may be misdiagnosed as having APS due to a false-positive aPL antibody identified using a nonspecific method as the sole or primary test to identify APS. aCL antibodies are found frequently at low titer and positive results should be interpreted with caution. Some experts have questioned the relevance of aCL testing in isolation due to a lack of compelling clinical evidence to support an association between isolated positive aCL testing and clinical outcomes (6, 16, 17).

2 Background

APS presents with a wide range of clinical symptoms. The clinical diagnosis of APS in a patient with symptoms and signs is strongly influenced by the presence of a positive antiphospholipid result. The classic clinical presentations include life-threatening thrombosis and obstetrical complications such as fetal loss and severe preeclampsia. The common thrombotic events are venous thromboembolism and ischemic stroke but thrombosis in any vascular bed may occur (2, 18). There are at least five clinical situations when testing for antiphospholipid seems appropriate: arterial or venous thrombosis that is not readily explained, history of pregnancy morbidity, unexplained cutaneous circulation disturbances, major autoimmune disease, and evidence for nonbacterial thrombotic endocarditis (4).

aPL antibodies are clinically associated with thrombocytopenia, skin lesions such as ulcerations and livedo reticularis, and non-stroke neurologic conditions such as transverse myelopathy. APS may affect organs such as the lungs, heart, kidneys, adrenal glands, and liver (1, 13, 19). There are many explanations as to how the aPL antibody triggers or is associated with thrombotic events. Thrombosis may be caused by aPL-associated changes in coagulation such as coagulation factor inhibitors, impairment of the fibrinolytic system, interference with complement or with coagulation factors including prothrombin, protein C, protein S, and annexins. Antibodies may develop due to the activation of platelets to enhance endothelial adherence; the activation of vascular endothelium, which, in turn, facilitates the binding of platelets and monocytes; and the reaction of autoantibodies to oxidized low-density lipoprotein. Alternatively, the direct effect of aPL antibodies on cell function might cause a defect in cellular apoptosis that exposes membrane phospholipids to the binding of various plasma proteins, such as beta 2 glycoprotein. Once bound, a phospholipid–protein complex is formed and a neoepitope is uncovered, which becomes the target of autoantibodies (1, 2, 4, 11, 13, 20).

Depending on the assay, aPL antibodies are reported in up to 10% of healthy individuals and in 30–50% of patients with SLE (20, 21). aCL antibodies tend to be found more frequently in isolation, particularly in older patients (males >55 years of age and females >65 years of age) due to competing alternative causes for thromboembolic disease; therefore a positive titer result should be interpreted with caution (17, 22).

In clinical laboratory practice, aPL antibodies are assayed using one or a combination of the following: aCL antibody assay, anti-β2GPI antibody assay, and lupus anticoagulant (LA) assays (13). With regard to lupus anticoagulant testing, the evaluation must consist of at least two laboratory assays that have adequate lupus sensitivity with an appropriate confirmatory test (see Chapter 7) (8). The patient must have experienced a clinical occurrence and had at least one consistently positive aPL antibody test on at least two occasions 12 weeks apart. The titer of the antibody must be moderate or high, as low-titer antibodies are common (detected in up to 5% of tests), of questionable significance, often transient, and may be found in a range of other inflammatory, infectious, and malignant disorders. The 12 weeks between testing is required to eliminate the possibility of a false-positive result due to transient antibodies (16, 22). Similarly, it is suggested not to classify a patient as having APS when the time interval between the clinical event and the positive laboratory test is greater than five years.

Published recommendations on assay standardization for aCL, anti-β2GPI antibody, and LA tests include a large or predominant amount of expert opinion due to lack of a "gold standard" confirmatory test for APS (4, 13, 23). Experts base their opinions on anecdotal, oftentimes biased, assessments of evidence; thus varying views will exist. Guidelines and consensus statements derived and formulated independent of one another have been published to help determine appropriate testing and interpretation of APS (6, 24). In 1999, the Sapporo criteria were published which detailed the clinical and laboratory classification for APS (13, 25). In 2004, a European forum was held in which the outcome was to propose minimal requirements considered useful to decrease the interlaboratory variability. In the years following, new insights regarding clinical and laboratory findings were acquired and in 2006 the Sydney classification criteria was published. This led to improvement; however further debate remained such as serological criteria (16, 22). In 2008, the Australasian Anticardiolipin Working Group published a consensus approach to formulation of guidelines on aCL and anti-β2GPI antibody testing and reporting. In 2009, the Scientific Standardisation Subcommittee (SSC) of the International Society of

Thrombosis and Haemostasis (ISTH) provided updated guidelines obtained through consensus statements (14).

The criteria for APS revised in Sydney, Australia, in 2004 and published in 2006 noted that APS requires the combination of at least one clinical and one laboratory criterion. Patients are categorized into classes that are defined by antibody profiles including the number and type of positive test: more than one laboratory criterion in any combination, only lupus anticoagulants, only aCL antibody, and only anti-β2GPI antibody (16, 22). Clinical studies have confirmed the importance of triple positivity (lupus anticoagulant, aCL, and anti-β2GPI antibodies). Patients with this laboratory pattern appear at particularly high risk of developing future thromboembolic complications (5, 7, 15, 26, 27). Oral anticoagulant therapy significantly reduces recurrent thromboembolism, although it may not be sufficient in all cases (14, 27). Positive aCL and anti-β2GPI antibodies have been described in the setting of infectious diseases, including leprosy, parvovirus B19, syphilis, HIV, and acute Q-fever (16, 24, 28). As noted earlier, the clinical importance of isolated aCL or anti-β2GPI antibody positivity has been called into question by some authors.

The group of aPL antibodies is rapidly expanding; these antibodies include antiprothrombin/antithrombin antibodies (aPTs), a heterogenous group, including antibodies directed against prothrombin (aPT) and antibodies to the phosphatidylserine–prothrombin complex (aPS/PT). These antibodies were not included in the Sydney criteria as there was little evidence to support their clinical relevance. Some studies show that antibodies against aPS/PT, rather than against aPTs alone, are closely associated with APS and the presence of lupus anticoagulants (2, 3, 25, 29).

Treatment of aPL antibodies is difficult because of lack of standardized laboratory tests to confirm the diagnosis, limited data on its natural history, and a lack of randomized treatment trials. Further complicating this is the balance between thrombosis and hemorrhage in a patient with APS, who may have concomitant thrombocytopenia and other issues contributing to increased bleeding risks (30).

2.1 Anticardiolipin Antibody

aCL antibodies are a class of antibodies that may be of the IgG, IgM, or IgA isotype. Cardiolipin is a protein isolated from bovine heart: it shares epitopes with endogenous proteins that are the target for aCL antibodies (13). The aCL assay depending on design detects a wide range of aPL antibodies that may include clinically relevant antibodies associated with thrombosis such as anti-β2GPI antibodies and/or a large number of clinically irrelevant antibodies of which some are associated with infection. Of note, the aCL may detect antibodies potentially clinically important and directed against other phospholipid/cofactor complexes not yet defined by current testing (6, 28).

In 1983, Harris and coworkers developed a radioimmunoassay for detection of aCL and soon after developed (in 1985) the first quantitative ELISA to identify various isotypes (usually IgG, sometimes IgM, and rarely IgA) of antibodies directed to phospholipids or their cofactors. Using the assay, it was determined that SLE patients with positive aCL testing appeared to have a higher incidence of thrombosis and fetal death (1, 13). In 1985, Hughes introduced the term APS to characterize a group of patients with thrombosis and/or recurrent complications of pregnancy who had aPL within their plasma. In 1990, it was reported that aCL in patients with autoimmune disease were directed toward a complex formed by cardiolipin and a protein cofactor, beta 2 glycoprotein I (1). Given knowledge of the epitope specificity, a variety of ELISA-based assays for aCL antibodies were developed.

With the addition of anti-β2GPI antibodies to the APS test menu it was decided in the 2006 Sydney revision that the aCL antibody ELISA performed in a β2GPI-dependent manner be dropped from the criteria. This testing practice provides two potentially independent ELISA-based assays, one for aCL antibodies and one for anti-β2GPI antibodies. The revision allows detection of thrombosis risk but also detection of antibodies that recognize other phospholipid-binding plasma proteins, as well as infection-related antibodies against cardiolipin which are essentially false-positive tests in the setting of suspected APS (3, 6, 7).

The aCL assay is not reproducible as illustrated by interlaboratory comparisons of a panel of samples showing wide disagreement in results, in particular using samples with low-titer antibodies (2, 3, 6). An isolated positive test in the absence of clinical manifestations, thrombosis, or fetal loss does not support a diagnosis of APS; however, in contrast, a positive result in the presence of clinical manifestations does support a diagnosis of APS (with the caveats expressed elsewhere in this chapter) (3, 31, 32). IgA aCL testing is of questionable importance and might only be recommended in cases where the IgG and IgM assay are negative and there is a very strong suspicion of APS (6, 24).

Concerns with aCL assay occur as a result of pre-, post-, and analytical issues. To minimize these concerns, it is important to identify what the kit is measuring, specifically whether the manufacturer has added both cardiolipin and β2GP1, thereby increasing the potential specificity of the test. In addition, the use of an appropriate cutoff value is a critical requirement as only medium and high titer (i.e., >99th percentile or >40 U IgG and/or IgM phospholipid antibody) of aCL antibodies satisfy diagnostic criterion (2, 5, 13, 22, 24, 26). Claims vary regarding correlation between increased aCL antibodies and thrombosis or fetal loss. Some studies have reported that patients with additional risk factors for clinical complications, such as those with a simultaneous lupus anticoagulant, appear to be at a higher risk for thromboembolism. However, APS should not be diagnosed solely on the basis of a single positive ACL test result. The patient should present with appropriate clinical manifestations of APS, plus some other confirmatory laboratory finding such as persistent moderate to high positive aCL titer on multiple testing at least 12 weeks apart or positive anti-β2GPI antibodies and/or LA testing (6, 13, 16, 31).

IgG isotype aCL should be performed when "aCL antibody" or "aPL antibody" testing is requested and the isotype is not specified. It has been suggested that if IgM isotype is routinely performed on all requests then a comment should be provided indicating the lower specificity of positive IgM aCL results compared to IgG aCL results for APS (33).

2.2 Anti-beta 2 Glycoprotein I Antibody

β2GPI, also known as apolipoprotein H, is a 50-kDa glycoprotein plasma protein, which occurs in plasma at a level of 200 μg/mL. It is mainly synthesized in the liver and to a lesser extent by endothelial cells and placental cells. It consists of five homologous complement-binding repeats, designated as domain I to domain V, of which domain V is slightly aberrant. Domain V contains a large positively charged patch with a phospholipid insertion loop, which is responsible for binding to anionic phospholipids (1, 2, 4, 34). In an effort to improve the diagnostic utility of aCL antibody assays it was determined that a subset of patients harbored antibodies directed against a circulating glycoprotein of unknown clinical significance known as β2GPI. In 1992, antibodies directed toward β2GPI in the absence of cardiolipin or other phospholipids were reported. Anti-β2GPI antibody testing was not included in the 1999 Sapporo criteria but was added to the 2006 Sydney laboratory criteria for the diagnosis of APS (5, 22).

The proposed mechanisms of thrombosis in APS and the role of anti-β2GPI antibodies in the process include the following (5, 30):

1. Anti-β2GPI antibody complexes may interfere with endogenous anticoagulant mechanisms such as crystallization of annexin A5 anticoagulant shield, fibrinolysis triggered via annexin A2 and mediated via plasmin, the protein C and protein S mechanism, tissue factor pathway inhibitor, and others.
2. Anti-β2GPI antibody may trigger signaling events on cells such as blood leukocytes, endothelium, platelets, and trophoblasts that may lead to the expression of prothrombic and pro-adhesive phenotypes.
3. Anti-β2GPI antibody may activate complement and trigger inflammatory reaction on the vascular and/or trophoblast surface.

Anti-β2GPI antibodies are found in a subset of patients with aCL antibodies and rarely in patients who are aCL antibody negative but in whom the presence of an aPL antibody is suspected. In 2003, following a literature review, Galli et al. concluded that anti-β2GPI antibodies are more strongly related with venous thrombosis than aCL (25). In addition, studies by de Groot et al. showed that a lupus anticoagulant caused by antibodies directed against anti-β2GPI antibodies has a stronger correlation with thromboembolic complications than does a lupus anticoagulant caused by antibodies with a reactivity toward other plasma proteins. The subset of anti-β2GPI antibodies that have lupus anticoagulant activity are directed against domain I of the β2GPI molecule (3).

Anti-β2GPI antibodies are assessed using ELISA-based assays and have performance characteristics similar to aCL antibodies. IgG anti-β2GPI antibody should be performed on all requests for "anti-β2GPI antibody" where isotype is not specified. If both IgG and IgM anti-β2GPI antibody testing is routinely performed on all requests then it has been suggested that a comment should be provided indicating that the association between isolated positive IgM anti-β2GPI antibody results and thrombosis is uncertain but appears to be lower than for IgG anti-β2GPI antibody. In selected patients where the clinical suspicion of APS is high but all other antiphospholipid tests are negative testing for IgA anti-β2GPI antibody may be clinically useful (35).

In the case where two patients have comparable high levels of IgG anti-β2GPI antibody, there may be significant differences between their antibody epitope specificity and IgG subclass. Studies have shown that patients with anti-β2GPI antibodies specific for epitope Gly40-Arg43 in domain 1 of β2GPI are more likely to exhibit a clinical manifestation than other anti-β2GPI antibodies (15, 34).

2.3 Standardization of Assays

Given their potential clinical importance, it is essential that aPL assays are reliable. However, there remains a lack of reliable, reproducible, and standardized assays (3, 6, 19). Different assays, either commercial or in-house, using the same sample, produce different values for both aCL antibody and anti-β2GPI antibody in interlaboratory comparisons and external quality control exchange programs due to variation in testing practice, determination of cutoff values, and reporting of results (2, 3, 12, 24).

Issues with standardization are illustrated by noting that most antibodies detected by anti-β2GPI antibody assays may not provide a positive aCL assay when tested using a β2GPI-dependent method. The reason for the discrepancy is not clear but may include the variety of antibodies, methods, and assay formulations available and used by laboratories. Early on, when laboratories were using in-house assays, attempts were made to standardize the method by using a common calibrator, derived from a pool of positive patient samples, and defined according to the presence of a standard amount of IgG or IgM antibody (resulting in the Louisville GPL or MPL units) (3, 6, 31, 36). Later, monoclonal antibodies for aCL, primarily targeting β2GPI, were developed, these being

HCAL, a chimeric IgG and EY2C9, an IgM antibody. These standards were found to reduce variability but have not been widely accepted or utilized (16, 28, 36).

Diagnostic laboratories use a wide diversity of commercial assay kits with different formulation protocols. Performance varies due to type of microtiter plates, the charge on the plates, the source of cardiolipin, the solvent used to apply the cardiolipin onto the plates, the orientation and presentation of cardiolipin on the plate, the use of bovine versus human plasma, the specific use of particular cofactor components, and the nature of the calibrator whether it be a primary or a secondary standard (6, 9, 28).

Unfortunately, commercial test kits may be chosen based on cost and preexisting supplier arrangements or adaptation to existing instrumentation, rather than through an evidence-based validation process. In addition, regulatory pressures force laboratories to adopt approved "in vitro diagnostics" products. This may result in production of assay kits to a regulatory approved "standard of uniformity" rather than to a standard based on improved clinical utility. In addition, manufacturers may modify their test kit's cutoff values to better compare with that of a competitor. Due to proven variation of interlaboratory results and external control exchange programs it is clear that different kits do not identify aCL and anti-β2GPI antibodies in exactly the same way (2, 3, 6, 16).

2.4 Anticardiolipin Antibody Assay

The aCL antibody ELISA method measures the interaction of antibodies with β2GPI bound to cardiolipin (CL) or to other anionic phospholipids coated on the microplate (37). The ELISA involves the assessment of diluted patient serum binding to a CL-coated plate in the presence of bovine serum. It will detect antibodies that bind CL alone and those that bind CL-bound bovine β2GPI. Both types are termed aCL antibodies. A weakness of this assay is that there remains a potential to miss patients with antibodies that bind human but bovine β2GPI. Therefore, some assays now use human β2GPI in the aCL ELISA (28).

Standardization of this assay has challenges due to the following important factors affecting results (36):

1. The type of hydrophobic surface required to bind cardiolipin of the ELISA microplate.
2. The microplate coating procedure (mainly the extent of CL oxidation).
3. The source and amount of β2GPI in serum (e.g., diluted calf serum [fetal or newborn], adult bovine, or goat serum).
4. The presence in the serum of other phospholipid-binding proteins that bind immobilized cardiolipin. As a result, antibodies other than those directed to cardiolipin–β2GPI complex may be measured.

2.5 Anti-beta 2 Glycoprotein I Antibody Assay

The anti-β2GPI ELISA method uses β2GPI as the antigen directly coated on the ELISA microplate.

Standardization of this assay has challenges due to the following important factors affecting results (36):

1. The binding of the β2GPI requires a microplate surface with a high density of negative charges.
2. Microheterogeneity in the final product may occur depending on the method of antigen purification. Several isoforms of β2GPI with different isoelectric points are present in the plasma. These may cause differences in anti-β2GPI antibody binding.

2.6 Anticardiolipin Antibody and Anti-beta 2 Glycoprotein I Antibody Assays

Standardization of these assays has challenges due to the following important factors affecting results (36, 37):

1. The lack of worldwide reference calibrators (e.g., monoclonal vs. polyclonal). This is illustrated in the difference in sample results, when expressed in GPL or MPL units between commercial kits. Sample classification as low, medium, and high positive results is different depending on the kit.
2. The statistical method used to calculate the cutoff value (e.g., ±SD vs. percentiles) and the use of cutoff values.

The lack of worldwide reference calibrators influences the interpretation of the patient's result. First, due to the lack of standardization in the calibrators for both aCL and anti-β2GPI antibody assays, the ELISA titers from different manufacturers are not interchangeable (3). Given a lack of international consensus and a lack of consistent and large-volume calibrator serum between laboratories, reliability of these assays is generally poor. An alternative has been proposed to produce calibrators by "spiking" human monoclonal antibodies into control serum to improve standardization and interlaboratory quality. However these monoclonal antibodies do not bind consistently to current aPL assays, in particular aCL and anti-β2GPI antibody assays, and there is an uncertainty that the assays that best bind these monoclonal antibodies represent clinically significant assays. In addition, use of monoclonal antibodies may limit future identification of clinically relevant new aPL assays. Lastly, a potential long-term issue with the use of monoclonal antibodies as the only source of assay calibrators is the commercial influence of a single supplier or manufacturer which could potentially impact cost and supply (6, 35, 36).

To deal with the above challenges the following improvements to the ACL and anti-B2GPI assays have been recommended (36):

1. Use of human purified β2GPI as a source of cofactor in the aCL assay.
2. Optimize the purification procedure (reducing glycosylation) for β2GPI for both assays.

3. Adopt monoclonal calibrators for both assays.
4. Obtain relevant information from manufacturers regarding cutoff assessment.
5. Assess the local cutoff whenever possible as manufacturers often set the cutoff value to fit with specificity and sensitivity values obtained with a "mode" assay. These limits may not be clinically appropriate for your facility. Cutoff values should be determined in conjunction with the laboratory director.
6. Build a close collaboration between manufacturers and laboratorians. However, difficulties for manufacturers occur in revising the composition of kits already approved by regulatory authorities or if the kit was originally designed to compare with peer manufacturers.

European experts have identified "minimal requirements" considered appropriate practice (38, 39):

1. Run the samples in duplicate.
2. Determine the cutoff level in each laboratory analyzing at least 50 samples from normal subjects, possibly age and sex matched with the patient population.
3. Calculate the cutoff level in percentiles.
4. Use stable external controls in the test.

2.7 Interpretation of Results

Clinicians from both general practice and specialties order tests for aPL antibody. There is a lack of understanding regarding the limitations and variation of laboratory assays and therefore inappropriate clinical decisions occur as a result of this testing. Laboratory reports should include interpretive comments to help guide clinicians. The diagnosis of the aPL antibody syndrome depends upon the demonstration of persistent positive tests for an aPL antibody in the setting of a compatible clinical history. The interpretation of these results is difficult due to the lack of standardization, reproducibility, and method specificity. It is strongly recommended that the testing be performed in a specialized coagulation laboratory where results can be interpreted by an experienced clinician who understands the relevant factors that may influence test results and subsequent patient treatment. Retesting is very important to identify transient aPL antibodies such as an IgM aCL which often is the result of intercurrent infection and seldom clinically relevant (2, 16, 24, 40).

Consensus recommendations have been published to assist in the interpretation of aPL antibody testing. These recommendations include that patients are generally only labelled as having aPL antibody syndrome (APS) if they have one positive test for an aPL (aCL antibody, anti-β2GPI antibody, or lupus anticoagulant) on two occasions, a minimum of 12 weeks apart in the setting of either prior, objectively confirmed thromboembolism or pregnancy morbidity.

The diagnosis of aCL antibodies requires the presence of IgG and/or IgM antibodies at medium or high titers (i.e., >40 GPL or MPL units or >99th percentile) and that of anti-β2GPI requires the presence of IgG and or IgM in titers >99th percentile (2, 16, 22). Of note, using the 99th percentile cutoff of a normal population makes by definition 1% of the "normal" population positive (37). Possible interference of cryoglobulins and rheumatoid factor should be considered in the interpretation of IgM for both aCL and anti-β2GPI antibodies (22). It has been suggested that laboratories comment that rheumatoid factor may produce false-positive IgM aCL/anti-β2GPI results whenever a positive IgM aCL/anti-β2GPI result is obtained (24).

Thrombosis, recurrent fetal loss, and thrombocytopenia appear to occur more frequently as the level of aCL increases. An aCL titer of >35 to 40 GPL units has been associated with an increased risk of thrombosis. IgG isotype appears to be more closely associated with clinical manifestations than are the IgM or IgA isotypes (14). Studies have shown a stronger relationship between thrombosis in the presence of multiple positive aPL tests when compared to a single positive result (5, 27).

Despite consensus recommendations, there remains considerable controversy around the diagnosis of aPL antibodies and the interpretation of the aPL antibody testing. Due to the variation in sensitivity and specificity of aPL antibody methods the false-positive and false-negative detection rate is relatively high. False-positive results may cause patients to receive unnecessary and extended anticoagulant treatment. Treatment therapy for APS must be individualized according to the patient's current clinical event and history of thrombosis (19).

3 Quality Assurance

3.1 Quality Control

A positive and negative control should be included with each run of patient samples and on each ELISA plate. The laboratory should use separate positive and negative controls, with the positive control(s) having a defined value and error range. In the event the value of the positive control falls outside the predefined range, the whole run should be rejected and repeated. Many commercial aCL and β2GPI ELISA kits provide pre-diluted positive and negative controls. It is suggested that laboratories prepare an in-house (non-kit) positive and negative serum control or a commercial non-kit control that can be processed in the same manner as the patient samples in the pre-analytical and analytical aspects of the ELISA method. This will allow kit comparison of between batch-to-batch or lot-to-lot variation and when changing manufacturers. One of the positive controls should have a titer in the clinically significant low/moderate positive cutoff range (20–40 GPL/MPL) and within the linear range of the assay illustrating that the positive control is within the linear range of the kit (6, 24, 33, 35).

Controls should be included on each ELISA run to monitor the inter-assay reliability of the assay, assess batch-to-batch variation, and the assay's uncertainty of measurement. Consensus guidelines on testing and reporting recommend an inter-assay inter-run coefficient of variation (%CV) value of less than 20% (24).

3.2 External Quality Assessment

External quality assessment (EQA) provides laboratories with an opportunity to assess and compare their own test process to peer laboratories. Although results may vary the median values provide some evidence of ongoing test validation. In addition, EQA improves laboratory practice and helps determine best practice standards (2, 6, 40). Participants are required to treat proficiency testing material in a similar manner as patient samples and therefore reflect the real-world situation (36). In addition, EQA provides useful information on the best available methods by reviewing methods with the lowest interlaboratory variability and best correlation to clinical details (6). Participants receive educational correspondence and reports showing their performance in relation to peers, and results are often grouped by the manufacturers of the ELISA kits. Some EQA providers assess the laboratories' responses against the assigned value (numerical or interpretive) while others, because of the lack of standardized methods, provide the frequency of results reported by participants (2, 6, 16, 41).

EQA aCL and β2GPI challenges have produced variable results, even between laboratories using the same commercial kit. The interlaboratory and inter-method variability are a matter of concern and point out the need for standardization. Greater consensus is observed in samples with higher amounts of antibody present (12, 36).

Qualitative or semiquantitative, rather than quantitative, EQA responses achieve better inter- and intra-laboratory agreement (16). Variation of results is due to lack of standardization of pre-analytic (quality of blood sample), analytic (sensitivity of microplates, quality and source of antibody, technical expertise, reagents, lack of common calibrators), and post-analytic (use of inappropriate cutoff values) factors (1, 12, 37, 38, 42, 43).

3.3 Reference Intervals/Cutoff Values

aCL antibodies and anti-β2GPI antibodies can be reported as a numerical value or a semiquantitative titer in addition to a qualitative (interpretive) result. Clinicians can compare the patient's result in relation to the laboratory's semiquantitative cutoff values. Laboratories using kits where the manufacturer does not provide a semiquantitative cutoff value would have to report numerical values or determine their own semiquantitative cutoff values. This process is hampered by the lack of a standardized calibrator serum and consensus on the definition of the "aPL antibody syndrome" which leads to important limitations in the availability of "positive" and "negative" serum for testing. Laboratories may establish different cutoff values causing further variation in semiquantitative results between different laboratories using the same assay kit. Subsequently, a comment may be required informing clinicians of the potential for variation in numerical and semiquantitative results by different laboratories, even using the same aCL kits, and therefore the need for caution when comparing aCL results (36, 38, 39, 41–43).

When establishing cutoff values the distribution of the optical density (OD) value is not Gaussian (non-normal distribution with a clear positive skew) and therefore it has be advised that cutoff values cannot be determined using standard deviations. Instead, the use of percentiles has been recommended as a better approach where the percentage of positive aCL results in the normal population ranges from 2 to 4%; therefore the cutoff should be set at the OD value that corresponds with the 97.5% percentile of the OD population to calculate an appropriate reference interval and negative/positive cutoff (36).

Many laboratories adopt commercial reference or "expert laboratories'" reference intervals/cutoff values. Such practice is problematic since the patient population analyzed and laboratory methods will vary between laboratories leading to important differences in reference intervals/cutoff values both between and within centers over time. It has been suggested that a comment indicating the potential for interlaboratory variation in values between manufacturers should be included in the laboratory report.

If an aCL or an anti-β2GPI antibody test is performed as a stand-alone investigation and not as part of a comprehensive thrombophilia investigation the report should include a comment indicating that if positive additional testing for a lupus anticoagulant is recommended. Testing should be repeated after 12 weeks to determine antibody persistence. If the result for either aCL or an anti-β2GPI antibody test is negative it is suggested that the report should comment that a portion of patients with aPL antibody syndrome have undetectable aCL or anti-β2GPI antibody test antibodies and testing for lupus anticoagulant is recommended (33, 35).

4 Reporting of Results

There is a lack of standardization regarding the post-analytical process including format and content of test reports, as well as the clinician's response to these reports. Different laboratories use different formats for test result reports, thereby impacting clinical follow-up and management of the patient. Some laboratories use a semiquantitative nominal scale for rating laboratory results for aCL including the following designations: negative, equivocal, moderate-positive, medium-positive, and high-positive; however others use fewer categories (16). Laboratories should provide interpretive comments and if aPL testing is performed in isolation of lupus anticoagulant testing, there should be integration of test reports and comments (6, 13, 33, 35, 40).

5 Method

5.1 Blood Collection

All patient laboratory specimens are treated as infectious and handled according to "standard precautions." Serum is the preferred specimen for both the aCL antibody and the anti-β2GPI antibody ELISA assays. Whole blood is collected into vacutainers containing no additives using approved phlebotomy procedures, avoiding hemolysis. Inversion of the tube is unnecessary and may activate platelets that can interfere with the assay.

A citrated plasma sample may be provided because the clinician has also requested lupus anticoagulant testing and this test requires citrated plasma. However, citrated plasma samples are not preferred for either of these ELISA assays due to the anticoagulation dilution artifact of approximately 10%. If citrated plasma is used a correction factor is required or alternatively a comment is required noting, "Testing of citrated plasma may yield results lower than with serum." Use of citrated plasma samples must only occur if the laboratory has validated the procedure and only when the platelet-poor plasma is prepared according to approved lupus anticoagulant testing procedures. Alternatively, concentrated thrombin can be added to the citrated plasma sample to convert the fibrinogen to fibrin, resulting in a serum sample. After incubation at 37°C, the sample is centrifuged and the serum is removed from the clot.

Laboratories must recognize that when they receive a sample in an aliquoted secondary tube, it is difficult to know the original sample type. It is possible that laboratories are unknowingly testing samples other than serum samples using their ELISA method (6, 24, 33, 35, 44).

5.2 Processing

Blood collected by vacuum draw should sit at room temperature, or may be incubated at 37°C, for a minimum of 30 min to ensure that the sample is clotted. The time to clot will be prolonged if the patient is on anticoagulant therapy. The sample is then centrifuged at 1,500 relative centrifugal force (RCF; g-force) for 15 min. The serum is removed as soon as possible to avoid hemolysis (44, 45).

5.3 Storage

Samples for aCL antibody and anti-β2GPI antibody ELISA testing should be stored at −70°C until ready to analyze unless the assays can be performed within 4 h. Samples are stable at −70°C for at least 6 months. Avoid repetitive freezing and thawing of serum sample which may result in loss of antibody activity. A frost-free freezer should not be used as the freeze–thaw cycle allows the temperature of the sample to increase and then drop when the sample refreezes (44, 45).

5.4 Thawing

Samples should be thawed in a circulating water bath at 37°C (±1°C); thawing should be assessed frequently beginning at 5 min. Samples must be removed from the water bath as soon as the last ice crystals have melted. Mix well to ensure homogeneity of sample prior to use (46).

6 Materials

6.1 Calibrators

Calibrators should be used according to manufacturer's instructions unless the laboratory has validated an alternate approach. Calibrators may be performed as a single specimen provided the inter-assay %CV of the assay was <20% (24, 33, 35, 38).

Commercial assays demonstrate substantial variation in results due to a lack of established calibrators for standardization causing interlaboratory variation of results (6).

6.2 Reagents and Reagent Preparation

Reagents should be prepared as per manufacturers' recommendations. Individuals must follow the safety precautions recommended by the manufacturer. Reagents should be at room temperature before use. If the reagent needs to be reconstituted, purified water with a pH 5.3–7.2 (distilled, deionized, or type 1 reagent grade) should be used for this procedure (47).

6.3 Samples

Dilutions of the serum samples should be prepared as per manufacturers' recommendations. Laboratories introducing these tests should run a patient's sample in duplicate; however once the test is established the laboratory may choose to run a single assay provided that the inter-run %CV of the aCL and anti-β2GPI antibody assay was <20% (24, 33, 35).

6.4 ELISA Techniques

aCL antibody and anti-β2GPI antibody testing are performed using ELISA-based assays and follow the same principle for measurement. The ELISA technology allows for batch testing and use of small volumes of serum and can be reliably repeated on frozen or shipped samples (48). The results are unaffected by coagulation factor deficiencies, immunoglobulin inhibitors of specific clotting factors, or anticoagulant therapy (2, 4, 24, 31).

6.5 Example of ELISA Anticardiolipin Antibody Assay

Diluted serum samples, pre-diluted calibrators, and controls are incubated in microwells coated with purified cardiolipin, allowing aCL antibodies present in the samples to react with the immobilized antigen. The samples of known antigen concentrations comprise a calibration curve used to calculate antigen concentrations of unknown samples. If antibodies are present in the serum, the antibodies bind to the cardiolipin on the microwell surface. After a washing procedure to remove unbound serum proteins, labelled antibodies specific for human IgG, IgM, or IgA cardiolipin are added resulting in the formation of an enzyme/antigen complex. After a second washing procedure, the bound enzyme/antigen complex is quantitated by the addition of a chromogenic substrate. The intensity of the color development in the microwell is directly proportional to the concentration of cardiolipin. Results are obtained by reading the OD (optical density or absorbance) of each microwell using a spectrophotometer. The titer of antibody is then reported by comparing the sample optical density to a calibration curve.

6.6 Example of ELISA for Anti-beta 2 Glycoprotein I Antibody Assay

Patient serum is diluted with sample diluent and incubated in microwells coated with human β2GPI. Antibodies to β2GPI present in the sample will bind to the coated wells. After washing, enzyme-conjugated anti-human IgG, IgM, or IgA immunoglobulin is added, the wells are washed again, substrate is added, and color development is measured in a spectrophotometer and quantitated as described above.

6.7 Sources of Error in the ELISA Technique

1. Incorrect washing procedures may result in falsely high or low titer.
2. Inadvertent drying of the reaction wells may result in falsely high or low titer.

7 Conclusion

Following the revision and publication of the Sydney criteria to improve the classification of aPL antibodies it is now thought that there is significant "overdiagnosis" of APS as not all aPLs detected are clinically relevant. Since there is insufficient information as to determine which antibody subpopulations are disease related patients may be at risk due to inappropriate anticoagulation treatment (3, 37).

As illustrated through interlaboratory studies and external quality assessment standardization of the various assays is required to provide further clarification regarding clinical relevance and the relationship between aPL populations. Manufacturers, laboratorians, and clinicians need to agree on the most effective combination of assays, reagents, and methods to provide optimal assay sensitivity and specificity (6). Future studies need to be supported and provided by a WHO-accredited laboratory with method validation performed in controlled cohort studies (3). In addition, guidelines should be updated as to pre-analytical, analytical, and post-analytic technical and clinical best practice. The ordering physician may believe that a positive aCL antibody or anti-beta 2 glycoprotein antibody defines the presence of APS and a negative result excludes the diagnosis but this confidence is misplaced due to a lack of method standardization. Positive results for aCL antibody or anti-beta 2 glycoprotein antibody should not be used in isolation to diagnose APS or an APS-like disorder but should be used as an adjunct to clinical, radiologic, and other laboratory findings (41).

References

1. Triplett DA (2002) Antiphospholipid antibodies. Arch Pathol Lab Med 126(11): 1424–1429
2. Kitchen S, Olson JD, Preston FE (eds) (2009) Quality in laboratory hemostasis and thrombosis. Wiley-Blackwell, West Sussex
3. de Groot PG, Derksen RH, de Laat B (2008) Twenty-two years of failure to set up undisputed assays to detect patients with the antiphospholipid syndrome. Semin Thromb Hemost 34(4):347–355
4. Arnout J, Vermylen J (2003) Current status and implications of autoimmune antiphospholipid antibodies in relation to thrombotic disease. J Thromb Haemost 1(5):931–942
5. Rand JH (2007) The antiphospholipid syndrome. Hematol Am Soc Hematol Educ Program 136–142
6. Favaloro EJ, Wong RC (2008) Laboratory testing and identification of antiphospholipid antibodies and the antiphospholipid syndrome: a potpourri of problems, a compilation of possible solutions. Semin Thromb Hemost 34(4):389–410
7. Andreoli L, Rizzini S, Allegri F, Meroni P, Tincani A (2008) Are the current attempts at standardization of antiphospholipid antibodies still useful? Emerging technologies signal a shift in direction. Semin Thromb Hemost 34(4):356–360
8. Moffat KA, Ledford-Kraemer MR, Plumhoff EA, McKay H, Nichols WL, Meijer P, Hayward CP (2009) Are laboratories following published recommendations for lupus anticoagulant testing? An international evaluation of practices. Thromb Haemost 101(1):178–184
9. Greaves M, Cohen H, Machin SJ, Mackie I (2000) Guidelines on the investigation and management of the antiphospholipid syndrome. Br J Haematol 109(4):704–715
10. Galli M, Luciani D, Bertolini G, Barbui T (2003) Lupus anticoagulants are stronger risk factors for thrombosis than anticardiolipin antibodies in the antiphospholipid syndrome: a systematic review of the literature. Blood 101(5):1827–1832
11. Hoppensteadt DA, Fabbrini N, Bick RL, Messmore HL, Adiguzel C, Fareed J (2008) Laboratory evaluation of the antiphospholipid syndrome. Hematol Oncol Clin North Am 22(1):19–32
12. Pengo V, Biasiolo A, Bison E, Chantarangkul V, Tripodi A (2007) Italian Federation of Anticoagulation Clinics (FCSA). Antiphospholipid antibody ELISAs: survey on the performance of clinical laboratories assessed by using lyophilized affinity-purified IgG with anticardiolipin and anti-beta2-glycoprotein I activity. Thromb Res 120(1):127–133
13. Devreese K, Hoylaerts MF (2010) Challenges in the diagnosis of the antiphospholipid syndrome. Clin Chem 56(6):930–940
14. Galli M (2010) The antiphospholipid triangle. J Thromb Haemost 8(2):234–236
15. Roubey RA (2010) Risky business: the interpretation, use, and abuse of antiphospholipid antibody tests in clinical practice. Lupus 19(4):440–445
16. Abo SM, DeBari VA (2007) Laboratory evaluation of the antiphospholipid syndrome. Ann Clin Lab Sci 37(1):3–14
17. Galli M (2003) Antiphospholipid syndrome: association between laboratory tests and clinical practice. Pathophysiol Haemost Thromb 33(5–6):249–255
18. Saidi S, Mahjoub T, Almawi WY (2009) Lupus anticoagulants and anti-phospholipid antibodies as risk factors for a first episode of ischemic stroke. J Thromb Haemost 7(7):1075–1080
19. Wong RC, Favaloro EJ (2008) Clinical features, diagnosis, and management of the antiphospholipid syndrome. Semin Thromb Hemost 34(3):295–304
20. Belilos E, Carsons S. Antiphospholipid syndrome [Internet]. Omaha (NE): WebMD LLC; c1994–2010 [updated 2009 Aug 3; cited 2010 July 20]. Available from: http://emedicine.medscape.com/
21. Lim W, Crowther MA, Eikelboom JW (2006) Management of antiphospholipid antibody syndrome: a systematic review. JAMA 295(9):1050–1057
22. Miyakis S, Lockshin MD, Atsumi T, Branch DW, Brey RL, Cervera R, Derksen RH, de Groot PG, Koike T, Meroni PL, Reber G, Shoenfeld Y, Tincani A, Vlachoyiannopoulos PG, Krilis SA (2006) International consensus statement on an update of the classification criteria for definite antiphospholipid syndrome (APS). J Thromb Haemost 4(2):295–306
23. Tripodi A (2008) Laboratory testing for lupus anticoagulants; diagnostic criteria and use of screening, mixing, and confirmatory studies. Semin Thromb Hemost 34(4):373–379
24. Wong RC, Favaloro EJ (2008) A consensus approach to the formulation of guidelines for

laboratory testing and reporting of antiphospholipid antibody assays. Semin Thromb Hemost 34(4):361–372
25. Galli M, Luciani D, Bertolini G, Barbui T (2003) Anti-beta 2-glycoprotein I, antiprothrombin antibodies, and the risk of thrombosis in the antiphospholipid syndrome. Blood 102(8):2717–2723
26. Swadźba J, Iwaniec T, Szczeklik A, Musiał J (2007) Revised classification criteria for antiphospholipid syndrome and the thrombotic risk in patients with autoimmune diseases. Thromb Haemost 5(9):1883–1889
27. Pengo V, Ruffatti A, Legnani C, Gresele P, Barcellona D, Erba N, Testa S, Marongiu F, Bison E, Denas G, Banzato A, Padayattil Jose S, Iliceto S (2010) Clinical course of high-risk patients diagnosed with antiphospholipid syndrome. Thromb Haemost 8(2):237–242
28. Giannakopoulos B, Passam F, Ioannou Y, Krilis SA (2009) How we diagnose the antiphospholipid syndrome. Blood 113(5):985–994
29. Oku K, Atsumi T, Amengual O, Koike T (2008) Antiprothrombin antibody testing: detection and clinical utility. Semin Thromb Hemost 34(4):335–339
30. Lim W (2009) Antiphospholipid antibody syndrome. Hematol Am Soc Hematol Educ Program:233–239
31. Pierangeli SS, Harris EN (2008) A quarter of a century in anticardiolipin antibody testing and attempted standardization has led us to here, which is? Semin Thromb Hemost 34(4):313–328
32. Nash MJ, Camilleri RS, Kunka S, Mackie IJ, Machin SJ, Cohen H (2004) The anticardiolipin assay is required for sensitive screening for antiphospholipid antibodies. J Thromb Haemost 2(7):1077–1081
33. Wong RC, Gillis D, Adelstein S, Baumgart K, Favaloro EJ, Hendle MJ, Homes P, Pollock W, Smith S, Steele RH, Sturgess A, Wilson RJ (2004) Consensus guidelines on anti-cardiolipin antibody testing and reporting. Pathology 36(1):63–68, Erratum in Pathology 2004;36(2):215
34. de Laat B, Derksen RH, Urbanus RT, de Groot PG (2005) IgG antibodies that recognize epitope Gly40-Arg43 in domain I of beta2-glycoprotein I cause LAC, and their presence correlates strongly with thrombosis. Blood 105(4):1540–1545
35. Wong RC, Favaloro EJ, Adelstein S, Baumgart K, Bird R, Brighton TA, Empson M, Gillis D, Hendle MJ, Laurent R, Mallon D, Pollock W, Smith S, Steele RH, Wilson RJ (2008) Consensus guidelines on anti-beta2 glycoprotein I testing and reporting. Pathology 40(1):58–63
36. Reber G, Boehlen F, de Moerloose P (2008) Technical aspects in laboratory testing for antiphospholipid antibodies: is standardization an impossible dream? Semin Thromb Hemost 34(4):340–346
37. Galli M (2008) Clinical utility of laboratory tests used to identify antiphospholipid antibodies and to diagnose the antiphospholipid syndrome. Semin Thromb Hemost 34(4):329–334
38. Tincani A, Allegri F, Balestrieri G, Reber G, Sanmarco M, Meroni P, Boffa MC (2004) Minimal requirements for antiphospholipid antibodies ELISAs proposed by the European Forum on antiphospholipid antibodies. Thromb Res 114(5–6):553–558
39. Reber G, Tincani A, Sanmarco M, de Moerloose P, Boffa MC (2004) Proposals for the measurement of anti-β_2-glycoprotein I antibodies. Standardization Group of the European Forum on Antiphospholipid Antibodies. J Thromb Haemost 2:1860–1862
40. Haemostasis and Thrombosis Task Force, British Committee for Standards in Haematology (2001) Investigation and management of heritable thrombophilia. Br J Haematol 114(3):512–528
41. Favaloro EJ, Wong RC, Jovanovich S, Roberts-Thomson P (2007) A review of beta2 -glycoprotein-1 antibody testing results from a peer-driven multilaboratory quality assurance program. Am J Clin Pathol 127(3):441–448
42. Ruffati A, Pengo V (2009) Antiphospholipid syndrome classification criteria: comments on the letter of Swadzba and Musial. J Thromb Haemost 7:503–504
43. Ruffatti A, Olivieri S, Tonello M, Bortolati M, Bison E, Salvan E, Facchinetti M, Pengo V (2008) Influence of different IgG anticardiolipin antibody cut-off values on antiphospholipid syndrome classification. J Thromb Haemost 6(10):1693–1696
44. Clinical and Laboratory Standards Institute (2008) Collection, transport, and processing of blood specimens for testing plasma-based coagulation assays and molecular hemostasis assays; approved guideline, 5th edn. CLSI document H21-A5, January
45. Clinical and Laboratory Standards Institute (2010) Procedures for Handling and processing of blood specimens for common laboratory tests; approved guideline, 4th edn. CLSI document H18-A4, May
46. Clinical and Laboratory Standards Institute (1997) Determination of factor coagulant activities; approved guideline. CLSI document H48-A, April
47. Clinical and Laboratory Standards Institute (2006) Preparation and testing of reagent water in the clinical laboratory; approved guideline, 4th edn. CLSI document C3-A4, June
48. Lockshin MD (2008) Update on antiphospholipid syndrome. Bull NYU Hosp Jt Dis 66(3):195–197

Chapter 33

Testing for Apolipoprotein(a) Phenotype Using Isoelectric Focusing and Immunoblotting Technique

Claus Langer, Bertram Tambyrayah, and Ulrike Nowak-Göttl

Abstract

Increased levels of lipoprotein(a) are known as an independent risk factor for atherosclerosis, heart disease, and stroke in man. Even in children it could show that elevated levels of Lp(a) are an independent thromboembolic risk factor.

Levels of Lp(a) are influenced by several factors like nutrition, kidney or liver function, or acute-phase reaction. But the most important factors are genetically determined. About 45% of genetic variation depends on polymorphisms and mutations in the promotor region. About 50% are dependent on the size polymorphism of Lp(a). The number of Kringle 4 domains varies between 12 and over 40. The number of Kringle 4 repeats correlates negatively with the level of Lp(a) in plasma. The determination of apo(a) phenotype is able to estimate thromboembolic risk due to this risk factor.

Key words Apolipoprotein(a), Phenotyping, Isoelectric focusing, Immunoblotting technique, Thromboembolic risk factor

1 Introduction

Lipoprotein(a) is a lipoprotein that consists of the apolipoprotein(a) and a low-density lipoprotein (LDL) particle. Apo(a) is connected via a disulfide bridge with the apolipoprotein B in the LDL particle (1).

Less is known about the physiological role and the metabolism of lipoprotein(a). Despite that several studies could show that elevated Lp(a) is an independent risk factor for atherosclerosis, coronary heart disease, and stroke. Lp(a) levels higher than 25–30 mg/dl are associated with an increased risk for atherosclerosis.

It could be shown that Lp(a) is also an independent thromboembolic risk factor in children (2). We have used the method described in this chapter to define age-dependent reference values for Lp(a) (Tables 1 and 2). In a study of 334 children aged from

Paul Monagle (ed.), *Haemostasis: Methods and Protocols*, Methods in Molecular Biology, vol. 992,
DOI 10.1007/978-1-62703-339-8_33, © Springer Science+Business Media New York 2013

Table 1
Mean apolipoprotein(a) concentrations and associated Kringle 4 repeats

Age	Lp(a) mg/dl (nmol/l)	Kringle 4 (*n*=334)
1–12 months	3	
1–18 years	10	
15–19 years	66	77
20–21 years	45	64
22–24 years	17	25
25–27 years	12 (29)	23 (55)
28–32 years	7	16
>33 years	9	9

Table 2
Age-dependent reference values for Lp(a)

Lipoprotein(a) in healthy controls (*n*=150) (90th upper percentiles)	
3–6 months	14 mg/dl 34 nmol/l
6.1–12 months	15 mg/dl 36 nmol/l
1.1–9 years	22 mg/dl 53 nmol/l
9.1–18 years	30 mg/dl 72 nmol/l

1 month to 18 years we could find that the mean Lp(a) concentration was 3 mg/dl for the group 1–12 months old. In the group 1.2–18 years old the mean value for Lp(a) concentration was 10 mg/dl.

One characteristic issue of apo(a) is its polymorphic structure. Apo(a) shows repetitive Kringle 4 domains from 12 Kringle 4 domains up to over 40 Kringle 4 repeats. The number of Kringle 4 repeats correlates negatively with the concentration oflipoprotein(a) in plasma.

The size polymorphism of apo(a) is strictly genetically determined and is responsible for about 50% of variation in Lp(a) levels. The determination of apo(a) phenotype is a possibility to estimate thromboembolic risk due to this risk factor.

The number of Kringle 4 repeats can be nicely measured by isoelectric focusing followed by immunoblotting which will be presented in this chapter.

2 Materials

2.1 Reagents

1. Agarose (ultrapure quality).
2. ß-Mercaptoethanol.
3. 0.5% bromophenol blue in 5% glycerol.
4. Western blot blocking reagent.
5. Biorad Submarine gel unit with 15×25 cm casting plate and comb.
6. Tank blotting device with cooling unit.
7. Polyclonal rabbit anti-human Lipoprotein(a) antiserum (Dako Cytomation).
8. Anti-rabbit IgG-biotinylated antiserum (Amersham Biosciences).
9. Streptavidin-biotinylated horseradish peroxidase complex (Amersham Biosciences).
10. Chemiluminescence substrate Lumi-Lite (Roche diagnostics).
11. FluorChemSystem Camera (Alpha Innotech).
12. AIDA software program for evaluation of size of detected bands.

2.2 Buffers

1. *Sample reducing buffer* (stored at 4°C): 50 µl ß-mercaptoethanol, 100 µl 0.5% bromophenol blue in 5% glycerol, 500 µl 5% SDS solution.
2. *Gel buffer*: 90 mM Tris 11.16 g/l, 90 mM boric acid 5.56 g/l, 2 mM EDTA 1.49 g/l, 0.1% SDS 1.00 g/l.

   Dissolve in 1 l aqua dest.
3. *Tank electrophoresis buffer*: 45 mM Tris 27.9 g/5 l, 45 mM boric acid 13.9 g/5 l, 2 mM EDTA 3.7 g/5 l, 0.1% SDS 5.0 g/5 l.

   Dissolve in 5 l aqua dest.
4. *Blot buffer*: 72.05 g glycine, 15.15 g Tris, 1,000 ml methanol.

   Dissolve in 5 l aqua dest.
5. *Wash buffer/PBS-Tween:* Phosphate buffer pH 7.4 with 0.05% Tween 20. 80 g $NaH_2PO_4{\cdot}2H_2O$, 160 g NaCl, 270 g $Na_2HPO_4{\cdot}2H_2O$.

   Dissolve in 20 l aqua dest.

   Add 10 ml Tween 20.

3 Methods

3.1 Isoelectric Focusing (3, 4)

1. Agarose gel is made with 150 ml of 1.5% ultrapure agarose dissolved in gel buffer and heated until boiling point by a microwave.
2. Dissolved agarose (after cooling for 5 min) is poured into a casting plate (15×25 cm) with comb for 20 wells (size for each slot:

5 mm wide and 2.5 mm deep; needed volume: about 60 μl; comb should be positioned 3 cm from the cathodic site of the gel).

Attention: Casting plate has to be equalized horizontally.

3. Samples are prepared by mixing 1–30 μl of sample EDTA-plasma with 30 μl reducing buffer and heating the mixture for 10 min at 95°C size standard (8 μl each) and control samples (10 μl each) are handled in parallel (see Note 1).
4. Sample amount is dependent on the lipoprotein(a) concentration according to the following:

Concentration (mg/dl)	Volume (μl)
<100	2
80–100	3
50–80	5
40–50	10
30–40	15
20–30	20
10–20	25
<10	30

5. Samples are brought to room temperature and used immediately or frozen for using the next morning.
6. Reduced samples are applied carefully into the slots on the cathodic site of the gel (see Note 2).
7. Each agarose gel contains at slot 1 and 20 human apolipoprotein(a) isoform standard or alternatively molecular weight standard for size determination.
8. Positions 2 and 19 contain known samples as control.
9. Electrophoresis is carried out in tank buffer for 12 h (overnight) at constant power of 10 W at room temperature.

3.2 Immunoblotting Technique (3, 4)

1. Next day gel slab is removed from the electrophoresis tank and placed on a glass plate and rinsed with aqua dest.
2. Gel is cut off 12.5 cm from running front, placed in a glass tray, and equilibrated with blotting buffer for 30 min.

   Commonly a small piece of gel is cut off from one corner and the relationship to slot numbers recorded in order to orientate the slot numbers on the gel for later interpretation.
3. Western blot is carried out on nitrocellulose transfer membrane (size 15 × 13 cm) for 4 h at 4°C with 400 mA constant current (power: 120 V).
4. After this period membrane is removed, placed in a glass tray containing wash buffer with 5% Tween 20, and washed on an orbital shaker for 5 min or at 4°C overnight.

3.3 Detection

1. Washed blotting membrane is put into a glass tray containing PBS-Tween buffer with 10% western blot blocking reagent and placed on an orbital shaker for 2 h.
2. First antibody incubation:

   Blot is incubated with polyclonal rabbit anti-human Lipoprotein(a) antiserum (Dako Cytomation) (1:4,000) in PBS-Tween buffer with 5% blocking reagent for 1 h at 37°C (alternatively at 4°C overnight).
3. Antibody incubation is followed by intensive washing with PBS-Tween buffer:

   Three times for 10 min each.
4. Second antibody incubation:

   Blot is incubated with anti-rabbit IgG-biotinylated antiserum (Amersham Biosciences) (1:4,000) in PBS-Tween buffer with 5% blocking reagent for 1 h at 37°C.
5. Second antibody incubation is followed by intensive washing with PBS-Tween buffer: Three times for 10 min each.
6. Third antibody incubation:

   Blot is incubated with Streptavidin-biotinylated horseradish peroxidase complex (Amersham Biosciences) (1:4,000) in PBS-Tween buffer with 5% blocking reagent for 1 h at 37°C (alternatively: 2 h at room temperature).
7. Third antibody incubation is followed by intensive washing with PBS-Tween buffer: Three times for 10 min each.
8. Blotting membrane is placed in a plastic bag and sealed.
9. 1,200 μl of chemiluminescent POD-substrate (600 μl of each component have to be mixed before injection) are injected carefully (avoid air bubbles).
10. After closing the injection hole the bag is rubbed to make sure that the substrate spread evenly on the membrane

    (Attention: Air bubbles can interfere with chemiluminescence detection).
11. The plastic bag is placed in a FluorChemSystem Camera (Alpha Innotech) and the luminous light from the bands measured. Time of measurement depends on the intensity of the bands (see Note 4).

3.4 Evaluation

The size of bands is determined using the AIDA software program.

- Therefore bands in lanes 1 and 20 (size markers) are detected and the bands for the samples/controls as well.
- Then you can draw horizontal lines to the positions of each band in the size marker lanes.

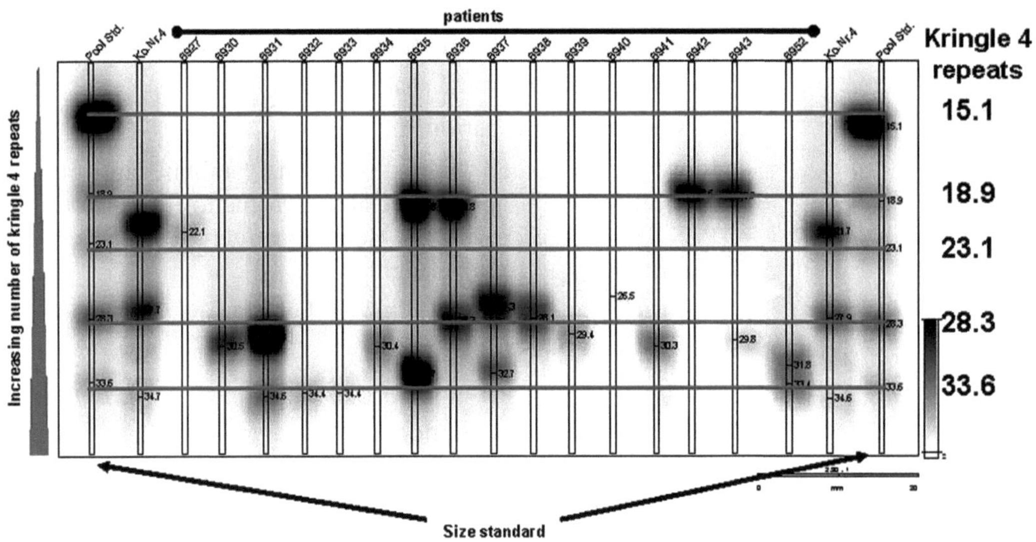

Fig. 1 Example of size determination of apo(a) isoforms

- According to the lines of the bands in the marker lines you can determine the size or the number of Kringle 4 repeats in each of your sample.
- Figure 1 shows a sample of an evaluation.

4 Notes

1. Determinations can be done with serum samples.
2. Reduced samples should be centrifuged shortly before application on the gel.
3. For blocking of the blotting membrane you can take bovine serum albumin as well.
4. If detection procedure with the chemiluminescence substrate was not successful you can repeat the procedure with injection of the substrate after washing the membrane several times.

References

1. Kostner GM (2002) Lipoprotein(a): metabolismus und beeinflussung des plasmaspiegels. J Kardiol 9:321–324
2. Nowak-Göttl U, Junker R, Hartmeier M, Koch HG, Münchow N, Assmann G, von Eckardstein A (1999) Increased lipoprotein(a) is an important risk factor for venous thromboembolism in childhood. Circulation 100:743–748
3. Marcovina SM, Hobbs HH, Albers JJ (1996) Relation between number of apolipoprotein (a) kringle 4 repeats and mobility of isoforms in agarose gel: basis for a standardized isoform nomenclature. Clin Chem 42:499–502
4. Kambouh MI, Ferrel RE, Kottke BA (1991) Expressed hypervariable polymorphism of apolipoprotein (a). Am J Hum Genet 49:1063–1074

Part VIII

Examples of Measures of Fibrinolysis

Chapter 34

D-Dimer and Fibrinogen/Fibrin Degradation Products

Linda J. Stang

Abstract

Although clinical requests for D-dimer are generally in the minority of assays in the routine clinical laboratory, they are an important aspect—especially if the laboratory supports an active emergency room and hematology service. Throughout the literature, D-dimer assays have been used for many purposes in the research setting; however it is generally the negative predictive value of the assay that is the most common piece of information being utilized from the standpoint of a clinician. Research or clinical needs will dictate the type of assay required—a qualitative, semiquantitative, or quantitative D-dimer assay may be appropriate for a particular purpose. Commonalities and differences between these assay types are outlined here, as well as universal concerns regarding standardization of D-dimer assay results.

Key words D-dimer, Fibrinogen/fibrin degradation products, Quantitative, Semiquantitative, Qualitative, Standardization

1 Introduction

D-dimer assays are used in the clinical setting mainly to aid in diagnosis of deep vein thrombosis (DVT) and pulmonary embolus (PE) (see Notes 1 and 2). These assays are also useful for detection of post-op thrombosis, and quantitative or semiquantitative assays (to a lesser degree) can be used as a continuous marker of thrombolytic activity in a patient who has been diagnosed with arterial and/or venous thrombosis. Elevated levels can also be seen in, but are not limited to, disseminated intravascular coagulation (DIC) and trauma, as well as liver disease, neoplasia, inflammation, or even normal pregnancy (1, 2). Increased levels have also, more recently, been associated with increased risk of a recurrent thrombosis following anticoagulation therapy (2).

In order for a patient's sample to have elevated levels of D-dimer present, a number of reactions must have taken place in vivo prior to sample collection. It all begins simplistically with fibrinogen being acted upon by thrombin, effectively releasing fibrinopeptide A (FPA),

Paul Monagle (ed.), *Haemostasis: Methods and Protocols*, Methods in Molecular Biology, vol. 992,
DOI 10.1007/978-1-62703-339-8_34, © Springer Science+Business Media New York 2013

and then fibrinopeptide B to produce fibrin monomer, which progresses to a polymer. Activated factor XIII can then begin to stabilize the polymer, by exchanging the hydrogen bonds for covalent cross-links (3). This stabilized fibrin network is almost immediately attacked for subsequent degradation. Plasminogen that has been activated to plasmin, via its primary activator—tissue plasminogen activator (tPA) (4), has the ability to cleave both the fibrin contained in the clot and its circulating precursor, fibrinogen. The fibrin mesh can bind both the tPA and plasminogen, and when bound, the rate of activation increases substantially. Through this mechanism, the plasmin is located right where it is needed—at the site of the fibrin clot, as opposed to being free in the circulating plasma (5). Only the fibrin that has completed the cross-linking step can produce fragments with the actual D-dimer configuration. When broken down, native fibrinogen produces fragments, although none of them share this unique D-dimer identity. Therefore, the fragments produced from fibrinogen alone should not cross-react with assay reagents containing antibodies that are specific for the D-dimer neo-epitope. The cross-linked polymer is of vast size, at least on a molecular level, and the plasmin can attack anywhere that D and E domains occur together (within the original fibrinogen molecule configuration), producing a heterogeneity of fragments. Of the cross-linked degradation products formed, the smallest fragment type that is resistant to further plasmin degradation is actually denoted as a DDE fragment and this fragment size alone is sometimes referred to as D-dimer, when in actuality all fragments containing the dimeric D domain collectively are D-dimer fragments.

1.1 Nomenclature and Terminology for Fibrinogen, Fibrin, and Fragments

The following is a simplified version of nomenclature and terminology commonly used in literature and texts to discuss the process of fibrin production and the fragments produced (4, 6).

A native fibrinogen molecule is usually referred to as (D-E-D); within this molecule the D domains, which are at opposite ends of the molecule, are not dimeric (or adjacent to one another).

The action of thrombin and F XIIIa on this molecule produces a stable polymer denoted as

(D-E-D)(D-E-D)(D-E-D)(D-E-D)(D-E-D)(D-E-D)
(D-E-D)(D-E-D)(D-E-D)(D-E-D)(D-E-D)

Plasmin has the capability to then act on this polymer, causing a breakage to occur only at the junctions denoted as (-) between the (D-E). Random breakage creates the possibility of the following fragments being generated, as well as various larger fragments:

Fragment Composition:	DD-E E-DD	E-DD-E DD-E-DD	DD E
Fragment name:	YD/DY	YY/DXD	DD/E

All of the degradation products are collectively referred to as D-dimer. Realistically, the lysis of a fibrin clot produces a very heterogeneous group of degradation products. These include X oligomers, YY/DXD, YD/DY, and DD/E, where (4):

Fragment X = D-E-D; an intermediate degradation product consisting of all three domain regions (resembles fibrinogen, but lacks fibrinopeptide A and B).

Fragment Y = D-E; contains a central E and one of either terminal D domains.

Initially large degradation products are released and only after a prolonged incubation with plasmin would the majority of fragments be DD/E, which is the smallest fragment resistant to further breakdown by plasmin (4). This is especially important when you consider the following: if a random group of patients were being tested for D-dimer, they would all be at different stages in the process of lysis. This fact, along with the different epitope specificity for the various antibodies in commercial kits, can produce slight variability in results between different assays.

Some publications also use the term fibrin degradation products (FDP), which occasionally can denote fibrinogen degradation products, as well. Another term sometimes used is XL-FDP, assumably in reference to "cross-linked FDP."

1.2 Detection of Fibrin/Fibrinogen Degradation Products

Fragments caused from plasmin breakdown of fibrinogen and fibrin can be detected using a commercially available fibrin/fibrinogen degradation product kit (Thrombo-Wellcotest, Remel, UK). This assay uses antibodies to the individual domains of D and E. Therefore the sample must be free of fibrinogen which *will* cross-react. A special collection tube containing *Bothrops atrox* venom and soya bean trypsin inhibitor will promote complete clotting of the fibrinogen, as well no further increase of D-dimer fragments should occur from the fibrin in the collection tube. Although not commonly used, this assay allows for testing for the breakdown products of fibrinogen and fibrin and has been particularly useful in DIC (7). When no pathological clot is present in other patient populations, this assay may be useful for detecting hyperactivity in a patient's fibrinolysis pathway. More specific assays relating to the root cause of the hyperactivity are available in specialized reference laboratories (plasminogen, tPA, PAI-1, etc.) and may be useful in these situations.

1.3 Differences in Assay Design

In order to choose an appropriate assay, the size of laboratory, type of equipment needed, acuity of patient population, and estimated frequency of the demand for D-dimer testing must be taken into consideration. Assays can be quantitative, semiquantitative, or qualitative (see Note 3). Quantitative assays would be more useful in situations where risk stratification is important or for ongoing monitoring in conditions such as DIC. The overall size of the measuring range of the assay is also important for this patient group as patient results can reach substantial values. For the primary purpose of exclusion of PE or DVT, a qualitative assay or one with a small measuring range is acceptable (8).

Commercially available D-dimer assays can be broken down roughly into four categories, all of which rely on antibodies and the ensuing agglutination, to assist in detection:

1. Slide tests:
   (a) Qualitative slide tests, usually known for having a very high negative predictive value; suitable for emergency room triage or similar situations where a negative or a positive result is adequate. Assay principles are somewhat similar to standard enzyme-linked immunosorbent assays (ELISA), using a modified sandwich antibody technique, or a modified antibody with essentially two Fab portions which allow the reaction to occur.
   (b) Semiquantitative assays for which general ranges of D-dimer are given as results (i.e., <0.5, 0.5–2.0, 2.0–4.0, and >4.0 μg/mL). The assay usually has a specific threshold over which a positive result will occur with a neat sample. The semiquantitative result is calculated by multiplying this threshold value by the reciprocal of the highest dilution of the sample which still produces a positive result. Slight modifications of the dilutions can usually be made to accommodate desired result ranges for these assays. When multiple dilutions are recommended by the manufacturer for more defined semiquantitative ranges, it may be more economic to omit one or more of the "middle" dilutions and only test the lower and higher of the recommended dilutions when a patient's neat sample is positive. Possibly at least one dilution can be omitted from the protocol without having any clinically significant differences produced in the semiquantitative result.

   Modifications to a qualitative slide test are sometimes included in the manufacturer's instructions to enable semiquantitative analysis using the same kit. Usually the instructions involve running preset-specific dilutions of patient's plasma to enable determination of the range in which a patient's D-dimer value falls.
2. Automated quantitative methods: These are usually immunoturbidimetric assays. Most automated methods are designed for the mid- to large-size coagulation analyzers, utilizing a monoclonal (or a combination of two monoclonals) antibody-coated (usually latex) microbead suspension, which aggregates proportionally to the concentration of D-dimer present in the patient's sample, producing an increase in light scatter or a decrease in transmitted light. One advantage to these assays is that quantitative results are available in minutes.

3. Quantitative ELISA: This assay type accommodates large batch analysis and is suitable for research studies (some commercial products are labelled "For research use only"). Standard ELISA methodology usually takes a few hours to generate results, making this assay type unsuitable in some clinical situations, where assay results are requested on a stat basis (see Note 4).
4. Small device or point-of-care quantitative analyzers: Suitable for smaller sites that desire a quantitative result; usually these sites use this result as a triage tool, transferring patients with positive results to larger institutions for active treatment.

1.4 Sample Requirements

Most standard assays for D-dimer contain antibodies that do not react with native fibrinogen; therefore plasma is a suitable specimen type. The commercially available assay that does contain antibodies which cross-react with fibrinogen requires a special serum collection tube, which is discussed in Subheading 1.2.

Platelet-poor plasma separated from a 3.2% sodium citrate vacuum collection tube (centrifuged at 1,700 × *g* for 10 min at room temperature) is generally the specimen required for a D-dimer assay. There are some variations to this, for particular commercially available assays. Some point-of-care analyzers require and some ELISA methods can substitute an EDTA (mauve top) sample in place of the citrate sample. The stability of an EDTA sample may be shorter, as some nonspecific agglutination may occur 4 h post collection (9). For some commercial assays, heparin primary collection tubes can also be a suitable sample replacement. It is important to verify and comply with the product insert specimen requirements for each specific assay.

Any Na citrate, EDTA, or heparin samples that are clotted should be discarded and recollected, as ex vivo sample clotting has the potential to cause a false positive result.

The sample stability for various commercially available D-dimer assays ranges from 4 to 8 h at room temperature, 2 weeks at −20°C, and 6 months at −70°C. Frozen samples should be vortexed after being thawed in a 37°C water bath for approximately 5–10 min, the length of thaw time being dependent on sample volume.

The in vivo half-life of D-dimer is approximately 12 h; thus timing of sample collection is not a critical issue, but this may be useful information when interpreting sequential quantitative or semi-quantitative results on the same patient over a given time span.

1.5 Difference in Antibody Specificity

Various kits use different clones of monoclonal antibodies, or combinations of clones of monoclonal antibodies. As a general rule, these antibodies have no cross-reactivity to the precursor molecule fibrinogen, FPA, or fibrin monomer.

The degradation products from fibrin clot lysis are a heterogeneous group of substances, as discussed earlier. Usually the term "D-dimer" is a collective term, in reference to this entire group of fragments. D-dimer-E, YD, DXD, and X oligomers are the individual items that make up this group. Specificity of the various antibodies used in commercial assays does cause slight variation between assays. Usually these variations are limited to the region of low positive values, or those near the predetermined cutoffs for clinical investigation. For the most part any comparison of patient samples containing a more robust amount of D-dimer will give results corresponding in the appropriate range (relative to the various reference ranges for those kits) on comparison between various commercial assays. As there currently is no international standard for D-dimer, each kit and therefore each antibody (or antibody combination) must be clinically validated and the values determined for a particular assay *cannot* be interchanged with another, without appropriate comparison studies.

Usually manufacturers have done robust studies to determine appropriate cutoffs associated with clinical situations (i.e., negative predictive value for DVT). It is a time-consuming and overwhelming project to replicate these studies and is not usually feasible in most clinical laboratories. Small in-house studies, that would alter the predetermined cutoff used for commercially available products, are not recommended, as they usually do not have the mathematical power necessary to convey significance (10).

1.6 Standardization of Assays, Including Fibrinogen Equivalent Units

Fibrinogen equivalent units or FEU are not referred to in the majority of commercially available package inserts. This nomenclature is somewhat historical in nature. When D-dimer was first quantitated in various laboratories, the vast differences in methodology (including Staphylococcus clumping assay or tanned red cell hemagglutination inhibition assay (6)) produced a large difference in reference ranges and clinically significant values amongst the various assays. In an effort to standardize the assays, the FEU was implemented. One FEU is the quantity of fibrinogen initially present that leads to the observed level of D-dimer. As the D-dimer fragments are a heterogeneous group, and each of the historical assays relied on a completely different principle, the FEU helped to make assays comparable. For the purposes of practicality, a positive cutoff of 0.5 μg/mL for FEU is generally equivalent to 0.25 μg/mL of D-dimer (11).

One of the problems plaguing this assay is that there is currently no reference standard available for antigenic D-dimer (12). Various manufacturers of commercially available products also cite this lack of an international reference standard for D-dimer contributing to the usage of FEU in some assay kits. In the determination of D-dimer standards by various manufacturers, the degree to which plasmin is allowed to act on the preset amount of fibrinogen initially measured for the standard may also play a role in the difference between commercially available products. Some manufacturers also use pools of affected patients, for standardization of the assay. High-molecular-weight fractions may also be more indicative of fibrinolysis occurring in a zone of flow (13) and can be associated with patients in DIC (14). To add to this already complex standardization situation, various manufacturers also do not use one common measurement unit for reporting. Some multi-assay comparison and standardization trials have increased our awareness and understanding of this complex problem (15); however at the time of this writing, the issue is still outstanding for the most part and must be considered when comparing data from various commercially available products.

2 Materials

The following is a table (Table 1) of common commercially available products for D-dimer and FDP. All required materials come with each kit. Patient values that fall below cutoff values are considered normal; for patients with levels above, suitable follow-up testing is usually recommended by the manufacturer (see Notes 1–6). Although the author attempted to include kits from all companies, this table may not be all inclusive for every product on the market. The intended objective is to leave an impression of the variability between assay values for commercial kits.

3 Methods

3.1 Slide Tests: Method and Procedural Notes

One of the downfalls of slide tests is the variability in the interpretation of the presence of agglutination by the end user; this is especially prominent if the lab does not do a large volume of slide tests. It is important to have good lighting by which to read the test and adhere to the product insert mixing instructions exactly. Some users have found that interpreting the agglutination present is easier if read from beneath a clear slide when the reaction is occurring; however this does present a safety hazard. Adequate proficiency testing for all staff performing the slide tests should be implemented to ensure quality results.

3.2 Method for Qualitative Slide Test

Qualitative slide methodologies vary between manufacturer with regard to sample amounts, speed and duration of slide rocking etc. Always use manufacturer's recommendations. For basic qualitative slide test instructions (see Table 2).

3.3 Semiquantitative Modification of Qualitative Slide Tests

The majority of qualitative slide tests can be modified to produce semiquantitative results. Serial (or other) dilutions of patient sample are made and tested in the same manner as for the qualitative slide test method above. The value of the patient's D-dimer is calculated using the threshold value for a positive result (on a neat patient sample), multiplied by the reciprocal of the dilution for the highest dilution of a patient that still tests positive in the reaction. For instance if the threshold value is 0.500 μg/mL and the highest

Table 1
Reference ranges and alert values

Product	Reference range or upper end of normal (NOTE: unit values differ)	Cutoff value for exclusion of DVT and/or PE, if different than reference range value
Qualitative or semiquantitative assays		
Clearview Simplify D-Dimer	<80 ng/mL	>80 ng/mL
AGEN Simplired D-Dimer	Not specified	>0.12 mg/mL
Diagnostica Stago D-Di Test	<0.5 μg/mL (FEU)	Not specified
HemosIL Dimertest	<0.20 mg/mL	Not specified
AMAX Accuclot D-Dimer	8–135 ng/mL	Not specified
Trinity Biotech Minutex D-Dimer	8–135 ng/mL	Not specified
Thrombo-Wellcotest FDP (serum sample)	4.9 ± 2.8 μg/mL	DVT—10–40 μg/mL PE—>40 μg/mL
Remel D-Dimer	<1 μg/mL	Not specified
Automated quantitative assays		
HemosIL D-Dimer HS	243 ng/mL	230 ng/mL
HemosIL D-Dimer (quant)	Dependent on analyzer models	230 ng/mL
Diagnostica Stago Liatest D-Di	<0.500 μg/mL (FEU)	>0.500 μg/mL (FEU)
AMAX Auto D-Dimer	Refer to instrument application	Not specified
Trinity Biotech Auto Dimer	<150 μg/mL	Not specified
ELISA quantitative assays		
American Diagnostica Imuclone	0–800 ng/mL	Not specified
Zymutest D-Dimer	<400 ng/mL	>500 ng/mL
Biopool/Trinity Biotech TintElize D-Dimer	130 ng/mL	Not specified
Small device or point of care		
MiniQuant d-Dimer	<250 μg/mL	Same as RR
Biosite Triage D-Dimer	0–600 ng/mL	Not specified
Vidas D-Dimer	<500 ng/mL (FEU)	>500 ng/mL (FEU)

dilution of a patient sample that still tests positive is a 1/8, then the patient's D-dimer level is greater than (0.500 × 8 = 4.00 μg/mL). It is important to check product inserts for specific dilution instructions and thresholds as there are differences between the various commercially available products. Product inserts should also provide the linear limit of a product over which a "greater than" value is resulted.

Table 2
Method for qualitative slide test

	Step	Details
1.	Allow reagents and QC to come to room temperature.	• This usually includes antibody-coated latex particles, test cards, and mixing rods and may include buffer. Some kit reagents may not contain latex. • Allow to stand for 30 min at room temperature.
2.	Label the test card for positive and negative controls and patient samples.	
3.	Place the specified amount of neat patient sample on the test card in the appropriate area.	• Follow manufacturer's recommendation for volume.
4.	Repeat step 3 for each of the controls.	• Mix controls prior to use. • QC may need to be reconstituted prior to first use.
5.	Place the appropriate amount of antibody-coated latex reagent (or other reagent) in the test area for each sample.	• The latex (or other) reagent should be adjacent to, but not mixed with, the samples. • Ensure that reagent is adequately resuspended.
6.	Using separate mixing rods, combine and mix each test area individually.	
7.	Rock the test card for the specified time.	• Adhere to manufacturer's mixing time and speed. • Manual or mechanical mixing may also be specified.
8.	Compare the test area of the patient sample with that of the negative and positive controls.	• Slide should be viewed macroscopically using a direct light source.
9.	Patient samples that show agglutination contain D-dimer levels above the cutoff value.	• Cutoff is specific for each commercially available kit; verify with insert and/or manufacturer.
10.	Discard the test card and mixing rods in the appropriate biohazard container.	• Cards are generally for single use only.

3.4 Quantitative D-Dimer Assays (Automated Analyzers)

Quantitative methods from the manufacturer for D-dimer are usually pre-set with important details (i.e., incubation times, reading wavelength, total read time etc.) in a particular instrument. For a general overview with basic instruction (see Table 3).

3.5 Interferences

As with most antibody-based lab assays, high levels of rheumatoid factor may cause interference, although some specific commercially available product inserts do state that there is no interference.

Interference by heterophile antibodies, although rare, can occur. Often the patient has an underlying malignancy such as prolymphocytic leukemia (16). This may be dealt with in a couple of

Table 3
Method for quantitative D-dimer assays (automated analyzers)

	Step	Details
1.	Bring reagents (usually latex suspension and buffer), controls, and calibrators to room temperature.	• Calibrators and controls and other reagents may need to be reconstituted; follow manufacturer's instruction. • Some commercial products have a calibration curve that has been predetermined for a specific lot number, and is reliable throughout the stability of that specific reagent lot.
2.	Load calibrators, controls, and reagents onto the analyzer.	• Ensure that all are well mixed. • Some reagents may require mixing bars to avoid precipitation while on the analyzer (see Note 5).
3.	Request a calibration to be done. A single calibration at the beginning of each lot number of reagent may be adequate, unless QC problems occur.	• The calibrator is assayed using various dilutions to prepare a standard curve (use manufacturer's recommendations).
4.	Request the positive and negative controls to be run.	• Verify that the results of the controls are acceptable.
5.	Load the patient sample and request the appropriate assays to be run (see Note 6).	• Some automated analyzers will reflex test to do a larger dilution if a patient sample is beyond the linearity of the standard curve. • This new assay dilution needs to be multiplied by the appropriate corrector factor to attain the correct result.

ways. Commercially available products to pretreat the sample removing the heterophile antibodies are used in some chemistry laboratories, and could be attempted as long as appropriate controls are assayed along with the patient sample. Also, some commercially available ELISA assays for D-dimer have a large excess of nonimmune mouse IgG in each well to minimize interference from the heterophile antibodies. Unspecified blocking agents are present in some automated methods.

Severely lipemic or hemolyzed samples may cause some interference, at least in the automated assays, as the rate of reaction is monitored as optical density or light scatter, over time. The original validation of the assay should include interference data if deemed necessary. For some assays, diluting the sample with saline, or other suitable diluent, may minimize interference (see Note 7).

The latex bead suspension for any type of assay should never be frozen. Agglutination of the suspension may occur and will be evident in the negative control.

Overmixing of the slide tests beyond the manufacturer's recommended time may result in the edges of the reaction zone drying out. The appearance of the drying slide may be judged in error to be positive.

3.6 Risk Stratification

Risk stratification, using quantitative D-dimer level as an indicator, has been investigated in a number of clinical contexts, including both acute myocardial infarction (17) and unstable angina/non-Q myocardial infarction (18). This may or may not be an important consideration, depending on the patient population being tested and the physician group interpreting the results. For dimer assays used in research studies especially, choosing an assay with a high linear limit may be useful, especially if risk stratification is considered to be a measured outcome of the study. The linear limit on some commercially available products is much higher than others. Each kit has its own defined maximum value for which a "greater than" value is assigned to all samples exceeding that value. Alternative dilutions, for some methodologies, may increase the maximum value allowed.

4 Notes

1. It is important to be careful when choosing a D-dimer assay, to consider the clinically significant cutoff value to use for that assay. This is the level above which a physician would likely expand the investigation on a patient who appeared at risk for a thrombosis. Careful review of the literature for a given product is necessary and this literature should include randomized control trials for the efficacy of the product in question. It is obviously most important to minimize false negative results, and if deemed necessary to "err on the side of caution" when choosing an appropriate cutoff value for recommendation to physicians.
2. It is very important to understand that cutoff values are strictly dependent on the assays used and are *NOT* interchangeable between various commercially available products.
3. When doing a side-by-side comparison of two or more assays, occasionally a patient will have differing results (i.e., positive or negative) for different assays, even after considering the various reference range values. The differences are likely related to the individual antibody clone(s) that is used by the manufacturer and the difference in reactivity with the various sizes of fragments. It is the author's experience that this occurs mostly at or around the cutoff level and for patients with a higher level of dimer present, usually concordance between assays is acceptable.
4. For the ELISA-based assays, the standard precautions that apply to these assays should be followed. The plate should not dry out during the assay. Both substrate and stop solution timings should be followed accurately to ensure optimal performance.
5. Some automated latex reagents do not need to have a stirring magnet present in order to remain in suspension. These reagents also have a long onboard stability, which would make

one think a stirring magnet is essential. Latex particles are sometimes so small that they will not precipitate out from suspension, even with routine centrifugation speeds and times.

6. Automated D-dimer assays are usually very costly and can usually be resulted from a single analysis after verification of the precision of the reagent/analyzer combination in use. In actual usage, the only results that one may choose to repeat are those close to the cutoff values. Values that are normal or very high usually do not make for cost-effective repeats in most cases.
7. Lipemic samples can interfere—most frequently in automated quantitative D-dimer assays. Basically the lipemia in the sample prevents the detector from perceiving that the bead agglutination is occurring. The amount of lipemia present in a sample that would cause interference can be quantitated in order for the front-line staff to have a quick indicator when unsure if a lipemic sample has reached the threshold past which interference is a problem. By spiking samples with various amounts of lipid (much like one would do for interference testing of a chemistry assay), the point at which interference occurs can be defined. Running "lipemic indexes" on chemistry equipment or "hemoglobin blanks" on hematology equipment on these same samples converts this defined threshold into a piece of attainable data when the staff member is questioning whether or not a patient's lipemic sample is producing interference on the particular quantitative D-dimer assay.

References

1. Hunt FA, Rylatt DB, Hart RA, Bundesen PG (1985) Serum crosslinked fibrin (XDP) and fibrinogen/fibrin degradation products (FDP) in disorders associated with activation of the coagulation of fibrinolytic systems. BJH 60(4):715–722
2. Adam SS, Key NS, Greenberg CS (2009) D-dimer antigen: current concepts and future prospects. Blood 113(13):2878–2887
3. Brown BA (1980) Coagulation. In: Hematology, 3rd edn. Lea & Febiger, Philadelphia, PA. p 115
4. Francis CW, Marder VJ (1994) Physiologic regulation and pathologic disorders of fibrinolysis. In: Colman RW, Hirsch J, Marder VJ (eds) Hemostasis and thrombosis: basic principles and clinical practice, 3rd edn. TB Lippincott Company, Philadelphia, PA, pp 1081–1083
5. Laffan M, Manning R (2006) Investigation of haemostasis. In: Lewis SM, Bain BJ, Bates I (eds) Dacie & Lewis practical haematology, 10th edn. Churchill Livingstone Elsevier, Edinburgh, p 386
6. Bockenstedt PL (2003) Laboratory methods in hemostasis. In: Loscalzo J, Schafer AI (eds) Thrombosis and hemorrhage. Lippincott Williams & Wilkins, Philadelphia, PA, pp 383–386
7. Ellman L, Carvalho A et al (1973) The Thrombo-Wellcotest as a screening test for disseminated intravascular coagulation. New Engl J Med 288:633
8. Dempfle CE (2006) D-Dimer assays: the current status and new assay technologies. Thromb Res 118:569–571
9. AMAX Accuclot D-Dimer product insert No. CRS116; revision 2003-02
10. Quantitative D-dimer for the exclusion of venous thromboembolic disease (2010) Proposed Guideline H59-P, Vol 30(No. 9)
11. Diagnostica Stago D-DI test package insert. REF 00454, 24552 02—Edition October 2003
12. Dempfle CE (2003) Evaluation of a new automated quantitative D-dimer, advanced D-dimer, in patients suspected of venous thromboembolism: a comment on correlation of D-dimer

assays. Blood Coagul Fibrinol 14: 313–317

13. Walker JB, Nesheim ME (1999) The molecular weights, mass distribution, chain composition, and structure of soluble fibrin degradation products released from fibrin clot perfused with plasmin. J Biol Chem 274:5201–5212
14. Pfitzner SA, Dempfle CE, Heene DL (1997) Fibrin detected in plasma of patients with disseminated intravascular coagulation by fibrin-specific antibodies consists primarily of high molecular weight factor XIIIa-crosslinked and plasmin-modified complexes partially containing fibrinopeptide A. Thromb Haemost 78:1067–1078
15. Dempfle CE, Zips S, Ergul H, Heene DL, and the FACT Study Group (2001) Evaluation of 23 quantitative D-dimer assays as basis for the development of D-dimer calibrators. Thromb Haemost 85:671–678
16. Hammouda W, Moroz LA (1987) False-positive reaction for fibrin degradation products due to a monoclonal (IgM lambda) cryoglobulin with warm-reactive antibody activity for rabbit IgG. Am J Med 82: 1263–1268
17. Demplfle CE, Kontny F, Abildgaard U (1999) Predictive value of coagulation markers concerning clinical outcome 90 days after anterior myocardial infarction. Thromb Haemost 81(5):701–704
18. Galvani M, Ferrini D, Ottani F, Eisenberg PR (1999) Early risk stratification of unstable angina/non-Q myocardial infarction: biochemical markers of coronary thrombosis. Int J Cardiol 68(Suppl 1):S55–S61

INDEX

Paul Monagle (ed.), *Haemostasis: Methods and Protocols*, Methods in Molecular Biology, vol. 992, DOI 10.1007/978-1-62703-339-8, © Springer Science+Business Media New York 2013

E

F

G

H

I

K

L

M

MIX
Papier aus verantwortungsvollen Quellen
Paper from responsible sources
FSC® C105338

If you have any concerns about our products,
you can contact us on
ProductSafety@springernature.com

In case Publisher is established outside the EU,
the EU authorized representative is:
Springer Nature Customer Service Center GmbH
Europaplatz 3, 69115 Heidelberg, Germany

Printed by Libri Plureos GmbH
in Hamburg, Germany